The Optic Nerve Head in Health and Disease

Surinder Pandav • Parul Ichhpujani
Michael A. Coote
Editors

The Optic Nerve Head in Health and Disease

Springer

Editors
Surinder Pandav
Advanced Eye Centre
Post Graduate Institute of Medical Education
Chandigarh
India

Parul Ichhpujani
Department of Ophthalmology
Government Medical College and Hospital
Chandigarh
India

Michael A. Coote
University of Melbourne and Latrobe University
Melbourne
Australia

ISBN 978-981-33-6837-8 ISBN 978-981-33-6838-5 (eBook)
https://doi.org/10.1007/978-981-33-6838-5

This Springer imprint is published by the registered company Springer Nature Singapore Pte Ltd.
The registered company address is: 152 Beach Road, #21-01/04 Gateway East, Singapore 189721, Singapore

Foreword

You see only what you look for.
You look for only what you know.

"What do you see there? Is that nerve damaged by glaucoma?" The teacher asks the student looking at the optic nerve. Some students see the damage; others do not. When examining patients, some doctors look but do not see. So, they miss things important to the health of patients. Rather than learn to see, many say to themselves, "ophthalmoscopy does not work," and turn to another method, such as optical coherence tomography (OCT). But the major issue is not with ophthalmoscopy or tomography, but rather with the learning. Those not able to see ophthalmoscopically are not likely to see using other methods. For example, they look at the printout of the OCT but do not understand what it means. At which point they either blindly follow an algorithm, without the thinking that is needed to give good care (and not as an aside, makes life worthwhile) or they say "OCT is not reliable" and switch to yet another method. To help patients, one has to learn what to look for. One also has to learn how to see. This book will help people learn those things.

Those with glaucoma— whether newborn infant, stressed young mother, hardworking farmer, busy bank president, or demented old man—are best cared for by a knowledgeable, skilled, wise person doing only what is necessary: taking a probing, empathetic, pertinent, honest, revealing history, carefully assessing visual function and pupillary responses, validly characterizing the anterior chamber angle and the optic nerve and retina. Yes, a rough idea of the intraocular pressure can give some guidance, but not much.

In a person being considered for glaucoma, the caregiver needs to determine if the person **already** has troublesome symptoms, and, if so, why; the answers to that question are likely to come most reliably from the history and the nature of the optic nerve. The caregiver and the patient will want to know whether troublesome symptoms *are likely to develop*: the history, the nature of the anterior chamber angle, and the nature of the optic nerve help address that issue. Risk factors for the development of open-angle glaucoma, such as age, central corneal thickness, and family history, provide guidance related to the frequency of follow-up but are of little help in diagnosing or deciding the treatment, because they were developed by considering groups with certain characteristics and are not applicable to all individuals. Consider two patients: one is an 85-year-old man with an intraocular pressure of 30 mm Hg, central cornea thickness of 450 microns, a positive family history, and a cup/disc ratio of 0.6; the other patient is a 25-year-old woman with an intraocular pressure of 15mm Hg, central corneal thickness of 550 microns, a negative family history, and a cup/disc ratio of 0.4. Of these two people who is more likely to be helped with treatment? The answer is, we do *NOT* know. Both have the same likelihood of becoming disabled from glaucoma: either 100% or 0% but on the basis of the data given no one can predict accurately which will remain stable and which will get worse; people can have all the findings of the old man and remain stable or all the findings of the young woman and go blind from glaucoma. So, the information provided is *not* the essential information. Now, add the fact that the 85-year-old man has a disc damage likelihood score (DDLS) of 4 and the 25-year-old woman a DDLS of 6, and suddenly we know what to do! The 85-year-old man does not need any treatment, while the 25-year-old woman already has glaucoma with field loss that was missed earlier.

Having said that, however, a further comment is necessary, for it is not the assessment of the optic nerve and retina that is needed and helpful. It is the *accurate* assessment that is needed and helpful. Wrong data are worse than no data! This book importantly addresses this issue.

We need to recall that in 1976, Lichter found that glaucoma specialists agreed poorly with each other when evaluating photographs of optic discs [1]. But in 1992, in a similar study, Varma and colleagues found the agreement excellent [2]; in 1994, Abrams and colleagues reported concurrence was sometimes good and sometimes bad [3], while in 1917 Haslett and colleagues found excellent agreement among specialists regarding the character of the optic nerve when examined with a high + lens [4]. Which is correct? All are correct relative to the study performed. None can be generalized to answer "can clinicians evaluate the optic disc validly." The correct answer to that is not a "yes" or a "no." The correct answer is "some can and some cannot." The differences in the results were partly due to the different quality with which the assessments of the optic nerve were performed. Few physicians seem to understand that the value of a test is usually more related to *how well* a test is performed and interpreted, rather than *the type of test* performed. For example, ophthalmoscopy is helpful or not depending on how well it is performed and interpreted. OCT is helpful or not depending on how well it is performed and interpreted. Perhaps artificial intelligence can help. Perhaps. Will it further decrease clinical skills? Or enhance them?

A noted glaucoma specialist once said to me, "Why do you keep stressing looking at the nerve when you know few can look at it well?" His comment is right and it is wrong. (1) (right) few look at the nerve well, but (2) he is wrong in thinking that doctors *cannot* look at it well. Accurate ophthalmoscopic assessment of the optic nerve *is* possible. Seeing well demands correct examination skills, cognitive knowledge about the strengths and weaknesses of various examination methods, recognizing discs that are likely to mislead or are too atypical to categorize validly with one or more methods, but likely to be better understood by using another method.

The quality of the clinical examination seems to be getting even worse. As practitioners substitute technology for clinical examination, their examining skills plummet. Even the most renowned pianists practice daily; honest surgeons know that they will not be as sharp in the operating room after missing surgery for two weeks, so they start the day with cases that should not be challenging.

Maintaining a skill takes constant practice but the goal should not be just maintenance—it is improvement. Improving skills requires effort, will, and discipline- and practice, whether playing the piano, writing poetry, or examining the optic disc. And the quality of the practice is instrumental in affecting whether it is associated with improvement. For example, the disc must be examined and drawn *prior* to looking at the previous drawing; then the two are compared so the examiner can compare the two, not just to consider whether the patient's disc has worsened, but importantly to evaluate the validity of the drawing: how could it be done better?! Without masking oneself, one simply copies the prior drawing and learns nothing. By evaluating one's skills constantly, one can become better and better and better. These comments apply to all technologies; learning to determine whether the test was performed properly and how to tease meaning out of the seemingly objective but actually, subjective printouts take constant practice, designed to improve skills. The OCT's mechanics are relatively objective, the choice of subject and how the technician operates the machine are subjective. The printer prints objectively, but the content on the paper is subjective. However, it is not whether the test is objective or subjective that matters: it is whether the results are *valid, relevant, and important,* and those considerations are unrelated to objective or subjective.

All technologies, such as optical coherence tomography, ophthalmoscopy, or angiography, yield information not possible to obtain with other technologies, and no technology provides complete information. Before a test is done, expending the time and effort of the patient, the technician, and the doctor, and increasing the costs of care, the person ordering the test needs to consider whether the information intended to be gained will be *valid, relevant, and important***.** If not, why do the test?

New technologies may help the brain do its job. The technologies are not aware that there is never a perfectly correct answer in medical care. The wise clinician knows this and is constantly considering whether the data are valid enough, are truly relevant, and are necessary; if they are not valid enough, relevant, and important, they must be discarded, and the person ordering the test should say either "why did I get that test?" or "why were those test results not satisfactory?"

The present text will help clinicians obtain evidence that is valid, determine its relevance, and use it appropriately in making decisions, so that patients may be better able to celebrate their lives.

You see only what you look for.
You look for only what you know.

Truth lies within these lines. So also does inadequacy. Learning so that one can look better and see more is a good start. But more challenging, and also important to betterment of the world, is seeing what you do not know and then finding out what you have seen. The thoughtful reader of *The Optic*

Nerve in Health and Disease will learn much, and be stimulated to see even more, that which has still not been understood.

George L. Spaeth,
Wills Eye Hospital, Philadelphia, PA, USA

References

1. Lichter PR. Variability of expert observers in evaluating the optic disc. Trans Am Ophthalmol Soc 1976;74:532–72.
2. Varma R, Steinmann WC, Scott IU. Expert agreement in evaluating the optic disc for glaucoma. Ophthalmology 1992; 99:215–21.
3. Abrams LS, Scott IU, Spaeth G, Quigley HA, Varma R. Agreement among optometrists, ophthalmologists and residents in evaluating the optic disc for glaucoma. Ophthalmology 1994; 101:1662–7.
4. Haslett RS, Batterbury M, Cuypers M, Cooper RL. Inter-observer agreement in clinical optic disc measurement using a modified 60 D lens. Eye 1917;11: 692-697.

Contents

About the Editors

Surinder Pandav is Professor and Head of the department of ophthalmology at the Advanced Eye Centre, Postgraduate Institute of Medical Education and Research, Chandigarh, India. His main role is to organize glaucoma services including patient care, medical education, and research at his institute. He did his glaucoma fellowship at Royal Perth Hospital and Center for Ophthalmology and Vision Sciences, Lions Eye Institute, University of Western Australia in the years 2004–2006. He served as visiting professor at the Center for Eye Research Australia, University of Melbourne, Australia, in 2014–1016, where he coordinated the Glaucomatous Optic Neuropathy Evaluation (GONE) project, which is an internet-based system for evaluation of optic disc assessment skills among ophthalmologists and trainees and conducted research on understanding functioning of glaucoma drainage devices with the aim to develop newer drainage devices. He is keenly interested in glaucoma surgical research especially mechanisms of wound healing after surgery and effect of aqueous flow through the tissues. He is an avid researcher having contributed many articles in peer-reviewed publications and a number of book chapters. He also serves as a reviewer for a number of ophthalmology journals.

He regularly organizes training workshops for the ophthalmologists of the region and has established a support group to help glaucoma patients. He has conducted a number of glaucoma awareness campaigns to educate public. He has contributed significantly to a number of professional bodies. Currently, he holds the position of the President of the Glaucoma Society of India.

Parul Ichhpujani is currently a Professor at the Department of Ophthalmology, Government Medical College and Hospital, Chandigarh, India, where she is chiefly responsible for glaucoma and neuro-ophthalmology services. She completed her glaucoma training at the Advanced Eye Centre, Postgraduate Institute of Medical Education and Research, Chandigarh, India and a subsequent clinical research fellowship, under Dr George L Spaeth, at Wills Eye Institute, Philadelphia, USA. She currently serves on the education committee of the World Glaucoma Association and is the associate managing editor of the *Journal of Current Glaucoma Practice*, the official journal of the International Society of Glaucoma Surgery. She was ranked among the powerlist 2015 for the "best 40 ophthalmologists under 40."

An avid researcher, she has co-authored three books: Pearls in Glaucoma Therapy, Living with Glaucoma, and Smart Resources in Ophthalmology and has edited another eight: Expert Techniques in Ophthalmology, Glaucoma: Basic and Clinical Perspectives, Manual of Glaucoma, Clinical Cases in Glaucoma: An Evidence Based Approach, Glaucoma: Intraocular Pressure and Aqueous Dynamics, Current Advances in Ophthalmic Technology, Glaucoma, and Ophthalmic Instruments and Surgical Tools. She is also the Springer series editor for the Current Practices in Ophthalmology series. She has also contributed several research articles and book chapters in national and international books and serves as a reviewer for many ophthalmology journals.

Michael A. Coote is an Associate professor and senior glaucoma consultant at the Royal Victorian Eye and Ear Hospital Melbourne and was the previous Clinical Director of ophthalmology. He is also a board director of St Vincent's Health Australia and chairs the board subcommittee in research and education and is currently on the executive team of the International Society for Glaucoma Surgery.

He is an active glaucoma surgery researcher and has developed the CERA model of bleb porosity testing and has published over 50 peer-reviewed manuscripts, authored 8 book chapters, and has given over 50 international lectures.

He is the developer of the Glaucomatous Optic Neuropathy Evaluation (GONE) project, the largest online evaluation and teaching system for ONH evaluation ever created. He is the co-author of the World Glaucoma Association Teaching module for ONH evaluation (https://wga.one/wga/basic-course-in-glaucoma/). His subspecialty interests include glaucoma management and glaucoma surgery, complex and failed glaucoma surgery, minimally invasive glaucoma surgery, anterior segment repair, cataract, and complex cataract surgery.

1 What Is the Range of Normal Variations in the Optic Nerve Head Appearance?

Sahil Thakur and Suresh Kumar

The art of examining the optic nerve head (ONH) begins before you even look at the patient's eye. It is imperative to keep in mind the patient history, vision status, and systemic abnormalities before you can examine and classify a suspicious ONH. A wide array of presentations are possible as different pathological processes affect different parts of the ONH. While the presentation may differ, the examination of the ONH remains a systematic process. It entails evaluation of the disc morphology, cup characteristics, and finally the neuroretinal rim features that help in flagging the abnormal. Usually clinching a diagnosis will require ancillary testing, like visual field evaluation for glaucoma or a MRI for an intracranial space occupying lesion/demyelination disorder like multiple sclerosis; it is the initial ONH appearance that may be the only sign apparent in a potentially life threatening condition. However, a majority of the eyes examined by an ophthalmologist are normal or physiologically normal variants. Normal ONH morphology can be affected by factors like age, gender, ethnicity, spherical equivalent, axial length, and even by the examination/assessment modality used. This chapter will present the readers with a wide variety of 'normal' ONH variants and help them develop a method to evaluate the ONH with reliable accuracy and confidence. In this chapter we will however limit ourselves to evaluation of the ONH using slit lamp biomicroscopy and stereoscopic or conventional fundus photographs. Many of the entities discussed are elaborated or discussed with a different perspective in other chapters as well.

1.1 Normal ONH

A normal ONH is pink in colour, usually round or oval in shape, mildly elevated, with a central depression called as the cup (Fig. 1.1).

The optic disc represents the point of exit of the retinal nerve fibres and point of entry for the vascular supply of the eye. Thus, it is the connection between the eye and the brain. The horizontal diameter of the typical ONH is ~1500 μm or 1.5 mm but population-based studies have shown significant variation across the normal population (Table 1.1). It is always imperative to evaluate the normal ONH in conjunction with other ocular parameters like visual acuity, colour vision, contrast sensitivity, and visual fields as structural findings need to be correlated with functional parameters for making a reasonably sound diagnosis.

S. Thakur (✉)
Department of Ocular Epidemiology, Singapore Eye Research Institute, Singapore, Singapore

S. Kumar
Department of Ophthalmology, Government Medical College and Hospital, Chandigarh, India

S. Pandav et al. (eds.), *The Optic Nerve Head in Health and Disease*,
https://doi.org/10.1007/978-981-33-6838-5_1

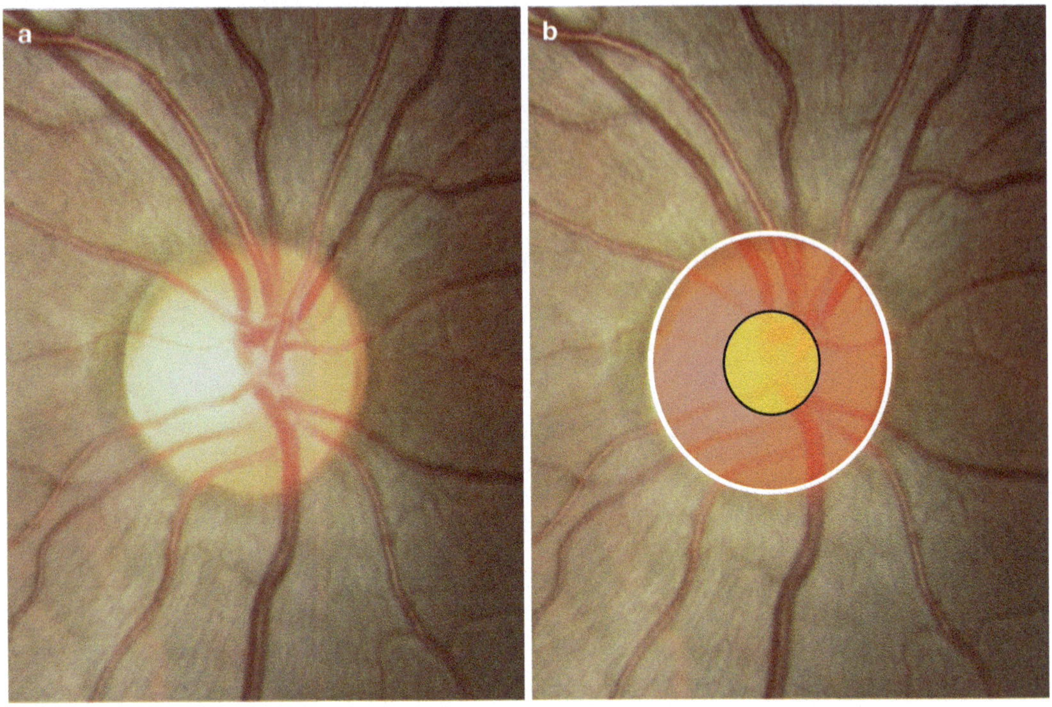

Fig. 1.1 (**a**) Normal ONH and (**b**) the schematic overlay of ONH features like the central cup (yellow), neuroretinal rim (red), and the peripapillary scleral ring of Elschnig (white ring)

Table 1.1 Normative disc diameter from selected population-based studies

Year	Study	Horizontal disc diameter (mm)	Vertical disc diameter (mm)
2001	Andhra Pradesh Eye Study [1]	1.97 ± 0.19	2.12 ± 0.23
2004	Blue Mountain Eye Study [2]		1.50 (50th percentile)
2008	Tanjong Pagar Eye Study [3]	1.58 ± 0.18	1.73 ± 0.19
2011	Chennai Glaucoma Study [4]	1.81 ± 0.19	1.94 ± 0.2

1.2 Evaluating the ONH

A wide variety of techniques and imaging modalities can be used to evaluate the ONH that are covered subsequently in the book. From the humble ophthalmoscope to optical coherence tomography angiography (OCTA) assisted evaluation, the features that define the normal ONH remain fairly consistent. Despite having a plethora of published literature, available textbooks and guides, observation of the ONH has remained a difficult art. In order to assist ophthalmologists in examining the optic nerve several online web-based platforms are now available that can help sharpen the observation skills for all clinicians. These offer educational features that are convenient and suitable for the learning needs of today's ophthalmologists. The glaucoma courses by the World Glaucoma Association [5] and the optic nerve examination course by the Glaucomatous Optic Neuropathy Evaluation [6] (GONE) project are two such excellent resources that can help readers develop good ONH observation skills at their own comfort and convenience. However, for those readers who prefer to have a conventional textbook approach, this chapter can serve as a primer for developing a systematic method of examining features of the ONH.

For clarity of presentation and also for aid in the systematic evaluation of the ONH, we have divided the ONH features into:

1. Disc morphology.
2. Cup characteristics.
3. Neuroretinal rim (NRR) and peripapillary retinal nerve fibre layer (RNFL) features.

In the subsequent sections of this chapter these features will be discussed in more detail.

1.2.1 Note on Magnification/ Correction Factors

As different lenses are available for assessment of the ONH using slit lamp biomicroscopy it is imperative to know the correction factor for measurements made on the slit lamp (Table 1.2).

1.2.2 Disc Morphology

The morphological features that define the outer limits of the ONH are often the ones that provide the most information about the underlying physiological state of the eye. Usually these morphological features show considerable range of normal findings in population-based studies (Table 1.3). These features are the peripapillary atrophy (PPA), disc size, disc shape, and the disc tilt (Fig. 1.2). This has been addressed in detail in Chap. 5.

1.2.2.1 Peripapillary Atrophy (PPA)

The PPA is the surrounding area that marks the boundary of the ONH and the peripheral retina. Classically two types of PPA have been described: the α (alpha) and the β (beta) PPA

Table 1.2 Correction factors for common fundus examination lenses

Lens	Magnification	Correction factor [7]	Working distance	Field of view (static/dynamic)
60D (Volk-Nikon)	1.15X	0.94–1.03	13 mm	$68^0/81^0$
78D (Volk)	0.93X	1.13	8 mm	$81^0/97^0$
90D (Volk-Nikon)	0.76X	1.36–1.59	7 mm	$74^0/89^0$
Super field® (Volk)	0.76X	1.50	7 mm	$95^0/116^0$

Table 1.3 Normative disc morphology parameters from selected population-based studies

Year	Study	Disc area (mm^2)	Neuroretinal rim area (mm^2)
1999	Rotterdam Eye Study [8]	2.42 ± 0.47	1.85 ± 0.39
2001	Andhra Pradesh Eye Study [1]	3.36 ± 0.68	2.79 ± 0.52
2003	Vellore Eye Study [9]	2.58 ± 0.65	1.60 ± 0.37
2003	Beijing Eye Study [10, 11]	2.65 ± 0.57	1.70 ± 0.30
2008	Tanjong Pagar Eye Study [3]	2.17 ± 0.46	1.43 ± 0.29
2011	Chennai Glaucoma Study [4, 12]	2.82 ± 0.52	2.29 ± 0.39

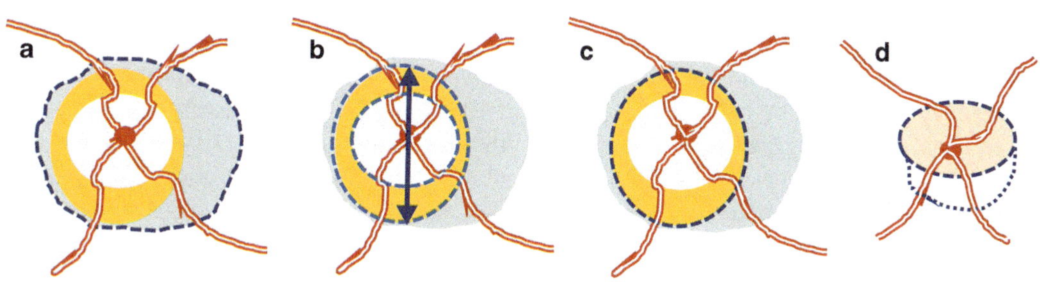

Fig. 1.2 Disc morphology features: (**a**) peripapillary atrophy (blue dotted line), (**b**) disc size, (**c**) disc shape, and (**d**) disc tilt/tort (adapted from the GONE [6, 13] project)

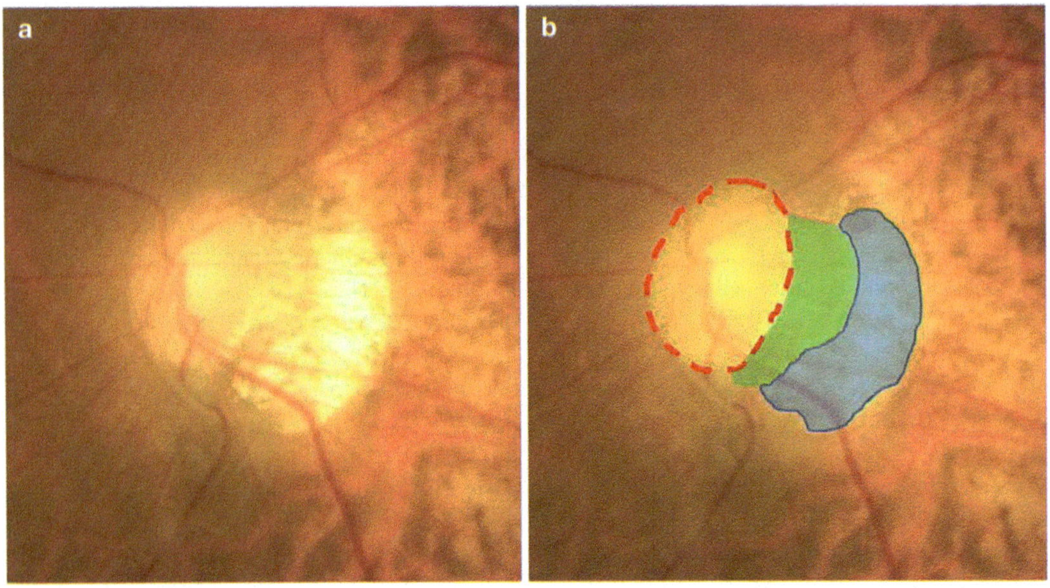

Fig. 1.3 (**a**) Tilted disc with extensive peripapillary atrophy and (**b**) classical α (alpha) zone: blue and the β (beta)zone: green peripapillary atrophy along with peripapillary scleral rim (red dotted line)

(Fig. 1.3a). The outer α zone is defined as the outermost/peripheral zone that occurs due to areas of hypo- and hyperpigmentation of the retinal pigment epithelium (RPE) layer, while the inner β zone is due to atrophy of the RPE leading to baring of the underneath choroidal and scleral tissue (Fig. 1.3b) [8]. Table 1.4 shows the normative PPA parameters from population-based studies. PPA is an important indicator of how much mechanical stretch the eye is under. Typically, in highly myopic eyes, PPA is larger and more apparent [14]. It is important to differentiate between the types of PPA and features of myopic degeneration in eyes with high myopia before starting anti-glaucoma therapy as these eyes may show fixed visual field defects due to morphological factors that can mimic glaucomatous damage [15–17].

Recently types of PPA have been expanded based upon the histological and OCT imaging-based data in highly myopic eyes [20–23]. Now there are 4 distinct types/zones of PPA: α, β, γ (gamma), and δ (delta). Fig. 1.4 shows a highly simplified scheme for understanding these four types of PPA. The δ zone corresponds to the peripapillary scleral flange which is the biomechanical anchor of the lamina cribrosa. It has been shown to be associated with increased risk of glaucoma in myopic eyes [23]. The γ zone corresponds to the peripapillary sclera without overlying choroid, Bruch's membrane, and deep retinal layers (details in Chap. 3). To differentiate between γ and δ zones, the blood vessels are an indicator. If vessels of at least 50 μm diameter and a minimal length of 300 μm are not detected, it is classified as δ zone [21, 22]. Typically, the arterial circle of Zinn–Haller lies in the γ zone [21].

1.2.2.2 Disc Size

Disc size is one of the most important morphological determinants of the ONH [24]. It is vital to classify the disc into small, normal, or large as it significantly affects evaluation of other ONH parameters like the cup–disc ratio (CDR) and the NRR. The discs can be classified on the basis of the disc diameter as: small (1.1–1.3 mm), medium (1.4–1.7 mm), and large (1.8–2 mm). Crowston et al. have shown that when compared for a small (1.2 mm) and large (1.9 mm) size optic disc, the 97.5th percentile CDR increased from 0.6 for small optic discs to 0.75 for large optic discs and from 0.62 to 0.83 for the 99th percentile [2]. This

Table 1.4 Peripapillary atrophy parameters from selected population-based studies

Year	Study	Sample	Prevalence/Progression		Area (mm²)		Remarks
			α	β	α	β	
1999	Rotterdam Eye Study [8]	1672 eyes, 894 subjects	58%	13%			α zone prevalence decreased 0.4% per decade ($P = 0.035$), β zone prevalence increased 1.3% per 1D myopia ($P < 0.001$)
2003	Vellore Eye Study [9]	70 subjects	98.6%	11.4%	0.84 ± 0.29	0.13 ± 0.38	α PPA usually temporal, correlates with disc and rim area
2007	Beijing Eye Study [18]	4003 subjects, 93 glaucoma				1.21 ± 1.92 mm² (glaucoma) versus 0.32 ± 0.99 mm² (normals); $P < 0.001$	β zone area increases with age ($P < 0.001$), myopia ($P < 0.001$), and glaucoma ($P < 0.001$)
2008	Beijing Eye Study [14]	4439 subjects	71.2%	19.9%	0.52 ± 0.64	0.46 ± 1.82	α and β usually temporal, size correlates with disc size ($P < 0.001$), age ($P < 0.001$), myopia ($P < 0.001$), and reduced visual acuity ($P < 0.001$)
2012	Beijing Eye Study (5 year follow up) [19]	3251 subjects	0.6 ± 0.1% progression	8.2 ± 0.5% progression			β progression associated with higher age, higher intraocular pressure, myopia, glaucoma, co-progression of α (all $P < 0.001$), rural region of habitation ($P = 0.002$), thicker central corneal thickness ($P = 0.02$), and absence of arterial hypertension ($P = 0.03$)

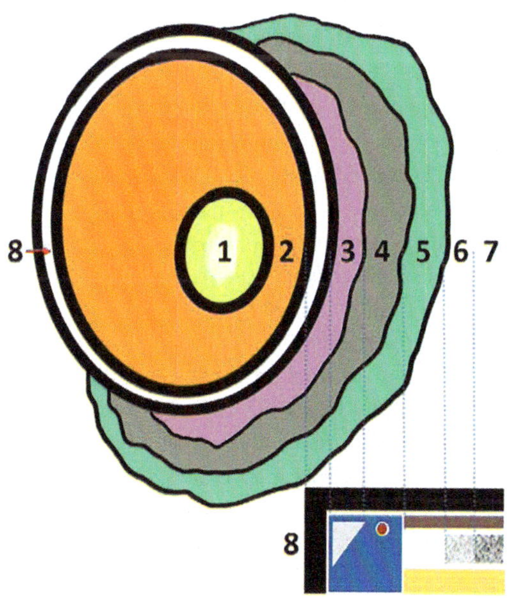

Fig. 1.4 Different types of peripapillary atrophy (PPA) in highly myopic eyes and the structures that define them. 1: optic cup, 2: neuroretinal rim, 3: δ (delta) zone, 4: γ (gamma) zone, 5: β (beta) zone, 6: α (alpha) zone, 7: peripheral retina, 8: parapapillary scleral ring of Elschnig (histologically: pia mater), blue box: peripapillary sclera without overlying choroid, Bruch's membrane, and deep retinal layers, white triangle: parapapillary scleral flange, red dot: arterial circle of Zinn–Haller, brown line: Bruch's membrane, black/white dotted box: retinal pigment epithelium, yellow box: choroid

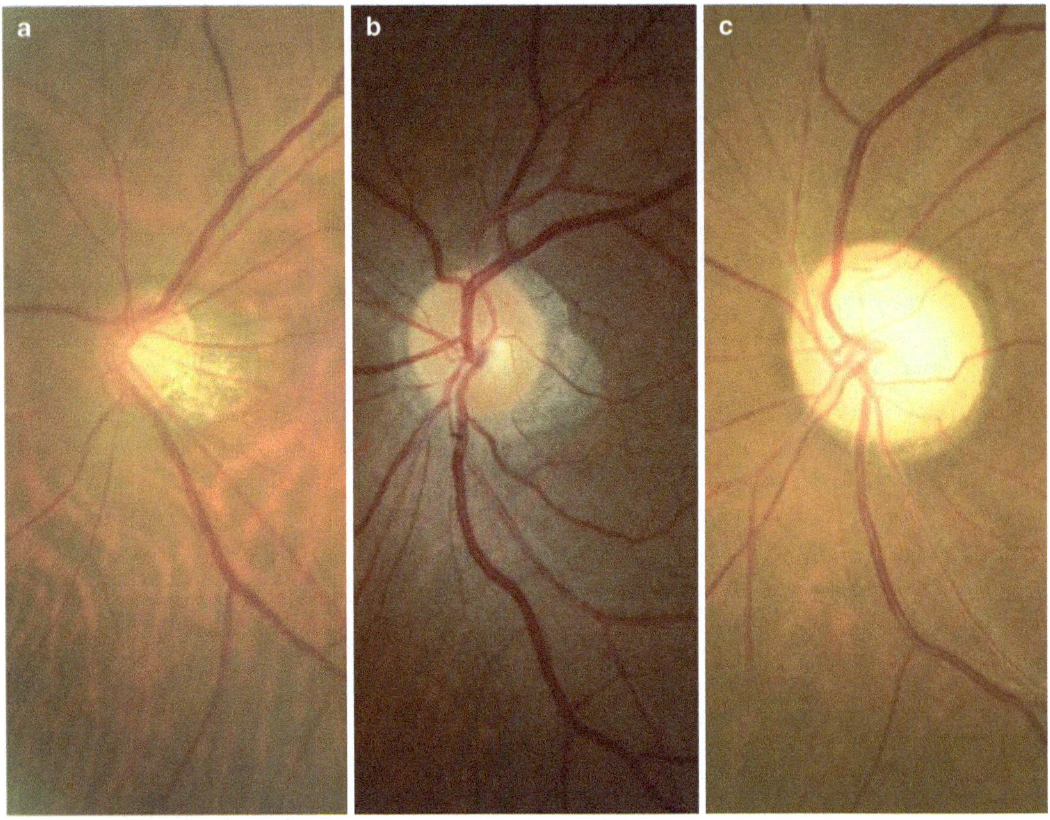

Fig. 1.5 Range of optic nerve head (ONH) size: (**a**) small, (**b**) medium, and (**c**) large

shows how the traditional CDR based diagnostic criteria can change significantly based on the disc size [25, 26]. If this is overlooked it can lead to overdiagnosis of glaucoma suspects and subsequently unnecessary visits for visual field and imaging tests. Thus, in order to classify a normal disc, it is vital to evaluate its features by corresponding them with the disc size (Fig. 1.5).

1.2.2.3 Disc Shape

The disc shape is another morphological parameter that can help identify the underlying physiological state and may get altered in pathological conditions. The disc shape also helps in defining the shape of the NRR and thus is vital in studies that evaluate structure function correlation. Garway-Heath et al. have previously described how visual field areas correspond to the ONH [27]. This map is now being incorporated in the OCT machines and is being increasingly used for structure function correlation studies [28, 29]. However, it is important to keep in mind that disc shape can significantly alter the representation areas in such analysis (Fig. 1.6).

1.2.2.4 Disc Tilt

The disc tilt helps in identifying the direction of the ONH as it enters the sclera. It can be traditionally classified as horizontally or vertically tilted (Fig. 1.7). Disc tilt is a vital parameter to record while disc evaluation, as conventional OCT machines cannot account for the impact of the disc tilt on automated measurements and thus may lead to incorrect observations about the pathological nature of the findings. Disc tilts can also lead to persistent scotomas on the visual field that can be misinterpreted as glaucomatous damage [15] (Fig. 1.6).

Disc tilt has also been defined based on the index of tilt and the angle of tilt which defines how torted the disc is (Fig. 1.8). Optic disc ovality is assessed using the ratio of minimum

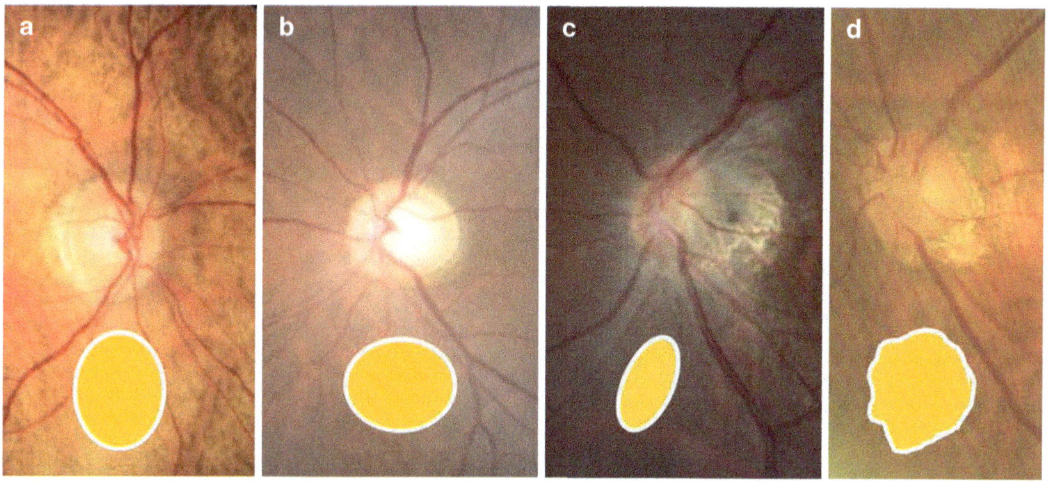

Fig. 1.6 Disc shapes: (**a**) vertical oval, (**b**) horizontal oval, (**c**) tilted oval, and (**d**) undefined/irregular

Fig. 1.7 Disc tilt: (**a**) horizontal tilt and (**b**) vertical tilt

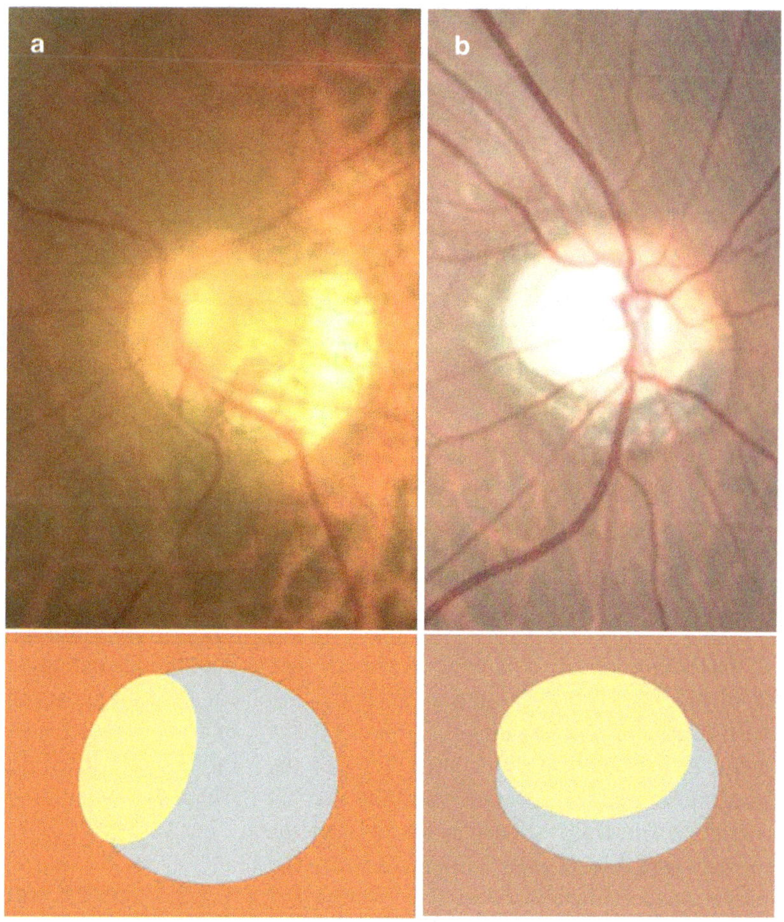

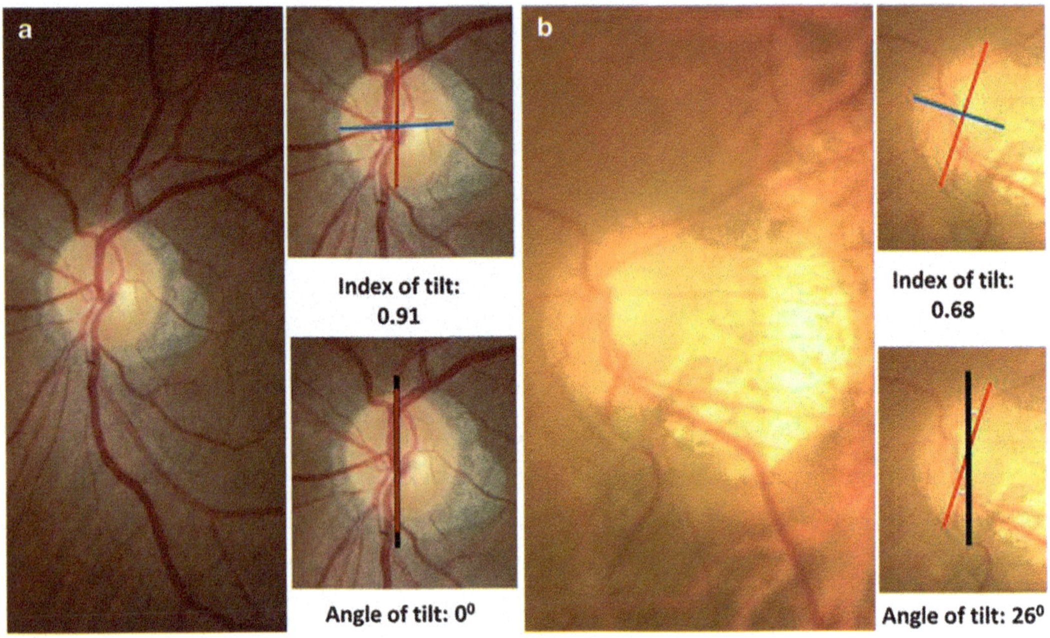

Fig. 1.8 Quantifying the tilted discs: (**a**) non-tilted, non torted disc and (**b**) tilted and torted disc

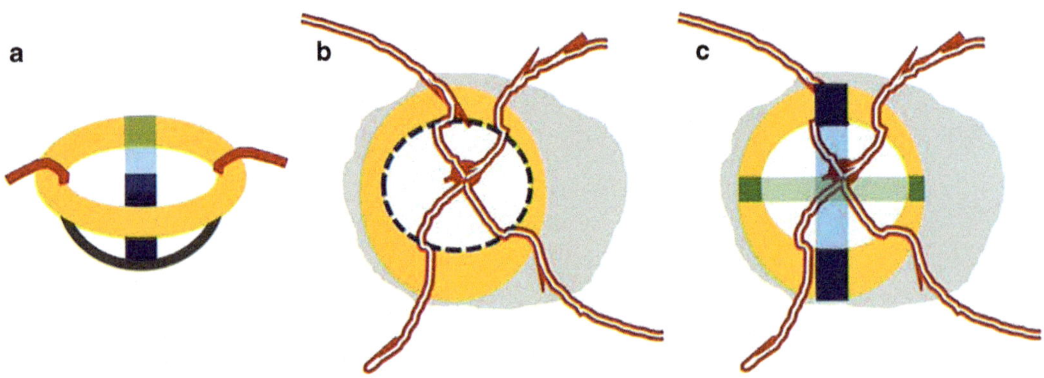

Fig. 1.9 Cup characteristics: (**a**) cup depth (blue rod); (**b**) cup shape (blue dotted line); and (**c**) cup–disc ratio (CDR) (adapted from the GONE [6, 13] project)

to maximum optic disc diameter (index of tilt). A tilted optic disc is defined as an optic disc with an index of tilt less than 0.75 [30, 31]. The angle of tilt is defined as the angle between the maximum optic disc diameter and the vertical meridian. The disc is graded as torted when the axis is rotated more than 15 degrees [32]. The prevalence of tilted discs in the Chinese has been reported as 3.5% and is higher than the 1.6% reported in the Australian population [32, 33]. Myopia is the most significant risk factor for associated tilted optic discs in the Chinese population and thus along with PPA complicates the diagnosis and monitoring of glaucoma in myopic subjects [32, 34]. How to assess neural tissue in tilted discs has been addressed in Chap. 7.

1.2.3 Cup Characteristics

The cup entails the central vacant space inside the ONH. Cup characteristics help us define the pathological state of the ONH (Fig. 1.9). A large deep sharply defined cup usually indicates a pathological process like glaucoma. Additionally, the shape of the cup helps in defining the NRR. Cup size also determines the CDR which is the most widely used parameter for glaucoma detection. In this section we look at the properties of the cup that help in evaluation of the ONH.

1.2.3.1 Cup Depth

The cup depth can be shallow or deep (Fig. 1.10). Shallow cups are usually difficult to evaluate as it makes the NRR less apparent. They are typically seen in small discs and are associated with hypermetropia. The cup base can also show features like the laminar dot sign, which is visibility of the lamina cribrosa fenestrations (pores in the scleral tissue) that allow passage of the retinal ganglion cell axons. In glaucoma, these pores can become enlarged and apparent indicating baring of scleral tissue due to loss of axons (Fig. 1.10b). Deep scalloped cups especially bean pot cupping are characteristic of glaucomatous damage and are often found in eyes with advanced glaucoma. To identify this kind of cupping the bending of the blood vessels is an obvious clue (Fig. 1.10c).

1.2.3.2 Cup Shape

The cup shape helps us to define the NRR and is perhaps the most important parameter for glaucoma evaluation. The cup shape is also vital as it defines the measurement boundaries for the CDR, which is the universal parameter used in glaucoma screening programs. The cup shape should always be classified on the basis of the vessel bending and never by the colour as it often leads to inaccurate detection of the cup boundary and underestimation of the CDR.

1.2.3.3 Cup–Disc Ratio (CDR)

The CDR is the parameter that is used to define a suspect disc; however, it has its own caveats and needs critical evaluation. Fig. 1.11 shows how despite having different CDR, the NRR may be equivocal among discs.

It is well known that CDR measurement is affected significantly by the disc size, it is underestimated in small discs and overestimated in large discs and thus makes the ONH examination error prone [35, 36]. It has been noted that trainees and comprehensive ophthalmologists tend to underestimate glaucoma likelihood in 22.1% and 23.8% discs in an internet-based assessment. It

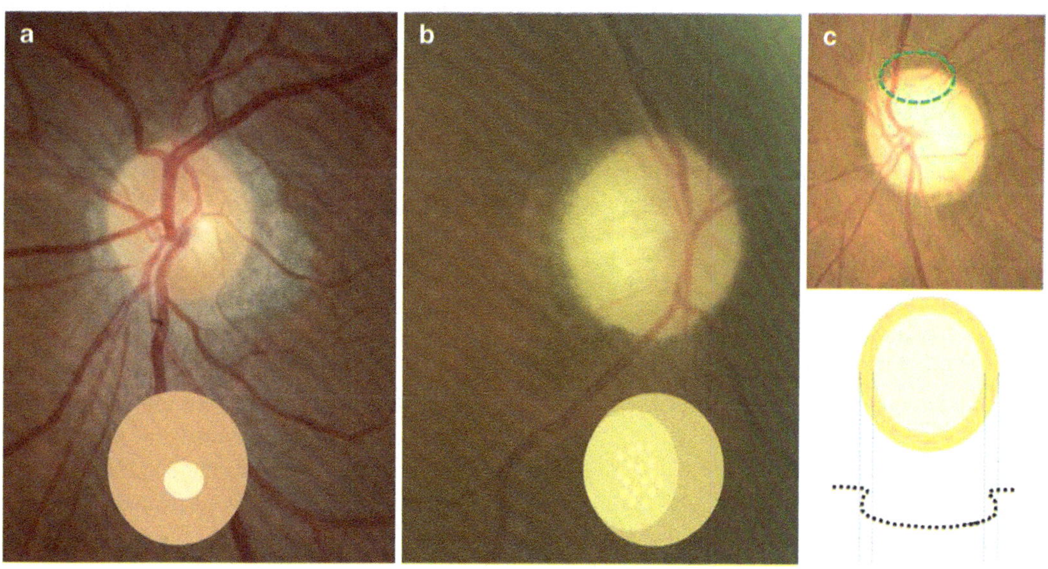

Fig. 1.10 Cup depth: (**a**) shallow cup; (**b**) deep cup (laminar dots at base of cup); (**c**) bean pot cupping (green circle: bending of vessels along the cup margin)

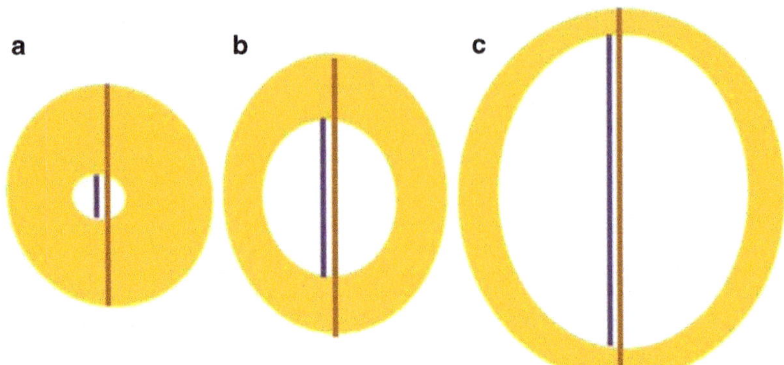

Fig. 1.11 Cup–disc ratio (CDR) and the neuroretinal rim (NRR): (**a**) vertical CDR = 0.2; (**b**) vertical CDR = 0.6; (**c**) vertical CDR: 0.9, however NRR (yellow area) is equivocal

Table 1.5 Normative (mean) cup–disc ratio (CDR) parameters from selected population-based studies

Year	Study	Horizontal CDR	Vertical CDR
1999	Rotterdam Eye Study [8]	0.40 ± 0.14	0.49 ± 0.14
2001	Andhra Pradesh Eye Study [1]	0.38 ± 0.09	0.36 ± 0.09
2003	Vellore Eye Study [9]	0.66 ± 0.07	0.56 ± 0.08
2004	Blue Mountain Eye Study [2]		0.43 ± 0.14
2008	Tanjong Pagar Eye Study [3]		0.55 ± 0.10
2011	Chennai Glaucoma Study [4, 12, 41]	0.39 ± 0.19	0.36 ± 0.18, 0.43 ± 0.17 [41]
2020	Singapore Epidemiology of Eye Diseases Study [42]		0.41 ± 0.1

was further noted that underestimating the vertical CDR was one of the key errors [37]. However, it has also been shown that with practice and training even non-physician graders can perform reliably well and with greater agreement [38, 39]. It is also important to note that out of all the ONH features it is the cup–disc ratio that has been most consistently shown to be associated with glaucomatous visual loss [40]. Thus, it is imperative that a lot of population-based studies have given the normative CDR values that can be helpful while classifying a normal disc (Table 1.5).

1.2.4 Neuroretinal Rim (NRR) and Peripapillary Retinal Nerve Fibre Layer (RNFL) Features

The NRR helps us quantify the reserve of neural tissue that the eye has for signal conduction. Glaucomatous damage can often be identified by observing the NRR features (Fig. 1.12).

The confirmatory feature for glaucoma diagnosis is usually a wedge shaped RNFL defect that becomes apparent in the red-free (green) illumination. Usually this is accompanied by thinning of the NRR and sometimes with a typical notch in the continuity of the rim (Figs. 1.13a, b) and a corresponding visual field defect (Fig. 1.13c). The rim has been traditionally classified using the ISNT rule which however has been shown not to be exceptionally reliable for normal eyes and myopes [43, 44]. OCT machines use the TSNIT (temporal-superior-nasal-inferior-temporal) curve that represents the physiological double hump distribution of the RNFL and can be considered an extension of the ISNT rule. The machines then represent the averaged data as the extremely popular 'traffic light' colour coded normative data that can be used to classify suspicious ONH's. In clinical practice, however, it is better to rely on rim specific parameters like the disc damage likelihood scale (DDLS) that can classify suspect discs on slit lamp biomicroscopy [45, 46]. In addition to this classification consistency of the NRR, symmetry between the two eyes and focal notching are factors that need to be considered while evaluating the NRR.

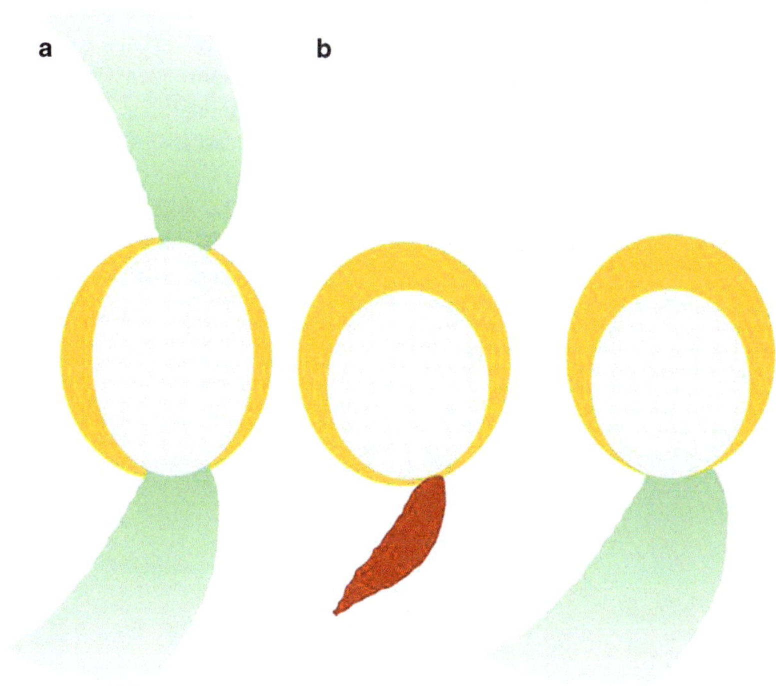

Fig. 1.12 Neuroretinal rim (NRR) features: (**a**): retinal nerve fibre layer wedge (green) defect, (**b**) disc haemorrhage (red) and corresponding visual field defect (green), usually seen on longitudinal follow-up

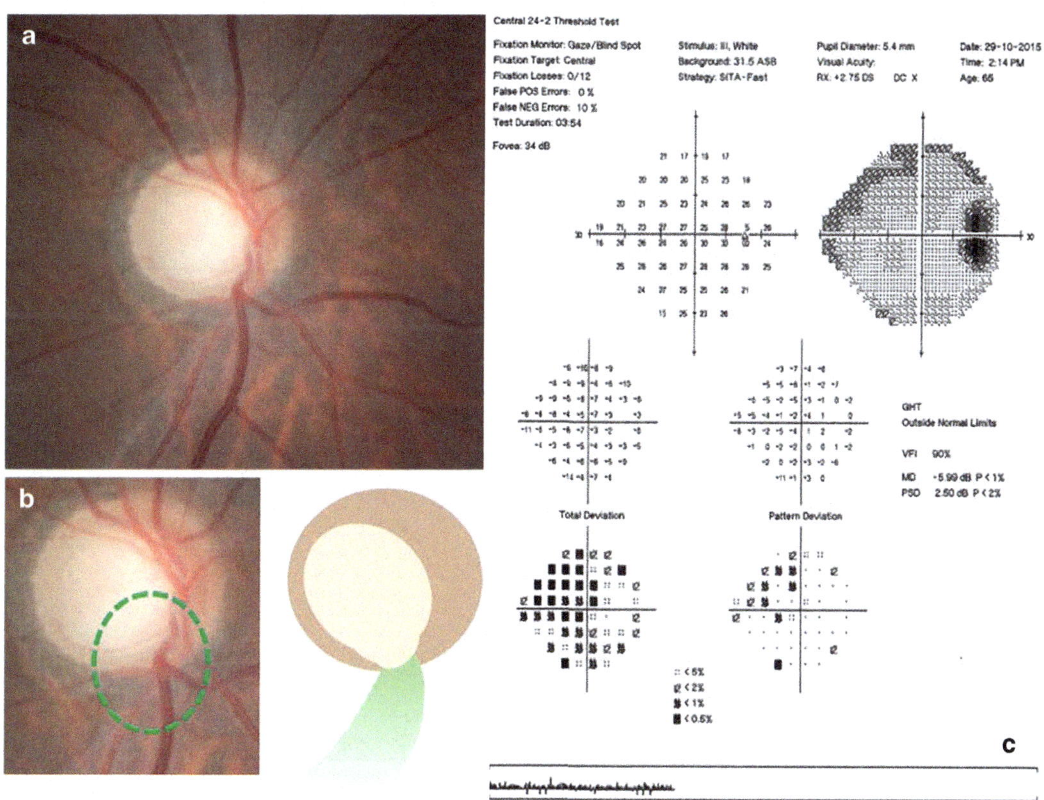

Fig. 1.13 (**a** and **b**) Typical notch in the inferior neuroretinal rim (NRR) and (**c**) corresponding superior visual field defect

1.2.4.1 Peripapillary RNFL Defect

The typical RNFL wedge defect is the most sensitive parameter that can confirm glaucomatous damage on the ONH examination. However, observing the RNFL in pigmented eyes, eyes with PPA, and as the eye ages becomes quite difficult (Figs. 1.14a–e).

Red-free illumination can help but sometimes these defects may be missed by even expert ophthalmologists. This is where complete dilated, systematic evaluation of the ONH comes into play. Subtle signs of glaucomatous damage like rim notching, localised rim thinning, and disc haemorrhage can assist diagnosis in these eyes. Subsequent evaluation with appropriate imaging modalities may however be needed in difficult cases.

1.2.4.2 Disc Haemorrhage

Disc haemorrhages have been found to be associated with low tension glaucoma (Fig. 1.15). These haemorrhages usually are followed by a RNFL defect indicating a focal vascular deficit (Fig. 1.12b). Quite often these show recurrence

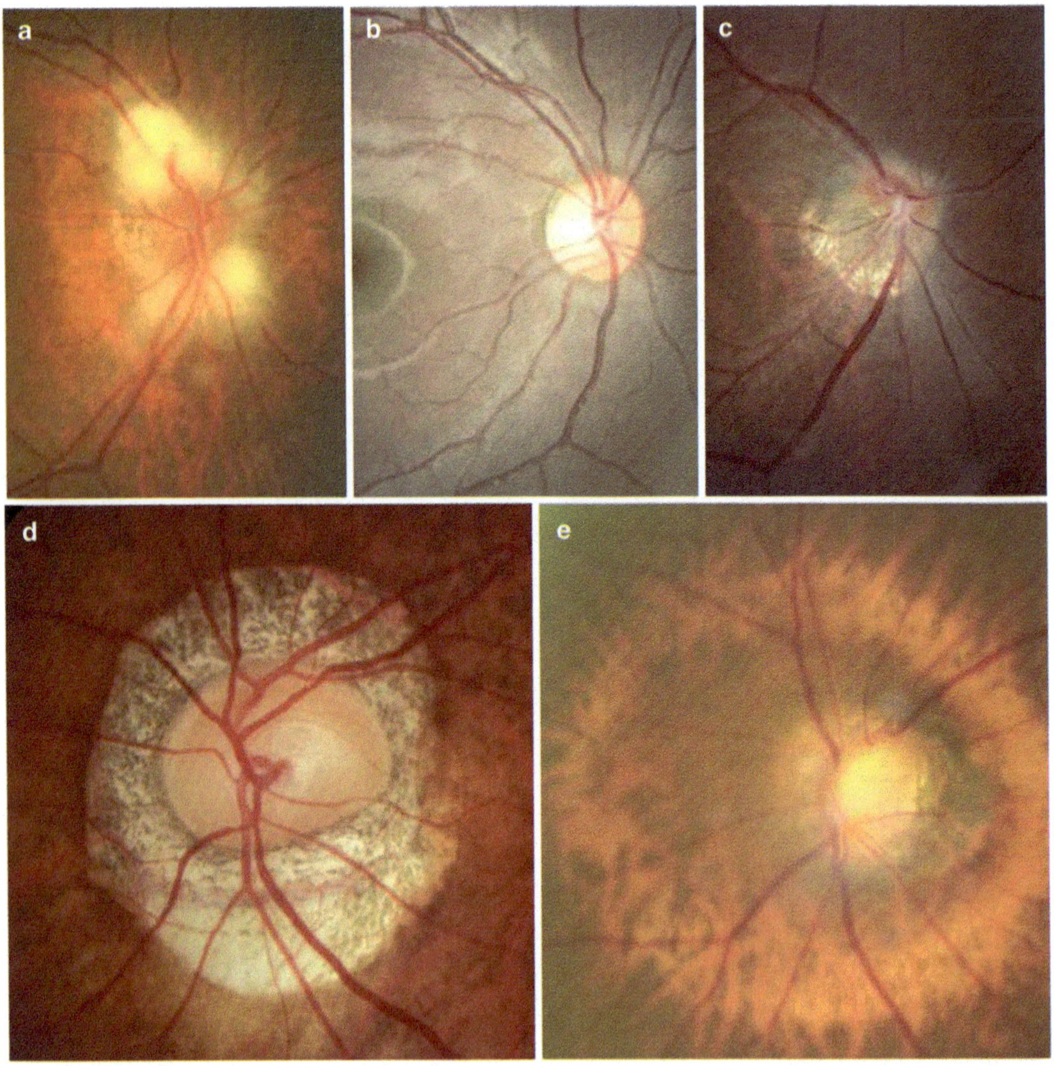

Fig. 1.14 Cases with difficult estimation of peripapillary RNFL: (**a**) myelination, (**b**) striations, (**c**) hypoplastic disc, (**d**) disc coloboma, and (**e**) staphyloma

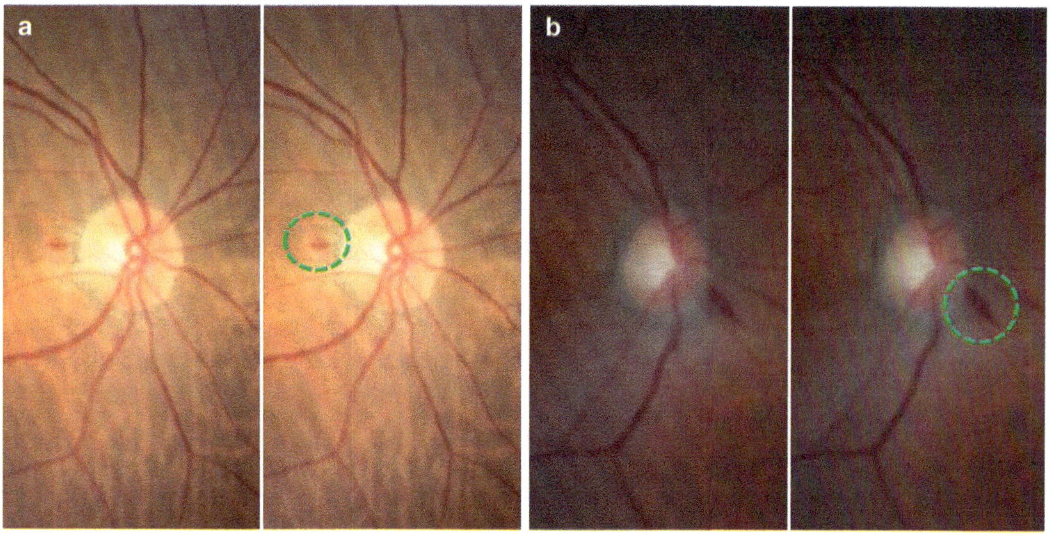

Fig. 1.15 Disc haemorrhages: (**a**) subtle and (**b**) obvious/classical

Table 1.6 Disc haemorrhage data from selected population-based studies

Year	Study	Subjects	Prevalence	Risk factors/Associations
1998	Blue Mountain Eye Study [47]	3654	1.4% Overall prevalence in POAG (high: 8%, low: 25%, OHT: 1.5%)	Higher prevalence in women (OR: 1.9), elderly (OR: 2.2/decade). Associated with higher IOP (OR: 1.7/5 mm/Hg), diabetes (OR: 2.9), pseudoexfoliation (OR: 3.5), and higher systolic BP (OR: 1.1/10 mmHg). In subjects without POAG, associated with larger VCDR and subjects with h/o migraine (OR: 2.2)
1999	Gifu Health Center Study [48]	5967	0.6%	Associated with female gender and peripapillary atrophy
2004	Tajimi Eye Study [49]	13,965	0.3% per eyes, 0.6% per subjects	74% associated with glaucomatous eyes. Associated in females and elderly. IOP for all glaucoma cases less than 20 mmHg
2006	Beijing Eye Study	4439	1.24%	Associated with glaucoma (OR: 9.3), age (1.01), however, only 8.8% glaucomatous eyes (20/226) had disc haemorrhage. Systemic factors not evaluated
2013	Central India Eye and Medical Study	4570	0.19% per eyes 0.35 ± 0.09% per subjects	65% associated with glaucomatous eyes. However, only 5.7% glaucomatous eyes (11/193) had a disc haemorrhage

and patients may progress rapidly. It is vital to evaluate all such patients for systemic disease as these haemorrhages are associated with a wide spectrum of diseases. However, it can be seen that normal populations can also have disc haemorrhages and careful evaluation of other patient parameters is required before concluding on a diagnosis (Table 1.6).

Despite having excellent tools available for learning how to examine the ONH, it has been shown that there is still a considerable lack of agreement between expert trainers and ophthalmology residents [50]. This indicates a need for soul searching in all glaucoma experts; so that the future generation of ophthalmologists can also be trained to have the same joy in observing the ONH rather than simply interpreting printouts from the multitude of machines that are crippling the traditional history, examination, and diagnosis approach.

References

1. Sekhar GC, Prasad K, Dandona R, John RK, Dandona L. Planimetric optic disc parameters in normal eyes: a population-based study in South India. Indian J Ophthalmol. 2001;49(1):19–23.
2. Crowston JG, Hopley CR, Healey PR, Lee A, Mitchell P. The effect of optic disc diameter on vertical cup to disc ratio percentiles in a population based cohort: the Blue Mountains eye study. Br J Ophthalmol. 2004;88(6):766.
3. Bourne RR, Foster PJ, Bunce C, et al. The morphology of the optic nerve head in the Singaporean Chinese population (the Tanjong Pagar study): part 1—optic nerve head morphology. Br J Ophthalmol. 2008;92(3):303–9.
4. Arvind H, George R, Raju P, et al. Optic disc dimensions and cup-disc ratios among healthy South Indians: the Chennai glaucoma study. Ophthalmic Epidemiol. 2011;18(5):189–97.
5. Glaucoma Online Courses by WGA [Internet]. 2020 [cited 2020/08/05/]. Retrieved from https://wga.one/wga/online-courses.
6. GONE—Glaucomatous Optic Neuropathy Evaluation Project [Internet]. 2020 [cited 2020/08/10/]. Retrieved from https://gone-project.com/newgone.
7. European Glaucoma Society Terminology and Guidelines for Glaucoma, 4th Edition—part 1. Br J Ophthalmol. 2017;101(4):1–72.
8. Ramrattan RS, Wolfs RC, Jonas JB, Hofman A, de Jong PT. Determinants of optic disc characteristics in a general population: the Rotterdam study. Ophthalmology. 1999;106(8):1588–96.
9. Jonas JB, Thomas R, George R, Berenshtein E, Muliyil J. Optic disc morphology in South India: the Vellore eye study. Br J Ophthalmol. 2003;87(2):189–96.
10. Wang Y, Xu L, Zhang L, et al. Optic disc size in a population based study in northern China: the Beijing eye study. Br J Ophthalmol. 2006;90(3):353–6.
11. Xu L, Wang Y, Yang H, Zhang L, Jonas JB. Size of the neuroretinal rim and optic cup and their correlations with ocular and general parameters in adult Chinese: the Beijing eye study. Br J Ophthalmol. 2007;91(12):1616–9.
12. Arvind H, George R, Raju P, et al. Neural rim characteristics of healthy South Indians: the Chennai glaucoma study. Invest Ophthalmol Vis Sci. 2008;49(8):3457–64.
13. Kong YX, Coote MA, O'Neill EC, et al. Glaucomatous optic neuropathy evaluation project: a standardized internet system for assessing skills in optic disc examination. Clin Exp Ophthalmol. 2011;39(4):308–17.
14. Wang Y, Xu L, Zhang L, et al. Peripapillary atrophy in elderly Chinese in rural and urban Beijing. Eye (London). 2008;22(2):261–6.
15. Vuori ML, Mäntyjärvi M. Tilted disc syndrome may mimic false visual field deterioration. Acta Ophthalmol. 2008;86(6):622–5.
16. Law SK, Tamboli DA, Giaconi J, Caprioli J. Characterization of retinal nerve fiber layer in nonglaucomatous eyes with tilted discs. Arch Ophthalmol. 2010;128(1):141–2.
17. Kumar RS, Baskaran M, Singh K, Aung T. Clinical characterization of young Chinese myopes with optic nerve and visual field changes resembling glaucoma. J Glaucoma. 2012;21(5):281–6.
18. Xu L, Wang Y, Yang H, Jonas JB. Differences in parapapillary atrophy between glaucomatous and normal eyes: the Beijing eye study. Am J Ophthalmol. 2007;144(4):541–6.
19. Guo Y, Wang YX, Xu L, Jonas JB. Five-year follow-up of parapapillary atrophy: the Beijing eye study. PLoS One. 2012;7(5):e32005.
20. Hu X, Shang K, Chen X, Sun X, Dai Y. Clinical features of microvasculature in subzones of parapapillary atrophy in myopic eyes: an OCT-angiography study. Eye (London). 2020. https://doi.org/10.1038/s41433-020-0872-6.
21. Jonas JB, Jonas SB, Jonas RA, et al. Parapapillary atrophy: histological gamma zone and delta zone. PLoS One. 2012;7(10):e47237.
22. Jonas JB, Ohno-Matsui K, Spaide RF, Holbach L. Panda-Jonas S. Macular Bruch's membrane defects and axial length: association with gamma zone and delta zone in peripapillary region. Invest Ophthalmol Vis Sci. 2013;54(2):1295–302.
23. Jonas JB, Weber P, Nagaoka N, Ohno-Matsui K. Glaucoma in high myopia and parapapillary delta zone. PLoS One. 2017;12(4):e0175120.
24. Hoffmann EM, Zangwill LM, Crowston JG, Weinreb RN. Optic disk size and glaucoma. Surv Ophthalmol. 2007;52(1):32–49.
25. Foster PJ, Buhrmann R, Quigley HA, Johnson GJ. The definition and classification of glaucoma in prevalence surveys. Br J Ophthalmol. 2002;86(2):238–42.
26. Prum BE Jr, Lim MC, Mansberger SL, et al. Primary open-angle glaucoma suspect preferred practice pattern guidelines. Ophthalmology. 2016;123(1):112–51.
27. Garway-Heath DF, Poinoosawmy D, Fitzke FW, Hitchings RA. Mapping the visual field to the optic disc in normal tension glaucoma eyes. Ophthalmology. 2000;107(10):1809–15.
28. Shin JW, Lee J, Kwon J, Choi J, Kook MS. Regional vascular density-visual field sensitivity relationship in glaucoma according to disease severity. Br J Ophthalmol. 2017;101(12):1666–72.
29. Ferreras A, Pablo LSE, Garway-Heath DF, Fogagnolo P, García-Feijoo J. Mapping standard automated perimetry to the peripapillary retinal nerve fiber

layer in glaucoma. Invest Ophthalmol Vis Sci. 2008;49(7):3018–25.
30. Giuffrè G. Chorioretinal degenerative changes in the tilted disc syndrome. Int Ophthalmol. 1991;15(1):1–7.
31. Jonas JB, Kling F, Gründler AE. Optic disc shape, corneal astigmatism, and amblyopia. Ophthalmology. 1997;104(11):1934–7.
32. How ACS, Tan GSW, Chan Y-H, et al. Population prevalence of tilted and torted optic discs among an adult Chinese population in Singapore: the Tanjong Pagar study. Arch Ophthalmol. 2009;127(7):894–9.
33. Vongphanit J, Mitchell P, Wang JJ. Population prevalence of tilted optic disks and the relationship of this sign to refractive error. Am J Ophthalmol. 2002;133(5):679–85.
34. Lee JY, Sung KR, Han S, Na JH. Effect of myopia on the progression of primary open-angle glaucoma. Invest Ophthalmol Vis Sci. 2015;56(3):1775–81.
35. Varma R, Steinmann WC, Scott IU. Expert agreement in evaluating the optic disc for glaucoma. Ophthalmology. 1992;99(2):215–21.
36. Hong SW, Koenigsman H, Ren R, et al. Glaucoma specialist optic disc margin, rim margin, and rim width discordance in glaucoma and glaucoma suspect eyes. Am J Ophthalmol. 2018;192:65–76.
37. O'Neill EC, Gurria LU, Pandav SS, et al. Glaucomatous optic neuropathy evaluation project: factors associated with underestimation of glaucoma likelihood. JAMA Ophthalmol. 2014;132(5):560–6.
38. Addis V, Oyeniran E, Daniel E, et al. Non-physician grader reliability in measuring morphological features of the optic nerve head in stereo digital images. Eye (London). 2019;33(5):838–44.
39. Wang X, Mudie LI, Baskaran M, et al. Crowdsourcing to evaluate fundus photographs for the presence of glaucoma. J Glaucoma. 2017;26(6):505–10.
40. Jonas JB, Bergua A, Schmitz-Valckenberg P, Papastathopoulos KI, Budde WM. Ranking of optic disc variables for detection of glaucomatous optic nerve damage. Invest Ophthalmol Vis Sci. 2000;41(7):1764–73.
41. Vijaya L, George R, Baskaran M, et al. Prevalence of primary open-angle glaucoma in an urban south Indian population and comparison with a rural population. The Chennai glaucoma study. Ophthalmology. 2008;115(4):648–54 e1.
42. Da Soh Z, Chee ML, Thakur S, et al. Asian-specific vertical cup-to-disc ratio cut-off for glaucoma screening: an evidence-based recommendation from a multi-ethnic Asian population. Clin Exp Ophthalmol. 2020;48(9):1210–8.
43. Poon LY, Solá-Del Valle D, Turalba AV, et al. The ISNT rule: how often does it apply to disc photographs and retinal nerve fiber layer measurements in the normal population? Am J Ophthalmol. 2017;184:19–27.
44. Qiu K, Wang G, Lu X, et al. Application of the ISNT rules on retinal nerve fibre layer thickness and neuroretinal rim area in healthy myopic eyes. Acta Ophthalmol. 2018;96(2):161–7.
45. Spaeth GL, Henderer J, Liu C, et al. The disc damage likelihood scale: reproducibility of a new method of estimating the amount of optic nerve damage caused by glaucoma. Trans Am Ophthalmol Soc. 2002;100:181–5. discussion 5-6
46. Henderer JD. Disc damage likelihood scale. Br J Ophthalmol. 2006;90(4):395–6.
47. Healey PR, Mitchell P, Smith W, Wang JJ. Optic disc hemorrhages in a population with and without signs of glaucoma. Ophthalmology. 1998;105(2):216–23.
48. Sugiyama K, Tomita G, Kawase K, et al. Disc hemorrhage and peripapillary atrophy in apparently healthy subjects. Acta Ophthalmol Scand. 1999;77(2): 139–42.
49. Yamamoto T, Iwase A, Kawase K, Sawada A, Ishida K. Optic disc hemorrhages detected in a large-scale eye disease screening project. J Glaucoma. 2004;13(5):356–60.
50. Rossetto JD, Melo LAS Jr, Campos MS, Tavares IM. Agreement on the evaluation of glaucomatous optic nerve head findings by ophthalmology residents and a glaucoma specialist. Clin Ophthalmol. 2017;11:1281–4.

2 What Are the Characteristic Changes to the Optic Nerve Head in Glaucoma and how Do they Evolve over Time?

Alp Atik, J. Crawford Downs, and Christopher Girkin

2.1 Introduction

The susceptibility of the optic nerve head (ONH) to intraocular pressure (IOP) related injury is a function of both the acute- and long-term response of its constituent tissues [1]. The ONH is a biomechanical structure in which IOP-related stress (force/cross-sectional area) and strain (local relative deformation of tissues) induced from IOP-related stress (force/cross-sectional area) is modulated by the morphometry and material properties of these tissues, which are both impacted by alterations in perfusion, cellular remodelling and other deleterious events in the milieu of the ONH [1–4]. Eyes with a particular combination of connective tissue geometry and stiffness, blood supply and cellular reactivity may be more susceptible to damage at normal levels of IOP, whereas others can withstand prolonged periods of relatively high levels of IOP without clinically significant detrimental effects. Moreover, strain-driven remodelling of these tissues due to age and glaucomatous disease may further alter these factors accounting for the increased susceptibility seen with aging and with advancing disease.

The mechanical properties of most soft biological tissues are dominated by an extracellular matrix (ECM) in which the connective tissue fibres (e.g. elastin and collagen) provide mechanical strength. The biomechanical properties of the ECM are tightly controlled by the specific composition and concentration of matrix components and by post-translational modifications such as glycosylation and cross-linking.

The continuous dynamic remodelling of the ECM with aging causes characteristic changes in the ONH, which play a central role in the IOP-related pathophysiology of glaucoma [1]. Additionally, IOP changes in glaucoma induce further alterations to the load-bearing ECM of the lamina cribrosa (LC) and peripapillary sclera, activate the resident cells of these tissues and damage the retinal ganglion cell (RGC) axons in the ONH [5]. It is unclear if the strain-driven remodelling in glaucoma is fundamentally different to aging, or an exaggeration of the same process.

2.2 Functional Anatomy of the Optic Nerve Head

Approximately 1.2–1.5 million RGC axons pass through the inner retina and converge at the ONH, where they exit the eye. The ONH can be divided into four anatomic regions: the superfi-

A. Atik (✉)
Department of Ophthalmology, Royal Victorian Eye and Ear Hospital, East Melbourne, VIC, Australia
e-mail: alp.atik@mail.harvard.edu

J. C. Downs · C. Girkin
Department of Ophthalmology and Visual Sciences, UAB Callahan Eye Hospital, Birmingham, AL, USA

S. Pandav et al. (eds.), *The Optic Nerve Head in Health and Disease*,
https://doi.org/10.1007/978-981-33-6838-5_2

cial nerve fibre layer (SNFL) followed, respectively, by the prelaminar, laminar and retrolaminar portions. The differences in these regions reflect the changing conditions to which the axons are exposed as they course through the ONH.

The entire passageway for the RGC axons passing through the eye wall has been termed the neural canal [6]. The neural canal extends from its internal opening at Bruch's membrane to its external opening at the posterior scleral canal. It is comprised of a pre-scleral and scleral component. The scleral canal portion of the neural canal extends from the anterior to the posterior surface of the sclera.

2.2.1 Superficial Nerve Fibre Layer

The SNFL is composed mainly of non-myelinated axons originating from the ganglion cells of the inner retina. They are interspersed with astroglial tissue. After travelling on the surface of the retina, the axons make an acute turn into the choroid. The vertical organisation of RGC axons within the retinal nerve fibre layer (RNFL) is retinotopic, depending on the proximity of the cell bodies to the ONH. Fibres from peripheral retina occupy the peripheral portions of the optic nerve while the more proximal axons lie centrally [7, 8]. Within the SNFL, the axons become progressively segregated into bundles by Müller cell processes and astrocytes.

2.2.2 Prelaminar Optic Nerve Head (Lamina Choroidalis)

The prelaminar portion of the ONH is the indistinct segment of axons surrounded by the outer retinal layers, choriocapillaris and choroid. It is composed primarily of astroglial cell bodies ordered into columns parallel to the axon bundles and interconnected by their processes in a basket-like arrangement. Extensions from these processes also enter the axon bundles, interdigitating and providing intimate contact with the axons [9].

2.2.3 Laminar Optic Nerve Head (Lamina Cribrosa)

The laminar portion of the nerve is contained with the lamina cribrosa (LC)—a fenestrated, three-dimensional network of load-bearing trabeculae that provides structural and nutrient support to the axons they pass from the relatively high-pressure environment in the eye to a low-pressure region in the retrobulbar cerebrospinal space [3, 10, 11].

The LC is a reticular structure filled with collagen fibrils and elastin fibres [12]. On cross-section, they form 500–600 pores of variable diameter (which convey the nerve fascicles arranged in bundles approximately 100 microns wide) and insert into the peripapillary sclera and/or pia mater [13]. The plates are lined by astrocytes resting on basement membranes, separating the ECM from the nerve fibre bundles. As in the prelaminar ONH, astrocyte processes extend into the axon bundles.

The LC is the main load-bearing connective tissue and acts as the primary source of structural stiffness in the ONH [4]. Its morphology can alter profoundly with aging and with progressive glaucomatous injury in which focal defects such as holes, pits and scleral disinsertions can develop [14].

2.2.4 Retrolaminar Optic Nerve Head

The retrolaminar portion of the ONH marks the posterior border of the LC and corresponds to the beginning of axonal myelination by oligodendrocytes. The posterior laminar beams are contiguous with the retrolaminar septa in this region with no distinct demarcation with the average beam orientation becoming less aligned with the scleral plane moving from the posterior laminar beams to retrolaminar septa [15]. The axon bundles are separated by collagenous septa, which (with axonal myelination) increases the thickness of the retrolaminar portion of the ONH to 3–4 mm.

2.2.5 Peripapillary Sclera

The LC and peripapillary sclera collectively form the connective tissues of the ONH. The peripapillary sclera is a 1–2 mm wide region bordering the neural canal opening. The superficial layers of the peripapillary sclera stromal connective tissue merge with the dural sheath of the optic nerve [12]. This forms the peripapillary scleral flange, which functions as a bridge between the sclera just outside the optic nerve meninges and the LC of the ONH. The deeper scleral fibres become continuous with the LC and provide the mechanical boundary conditions for the LC at its insertion into the scleral canal wall [16].

Scleral lamellae are comprised of collagen fibrils of various diameter with irregular spacing between them [17]. Collagen fibrils in the peripapillary sclera are more uniform in diameter, show greater spatial order and associate with increased numbers of elastin fibres compared to other regions of the posterior segment [18]. The diameter and organisation of collagen fibrils are significant determinants of scleral biomechanical properties. Collagen fibrils are oriented radial to the canal wall in the anterior sclera and more circumferential more posterior in the canal, while interwoven fibrils occur throughout the thickness [19]. The collagen fibres (90% of which are type I) form a layered, fibrous stroma embedded in a hydrated matrix of proteoglycans, elastin and fibroblasts [52].

2.2.6 Vascular Supply of the Optic Nerve Head

The blood supply of the ONH is a centripetal system, whose source varies according to segment. The SNFL is supplied mainly by branches of the central retinal artery. The remainder of the ONH is supplied by direct branches of the short posterior ciliary arteries (SPCAs) and the circle of Zinn-Haller—an intra-scleral vascular structure around the ONH, originating from the SPCAs. Small, end-arterial branches are sent from this circle to the ONH.

Anteriorly, the capillaries of the choroidal lamina are ensheathed by astrocytes within the glial columns. More posteriorly, capillaries are encased within the lamina beams of the LC and in the septa of the retrolaminar optic nerve. The intra-scleral and intra-laminar vasculature is unique in that it is encased in load-bearing connective tissue. Despite regional differences in the architecture of the non-fenestrated capillaries of the ONH, they are interconnected to form a continuous network.

Venous drainage from all levels of the optic nerve is into the central retinal vein.

2.3 Relevance of Optic Nerve Head Anatomy to the Pathophysiology of Glaucoma

Various anatomical features of the ONH make it susceptible to age- or pressure-induced damage, especially in eyes with a particular combination of tissue geometry and material properties. Axons must turn through 75–110° to exit the eye to maintain a retinotopic arrangement within the optic nerve. With age and IOP-related stress, the laminar beams actively remodel in a way that is likely to induce greater compressive force on axons (and their blood supply) lying in the peripheral part of the optic nerve [21].

The vasculature of the ONH has also unique aspects. It is an end-organ capillary bed encased in load-bearing connective tissue that is under continuous strain from the point these vessels penetrate the sclera. This anatomy intrinsically couples the vascular and mechanical pathophysiology models of glaucoma.

As such, in recent years, the ONH has been recognised as an integrated biomechanical structure. In this paradigm, variations in IOP-induced strain seen between individuals, with increasing age and glaucomatous injury, are distributed within the ONH according to the architecture and composition of its load-bearing connective tissues. This strain alters the perfusion and cellular behaviour in these tissues, which drives age-related and glaucomatous remodelling that further alters how IOP-related stress is experienced as strain by these tissues. Thus, perfusion, mechanical behaviour and tissue remodelling are intrinsic and inseparably intertwined within this biomechanical framework for the pathogenesis of glaucoma.

2.3.1 Lamina Cribrosa

The LC is commonly accepted as the principal site of RGC axonal injury in glaucoma [22, 23]. It is only approximately one-third of the thickness of the sclera at the scleral canal and its load-bearing connective tissues only comprise about 40% of the tissue volume in the laminar region of the ONH [10]. The LC beams have abundant connections between each other and form a compact three-dimensional array of pores through which axon bundles run [24]. The LC is an interconnected mesh-like structure in which any forces that result in distortion of one part will be transmitted throughout the structure.

The LC must provide structural support to the ONH by withstanding IOP-related mechanical strain while allowing the axons an open pathway to the brain. The LC also contains many of the capillaries that nourish the axons and cells in the laminar region and must resist the high mechanical strains that would otherwise reduce vessel size and blood flow [10].

The LC architecture is such that there is a lower density of support in the superior and inferior laminar pores (Fig. 2.1) [21, 24–26]. Local laminar strain has been correlated to local laminar density in primate eyes [27]. In these low-density segments, the pores tend to be larger and the laminar beams thinner, providing less support for the axon bundles. These LC features are also racially dependent, with an increase in LC pore size in the superior and inferior poles of the ONH and an increase in the number of pores in patients of African descent [28].

The number of laminar pores increases with increasing depth in the nerve. As a result, axons do not take a direct path out of the eye [29, 30]. This deviation can potentially make some axon populations more vulnerable as they pass between the LC plates [30, 31].

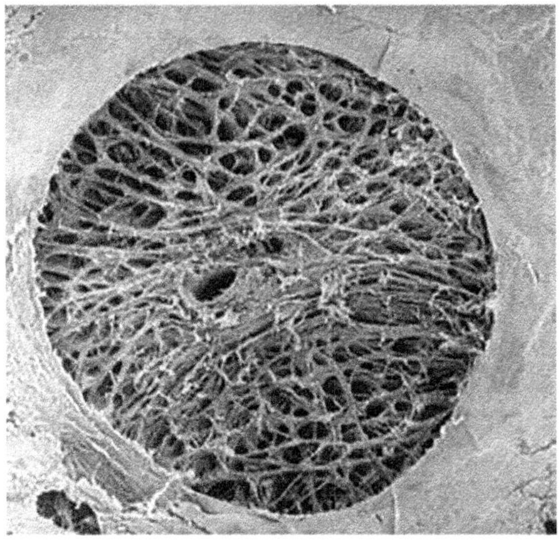

Fig. 2.1 Scanning electron microscopy of the normal LC. Note the smaller pores and denser collagen horizontally in contrast to the superior and inferior quadrants. Reproduced from Quigley et al. [24]

Axons within the LC don't have a direct blood supply. Axonal nutrition is dependent on diffusion of nutrients from the laminar capillaries, across the endothelial and pericyte basement membranes, through the extracellular matrix of the laminar beam, across the basement membrane of the astrocytes, into the astrocytes, across the astrocytic processes to the adjacent axons [32]. As such, axons are susceptible to changes in the laminar extracellular matrix and astrocyte basement membranes. Some recent evidence suggests that while many capillaries lie within the laminar trabeculae, there are also many that lie outside the beams themselves [33].

Individual beams of the LC are lined by astroglial components that vary throughout the laminar region [34]. Two types of astroglial cells populate the LC—astrocytes and LC cells [35]. Astrocytes in the LC line the laminar beams, resting on a basement membrane and extending cell processes into the ECM core to establish contact with processes of other astrocytes, axons and LC cells. They support and influence the ECM and RGC axons, and can become reactive astrocytes, changing their morphology, distribution and function with stress [36]. ONH astrocytes communicate via a network of gap junctions to form a syncytium, which may be a mediator of axonal injury [37]. They can generate harmful substances such as nitric oxide which can result in direct axonal damage [38]. Astrocytes lying at the myelin transition zone also have a phagocytic role by internalising axonal evulsions, which may be upregulated and contribute to axonal damage [39].

LC cells play an integral role in ECM remodelling [40]. They can upregulate expression of genes such as transforming growth factor-beta (TGF-β), which are important profibrotic modulators of ECM metabolism whose levels are elevated in glaucoma [40]. They share many similarities with myofibroblast cells, which are known to be associated with fibrotic disease [40, 41]. These include constituent expression of elastin, collagen type I and fibronectin. Both LC cells and ONH astrocytes exhibit actin microfilaments, which are involved in cellular contractility and can be remodelled by stress [42]. Contraction of these fibres takes place on a protracted time scale compared with muscle fibres and is thought to modulate cellular stiffness [43].

Integrins are especially prevalent in the LC and peripapillary sclera. These membrane-spanning proteins are capable of sensing external tissue forces and transmitting them into internal cellular responses, recruiting and activating matrix metalloproteinases (which dissolve the ECM) and allowing the migration of cells inherent in cell proliferation and tissue remodelling [44]. Integrins bind to ligands in the ECM and interact with the intracellular actin cytoskeleton [45]. In the setting of ECM stress, they activate intracellular domains, resulting in changes to cell motility, shape, survival and proliferation. Integrins also regulate force transmission from intracellular stress fibres to the local microenvironment, allowing for myofibroblast activation in the LC [46]. The individual LC beams are thus exquisitely sensitive to changes in the local biomechanical strain environment [10].

2.3.2 Peripapillary Sclera

The ONH is a discontinuation of the corneo-scleral shell and is thus considered a biomechanically weak spot within an otherwise strong corneo-scleral envelope [2]. Such discontinuities are considered weak spots in load systems as they can be a site of mechanical stress concentrations [47].

The peripapillary sclera surrounds the ONH and is thinnest at the posterior scleral canal opening [48]. It transmits IOP-related forces and deformations to the ONH at the scleral canal wall. Moreover, the penetrating branches of the short posterior ciliary arteries that perfuse the lamina cribrosa and the overlying peripapillary choroid mush traverse this region. Hence, the shape, thickness and material properties of the sclera have a significant impact on ONH biomechanical behaviour and perfusion.

The collagen comprising the scleral canal and peripapillary sclera shows a non-uniform (anisotropic) distribution [49]. There are also significant differences in collagen content and orientation that result in 'thin spots' with low collagen density [49]. There is likely higher strain in these areas within both the peripapillary sclera and adjacent LC at its insertion into the scleral canal wall [15].

Crimp is the 'waviness' of collagen fibres in the sclera and is a major determinant of tissue biomechanical behaviour [50]. Its parameters include amplitude and frequency (period). As a single fibre stretches, it loses its waves (uncrimps) and can only be stretched further by making the fibre longer using more force (and thus making it stiffer). At low IOP, collagen fibres in the sclera are initially crimped, making the sclera more compliant. As IOP increases, the scleral collagen fibres uncrimp and eventually become straight, resulting in a dramatic increase in scleral stiffness (Fig. 2.2a). The posterior sclera is thus highly non-linear (i.e. it gets stiffer as IOP increases) and anisotropic (i.e. the underlying collagen fibril distribution is non-uniform and changes throughout the scleral shell, thereby affecting directional stiffness) (Fig. 2.2b) [51]. The differences in the architecture of the scleral portion of the neural canal (large size, elliptical shape and thin peripapillary sclera) likely influence the level of IOP-related connective tissue stress for a given IOP [52].

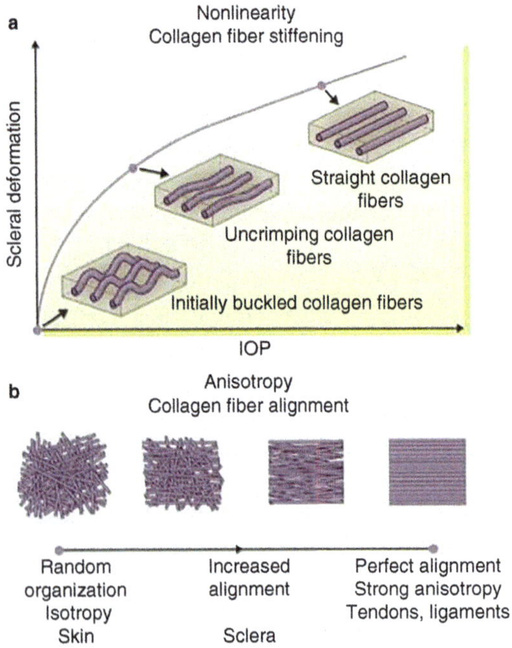

Fig. 2.2 Non-linearity and anisotropy are the two major biomechanical features that arise from the presence and organisation of the scleral collagen fibres. (**a**) Non-linearity occurs when the relationship between loading and deformation is not linear. At low IOP, collagen fibres are initially crimped, making the sclera more compliant. As a single fibre stretches, it uncrimps, requiring relatively little force until it loses all crimp. The straightened fibre can only be stretched further by making it longer, which requires increasing force and so the fibre appears stiffer. The stiffness of multiple fibres depends on the distribution of baseline crimp in the fibres. As IOP increases, the scleral collagen fibres uncrimp and become straight, resulting in increased scleral stiffness. (**b**) Schematic representation of planar anisotropy. A highly disorganised arrangement of collagen fibres resists loads in multiple directions, a property known as isotropy. In contrast, well-organised collagen fibres sustain loads differently along and across their length, a property known as anisotropy. Adapted from Sigal et al. [53]

2.4 Characteristic Changes to the Optic Nerve Head with Age

Even at physiologic levels of IOP, the load-bearing connective tissues of the peripapillary sclera, scleral canal wall and LC experience substantial mechanical stress and strain [54]. This exposure over time leads to a spectrum of changes in both the connective tissues and vasculature that comprises the biomechanical environment of the ONH and may underlie the increasing risk of glaucomatous injury seen with aging [55, 56]. These changes stiffen the connective tissues of the ONH, reduce compliance and diminish nutrient diffusion into the axons from the capillaries encased in the laminar beams [57], ultimately decreasing perfusion and leading to increased susceptibility to IOP-induced glaucomatous injury. It is thus important to appreciate that glaucomatous remodelling occurs in the context of changes associated with normal aging and that the aged eye (especially in certain races) may be more susceptible to IOP-related deformity due to these age-related alteration in biomechanical response.

2.4.1 Lamina Cribrosa

The ECM in the laminar beams is composed of collagen, elastin fibres, proteoglycans and other constituents [58]. During normal aging, profound changes have been observed in the LC ECM, including increased collagen, elastin and proteoglycan deposition [56, 59, 60]; change in the type of collagen, elastin and proteoglycans deposited [56, 60]; increased glycation cross-linking of collagen and elastin to produce advanced glycation end-products (AGE), thickening of astrocyte basement membranes [61, 62] and increased rigidity [56, 63].

The LC of younger eyes shows considerable elasticity and can, after a mechanical stress has been removed, return to its normal configuration. With older eyes, the elasticity of the tissue is lower and there is less of a tendency for the deformation to resolve with resolution of the impose pressure [63].

2.4.2 Peripapillary Sclera

Similar to the LC, the sclera has an extremely complex ECM microstructure with highly anisotropic collagen and elastin fibrils. The peripapillary sclera has been shown to stiffen with age [20, 55, 56, 64], possibly as a protective mechanism against mechanical strain. This stiffening results from age-related glycation cross-linking of the fibrillar extracellular matrix [65], a significant decrease in the degree of collagen fibre alignment, alterations in the content of scleral glycosaminoglycans [66], a significant increase in the matrix stiffness and a significant decrease in mechanical anisotropy [67]. Such age-related changes have been shown to occur more rapidly and over a larger area of the posterior scleral shell in people of African heritage [68]. These age- and race-related differences may be due to a higher collagen cross-linking density which reduces scleral collagen fibril solubility and/or loss of elastin-driven recoil [65].

All crimp parameters are significantly decreased with aging, consistent with progressive scleral stiffening [19]. Scleral stiffening decreases the elastic ability of the eye to absorb IOP energy, thus causing larger transient IOP fluctuations related to blinks, saccades and vascular filling [2]. Age-related scleral stiffening increases more dramatically in individuals of African descent who are at greater risk of disease progression. Stiffer sclera has also been shown to be associated with increased ganglion cell loss in animal models [69–71]. Other age-related morphologic changes in the peripapillary sclera include thinning [74] and changes in permeability [72].

The morphology of the peripapillary sclera is also altered by aging. The shape of the anterior peripapillary sclera is a characteristic v-shaped configuration, which becomes increasingly oblique with age [73]. This may be due to the degeneration of ONH connective tissues (e.g. elastin) and thinning of the sclera which occurs in the course of aging. An oblique peripapillary scleral boundary is associated with a more oblique neural canal [74]. This may contribute to damage and posterior deformation when IOP increases in susceptible eyes. A v-shaped configuration of the peripapillary sclera is also associated with a deeper cup of the ONH [73].

2.5 Characteristic Changes to the Optic Nerve Head with Early Glaucoma

A common clinical feature of early glaucoma is ONH cupping [47]. This cupping has two components: prelaminar and laminar [74, 75]. Prelaminar cupping of the ONH is characterised by the progressive loss of the prelaminar neural tissues. This increases both the depth and width of the cup and thus increases the cup-to-disc ratio [47]. In contrast, laminar cupping is connective tissue-based, with the LC progressively moving either anteriorly or posteriorly and excavating beneath the anterior scleral canal. In most cases, ONH cupping is a combination of these two components, reflecting both damage to and remodelling of laminar connective tissue and progressive loss of RGC axons.

Early glaucomatous cupping is principally the result of fixed deformation of the connective tissues of the neural canal wall and LC, rather than a manifestation of prelaminar neural tissue thinning due to axon loss [74]. In fact, there is evidence of prelaminar tissue thickening with animal models of early glaucoma, probably as a result of orthograde axoplasmic transport blockade within the RGC axons combined with prelaminar tissue oedema and gliosis [74].

The relationship between IOP and the deformations of the ONH (specifically the LC) and peripapillary sclera is complex (Fig. 2.3). The sclera deforms as IOP fluctuates, and these deformations create the boundary conditions which modulate strain within the LC in response to IOP [74, 76, 77]. As such, the ONH and peripapillary sclera behave as a mechanical system responding to IOP fluctuations.

From a biomechanical perspective, there are two components of acute IOP-induced deformation of the ONH in glaucoma (Fig. 2.4). The first is the effect of IOP on the anterior laminar surface, which deforms the lamina posteriorly. The second is the effect of IOP on the sclera, which causes expansion of the neural canal. These deformations are transmitted to the LC through its insertion into the canal wall, pulling the LC taut and displacing it anteriorly. As IOP increases, both components act simultaneously to varying degrees, depending on the material properties of the LC and sclera [27, 76, 78]. This results in a very small (under 10 μm) net anterior-posterior displacement of the LC [77, 79–81].

IOP is extremely variable, changing with blinks, saccades, ocular pulse and other eye movements [82, 83]. In fact, telemetry studies in non-human primates have revealed that the eye must

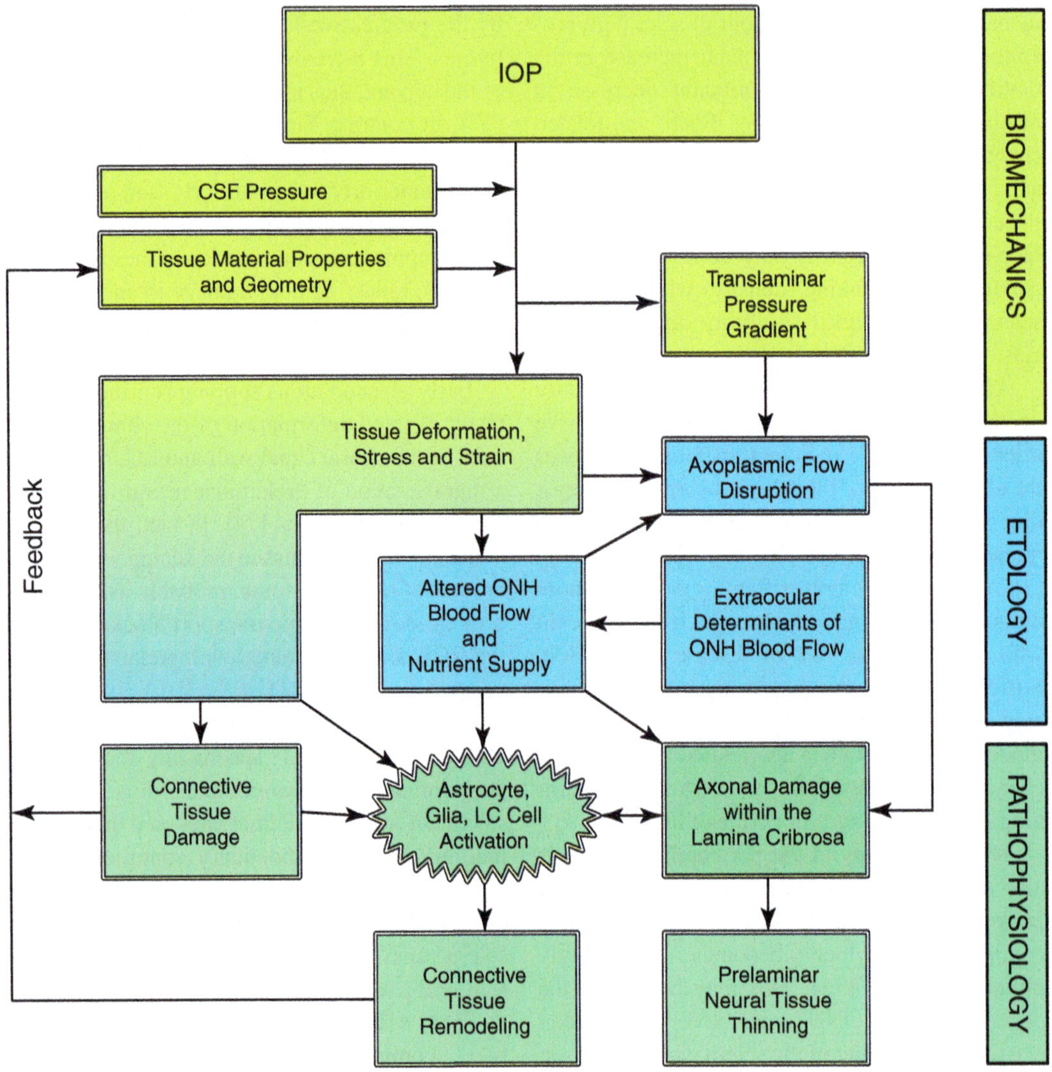

Fig. 2.3 IOP and cerebrospinal fluid act mechanically on the ONH, producing deformations and stress within the tissues. These deformations depend on the eye-specific geometry and material properties of the individual eye. In a biomechanical model, the stress and strain alters blood flow and the delivery of nutrients through chronic alterations in connective tissue stiffness and diffusion properties. IOP-related stress and strain also induces connective tissue damage via direct (laminar beam yield) and indirect (cell-mediated remodelling) mechanisms. This creates a positive feedback loop onto the mechanical effects of IOP. Reproduced from Downs [2]

absorb 2000–4000 transient IOP fluctuations per hour during waking hours, and 12% of the total IOP-related energy the eye must absorb during waking hours is due to these IOP fluctuations [84]. IOP-induced stress and strain in glaucoma causes pathologic changes in the ONH microarchitecture that exceed the effects of aging [2]. The eye can be considered an elastic pressure vessel that can expand and contract to absorb some of the energy associated with raised IOP [10]. Stiff ocular tissues absorb less energy and thus engender larger IOP transients [85], creating a cycle of progressive ECM remodelling and tissue stiffening consistent with progressive glaucoma.

The following anatomical changes in the ONH have been described in non-human primates with early glaucoma from moderate IOP elevation (Fig. 2.5):

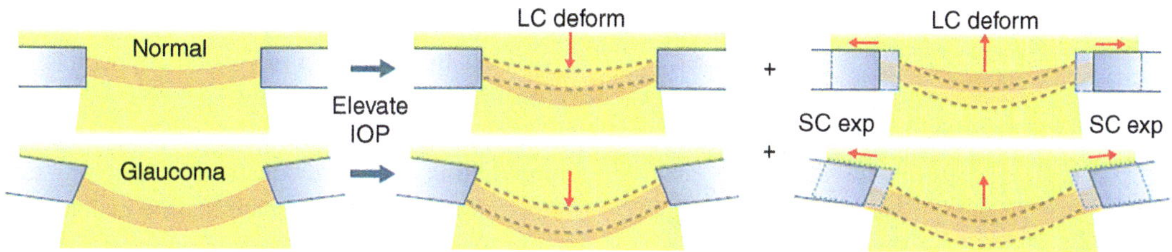

Fig. 2.4 Two biomechanical components of IOP-induced deformation of the LC in normal (upper) and glaucomatous (lower) eyes. One component is the effect of IOP on the anterior laminar surface, which deforms the LC posteriorly. The other component is the effect of IOP on the peripapillary sclera, which causes expansion of the scleral canal. Note that the glaucomatous eye has undergone permanent changes in ONH geometry including thickening of the lamina, posterior deformation of the lamina and peripapillary sclera and posterior scleral canal expansion. As IOP increases, the lamina displaces posteriorly due to the direct action of IOP. Much of this posterior deformation is counteracted as the lamina is pulled taut by the simultaneous expansion of the scleral canal. Even though the net result of the IOP-related deformation is a small amount of posterior LC displacement, substantial levels of IOP-related strain are induced in both the peripapillary sclera and LC. Reproduced from Downs et al. [32]

1. Lamina cribrosa
   - Posterior deformation and thickening of the LC [74] due to connective tissue synthesis and remodelling
   - Outward (posterior) migration of the posterior lamina insertion point [86]
   - Less pronounced outward migration of the anterior lamina insertion point [86]
2. Peripapillary sclera
   - Enlargement and elongation of the scleral canal [87]
   - Alteration in the elastic and viscoelastic material properties of the peripapillary sclera [16]

2.5.1 Lamina Cribrosa

LC strains in glaucoma are complex and arise from multiple sources of force [10]. Although IOP is the primer driver of ONH biomechanics, it is counterbalanced at the LC by the retrolaminar tissue pressure of the cerebrospinal fluid (CSF) surrounding the optic nerve [88]. As such, the mechanical stress in the LC is a combination of IOP acting on its inner surface, counteracted by CSF pressure on its outer surface. In addition, there are separate in-wall lateral forces imparted by the sclera at the LC insertion [10]. These forces are mediated by scleral mechanical behaviour, as well as the microarchitecture and local directional stiffness of the LC trabeculae [89–91].

2.5.1.1 Microarchitecture

The laminar microarchitecture of non-human primates with even early glaucoma demonstrates extensive remodelling. Characteristic changes include LC pore enlargement, LC beam thickening, increased laminar region volume and increased laminar connective tissue volume [92]. The increase in connective tissue volume fraction of 44–82% has been demonstrated in an early primate model of experimental glaucoma [93]. It is at least partly due to the recruitment of retrolaminar septa into the load-bearing LC, where they synthesise connective tissue. This strongly suggests that connective tissue remodelling and synthesis is active in the early stages of glaucomatous optic neuropathy [32]. Even though the LC adds a significant volume of connective tissue through modelling very early in the disease, the tissue is weakened considerably during this process [78]. The remodelling cascade in the laminar ECM thus likely begins with a reorganisation process that first weakens the tissues, followed by consolidation and stiffening.

As glaucoma progresses, the LC migrates either anteriorly or posteriorly in the scleral canal [86]. This migration can occur over a relatively short duration of glaucoma progression, starting even in the early stages of disease. Increasing laminar depth has been correlated in glaucoma patients with younger age, higher untreated IOP and lower RNFL thickness [94].

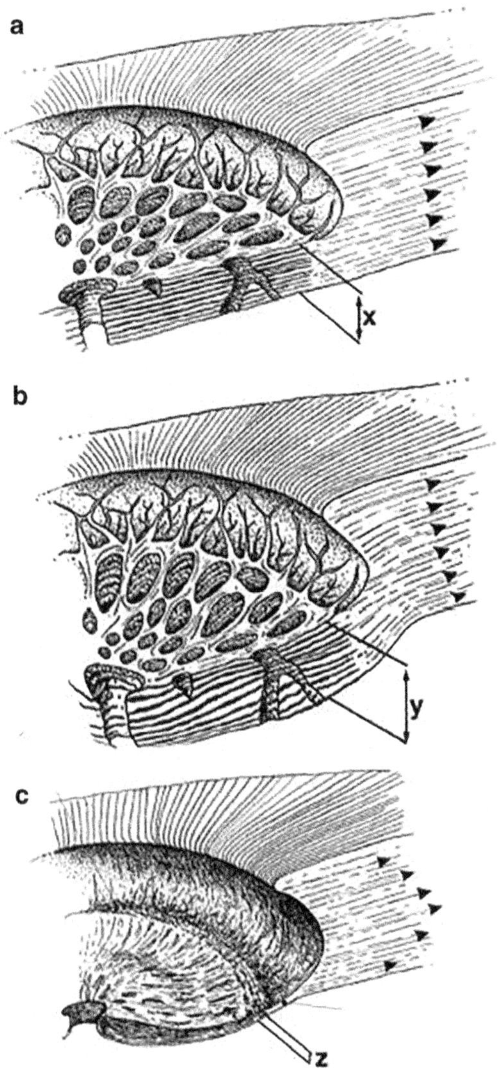

Fig. 2.5 Progression of ONH morphology from normal to early glaucoma to advanced glaucoma. (**a**) Normal ONH showing the thickness of the LC (x) and the stress created in the peripapillary sclera from raised IOP (arrowheads). (**b**) The ONH in early glaucoma with permanent posterior deformation and thickening (y) of the LC rather than failure of the laminar beams that occurs in permanent expansion of the posterior scleral canal. These changes suggest a combination of growth and remodelling of the connective tissues occur very early in glaucoma and are not yet accompanied by frank excavation. (**c**) As glaucoma advances, the lamina compresses (z) and scars, the lamina insertion into the sclera migrates further posteriorly and the scleral canal enlarges to the typical cupped and excavated morphology. Modified from Burgoyne et al. [52]

2.5.1.2 Cellular Changes

The cells that maintain the ocular connective tissues are biologically active and the ONH and peripapillary sclera are in a constant state of remodelling. Cells are constantly expressing factors that influence ECM degradation and synthesis to maintain biomechanical homeostasis [95].

ONH astrocytes and LC cells can sense their mechanical environment and respond to mechanical stimuli by remodelling the ECM [47]. Extensive remodelling of the ECM has been reported in the LC of eyes with early glaucoma. This remodelling includes reduction in the elastin content [96], buckling and disconnection of the elastin fibres from the ECM [18], loss of fibre-forming types of collagen [97, 98], proliferation of type-IV collagen in locations previously occupied by RGC axons [62, 99] and accumulation of chondroitin sulphate glycosaminoglycans [100]. These remodelling events in the LC affect the morphology and mechanical stiffness of these tissues and thus alter the load-bearing tissue response to chronic elevation of IOP, which drives further remodelling.

LC cells upregulate ECM and profibrotic gene expression (e.g. TGF-β1) in glaucoma [101]. Stress-induced glial cell activation after exposure of LC cells to strain involve major protein hubs (e.g. TGF-β1) and play an important role in ONH connective tissue remodelling [102]. In addition, LC cells can reorganise their cytoskeleton in response to stress to profoundly impact contractile properties and increase cell stiffness in response to biomechanical strains of the ONH [103].

ONH astrocytes can become reactive astrocytes in early glaucoma [36]. Reactive astrocytes increase the synthesis of ECM macromolecules [98], cell adhesion molecules and recognition molecules [36], a variety of growth factors and cytokines [104] and cell mediators and receptors [104]. An increase in the immunoreactivity for specific MMPs associated with astrocytes has been demonstrated in the glaucomatous ONH [105]. MMPs break down the ECM and allow profibrotic cells to migrate and rebuild the matrix

[106]. These changes contribute to the remodelling of the ONH and LC during glaucoma progression. ONH astrocytes can also migrate out from laminar cribriform plates in response to elevated hydrostatic pressure [107]. These astrocytic responses to elevated IOP may underlie cellular changes and several signal transduction pathways that lead to axonal damage and tissue remodelling in glaucoma.

A change in the location and alteration of integrin subunits of astroglial cells in the LC have been reported in glaucomatous eyes, creating an important link between LC stiffening and deformation and LC connective tissue remodelling in glaucoma [44]. The pattern of integrin alteration was similar between primary open-angle glaucoma and secondary glaucoma, suggesting that the responses observed are a generalised response of the ONH to altered stresses from IOP.

2.5.2 Peripapillary Sclera

The peripapillary sclera is a site of substantial stress and strain concentration in the ONH [76, 108]. As the main load-bearing tissue within the eye, it plays a central role in maintaining the mechanical integrity of the pressurised eye needed for pristine optics. It transmits the IOP-related forces and deformations to the LC [81, 109] and its mechanical properties (e.g. stiffness, collagen fibre organisation) have an influential role in governing the biomechanical environment of the ONH [1, 110].

The overall response of a tissue to a load is the combination of immediate (elastic) and time-dependent (viscous) responses, which are governed by its viscoelastic material properties of these tissues [111]. All ONH tissues are viscoelastic and their material properties are important to understanding their behaviour as load-bearing structures in response to short- and long-term changes in applied load.

The biomechanical properties of the peripapillary sclera are altered early in glaucoma. As scleral stiffness changes with aging and progressive glaucoma, the amount of deformation it experiences at a given IOP also changes. Since the other neural and vascular tissues in the retina and ONH are relatively more compliant compared to the sclera, scleral deformations are transmitted to all ONH tissues. As such, any changes to the scleral response to IOP (e.g. stiffness) significantly influences ONH biomechanics, especially within the peripapillary sclera (Fig. 2.6).

In addition to increased stiffening with age, the human sclera also shows significant stiffening in response to acute and chronic IOP exposure [16] and due to glaucomatous remodelling [20]. Stiffness of the peripapillary sclera has been shown to be a major material determinant of IOP-driven LC deformation [109, 112]. A compliant sclera allows the scleral canal to expand in response to elevated IOP, pulling the lamina taut within the canal and thereby increasing laminar resistance to posterior deformation. In contrast, a stiff sclera allows less IOP-driven

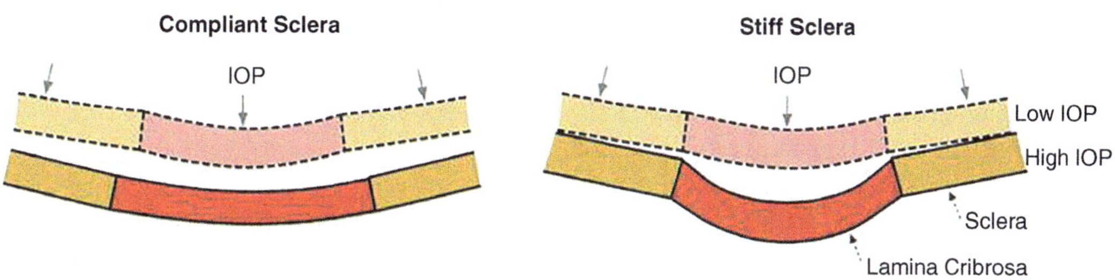

Fig. 2.6 Influence of scleral biomechanics on the ONH. IOP induces large scleral canal expansions in eyes with compliant sclera (left) that pulls the contained lamina taut despite the direct posterior force of IOP on the laminar surface. Conversely, a stiff sclera allows relatively little canal expansion with IOP elevation (right) and less stretching of the contained lamina. This causes the lamina to be displaced posteriorly by the direct action of IOP on its anterior surface. Reproduced from Sigal et al. [53]

expansion of the scleral canal, forcing the LC alone to bear the IOP-related stress [2].

2.5.2.1 Microarchitecture

The microstructure of the sclera consists of a complex load-bearing network of collagen fibres embedded in a proteoglycan matrix. The collagen fibres aggregate into lamellae that tend to be arranged within the plane of the sclera [113] and locally exhibit preferred orientations. Glaucoma is associated with decreased collagen density in the peripapillary sclera [18] and increased fibre and inter-fibre matrix stiffness in the peripapillary sclera [114–116], indicating the scleral ECM undergoes dynamic remodelling in response to IOP elevation.

The equilibrium modulus is a measure of a tissue's stiffness after it is fully relaxed following rapid deformation [111]. It is a measure of the long-term stiffness of the tissue. The peripapillary sclera exhibits an increased equilibrium modulus in early glaucoma [111], suggesting that its long-term elastic properties are altered via ECM damage or remodelling early in the disease. Variations in the degree of fibre alignment in the peripapillary sclera may determine the level of mechanical strains within the ONH [112, 117]. The increased fibre stiffening may be caused by accumulation of non-enzymatic glycation type cross-links of collagen fibrils [116].

Following acute IOP elevation, there is posterior bowing of the peripapillary sclera and expansion of the scleral canal [118, 119]. These acute changes signal a remodelling response that results in permanent alterations to the architecture of these load-bearing connective tissue that are present even at the earliest detectable stage of experimental glaucoma in the primate model [87]. All neural canal landmarks demonstrate at least regional radial expansion and axial elongation with raised IOP. The posterior scleral microstructure in glaucoma is organised such that there is increased scleral canal expansion with increased IOP [110, 120]. This is greatest in the external portions of the neural canal—the posterior laminar insertion point and the posterior scleral canal opening [87].

2.5.2.2 Cellular Changes

In comparison to ECM, less is known of the response of cells to eye pressure fluctuation. Cultured human scleral fibroblasts have been shown to be sensitive to their mechanical environment with altered expression levels of ECM molecules [121, 122], promotion of phenotypic changes such as differentiation into contractile myofibroblasts [123]. Animal models have shown a six-fold increase in cell proliferation in the sclera following IOP elevation [124].

2.6 Characteristic Changes to the Optic Nerve Head with Advanced Glaucoma

IOP-related deformations of the LC and peripapillary sclera are linked even in advanced glaucoma [110]. Excavational, deep laminar cupping of the ONH is the hallmark of advanced glaucoma, differentiating it from other axonal injuries. Characteristic features of the ONH associated with advanced glaucoma involve the following inter-related anatomical changes (Fig. 2.5) [24, 125]:

1. Prelaminar
   - Loss of neural rim axons
2. Lamina cribrosa
   - Deep posterior laminar deformation from elongation, stretching and collapse of the laminar beams
   - Profound excavation, thinning and scarring of the LC beneath the scleral canal rim (Fig. 2.7)
3. Peripapillary sclera
   - Progressive peripapillary scleral thinning and stiffening

2.6.1 Lamina Cribrosa

Strain-driven laminar remodelling resulting in migration of the LC is the likely central mechanism underlying the profound permanent deformation, thinning and scarring of the LC seen in advanced glaucoma [47].

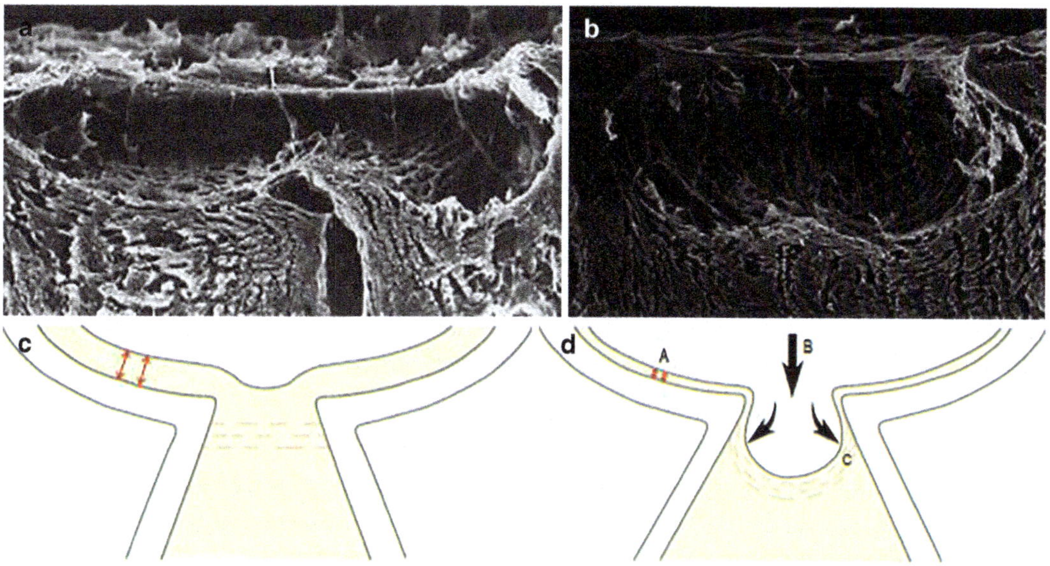

Fig. 2.7 Electron micrographs of the connective tissues of the ONH after trypsin digestion in (**a**) early glaucoma and (**b**) advanced glaucoma (reproduced from Quigley et al. [24]). As glaucoma excavation occurs, the LC takes on a W-shape and excavates beneath the scleral canal rim. (**c**) Schematic representation of a normal optic nerve head with the normally thick RNFL, minimal central cup and orientation of the laminar pores aligned with the curve of the posterior scleral wall. (**d**) Schematic representation of advanced glaucoma with thinning of the RNFL due to loss of neural rim axons (red arrows), posterior excavation and enlargement of the central cup (large black arrow) and posterior outward rotation of the LC with cupping (small curved black arrows). Reproduced from Stamper et al. [126]

Chronic IOP elevation induces remodelling-based stiffening of the LC [127], creating a feedback cycle that alters laminar stiffness as glaucoma progresses, which in conjunction with age-related connective tissue stiffening, remodels the eye to a state wherein the ONH is more susceptible IOP-related stress [2].

2.6.1.1 Microarchitecture

Loss of neural rim axons is associated with axonal atrophy in the retinal nerve fibre layer, prelaminar region, LC and retrolaminar region [128]. There is also associated overall tissue atrophy in the prelaminar region and retinal ganglion cell atrophy [128].

Thickening and recruitment of retrolaminar septa into the load-bearing LC in early glaucoma eventually leads to laminar deformation, collapse of the laminar beams and subsequent retrolaminar fibrosis [128]. At end-stage disease, there is total deformation, thinning and condensation of the LC [24, 129, 130]. There is also a significant decrease in collagen fibril density and regularity in the ECM of the LC in advanced glaucoma [106].

Thinning of the LC may increase glaucoma susceptibility by steepening the translaminar pressure gradient between the intraocular space and retrobulbar space (where the CSF is situated). This steepening of the gradient may impose additional compressive forces to the LC [131, 132], causing further deformation, which may at least partly explain why eyes with advanced glaucoma have a higher risk of progression than eyes with moderate stages of glaucoma [133].

The optic nerve volume shrinks with advanced glaucoma, decreasing the diameter of the optic nerve within the pia mater. This widens the part of the posterior LC surface directly exposed to the pia mater (and thus indirectly exposed to CSF). Since CSF does not resist a focally accentuated backward bowing of the LC, this can lead to a circumscribed herniation of the LC into the retrobulbar CSF space. This herniation may be enhanced by the anatomy of the LC itself, with its larger pores and less pronounced interpore connective tissue close to the optic disc border compared to the centre of the optic disc [21].

The posterior migration of the laminar insertion in advanced glaucoma is associated with physical disruption and remodelling of the laminar beams [1, 106, 129, 134] and their contained capillaries, providing the structural changes that lead to excavation [24, 129] and glaucomatous optic disc haemorrhage [135, 136]. This posterior laminar migration can be a distance greater than the full thickness of the LC [5, 86] or into the pia mater [13] as seen in acquired optic nerve pits.

2.6.1.2 Cellular Changes

Severe ONH damage from raised IOP in animal models is associated increased ONH cellularity and an increased expression of genes (e.g. TGF-β) associated with activation of microglia, immune response, ribosomes and lysosomes in a linear fashion [137].

Astrocyte basement membrane disruption and thickening, as well as damage to elastin and ongoing remodelling of the LC to become excavated, thinned and scarred are consistent phenomena in advanced glaucoma [21].

2.6.2 Peripapillary Sclera

Scleral geometric factors (e.g. thickness) influence ONH biomechanics in a similar way to scleral stiffness, through deformation transmitted to the peripheral ONH. Similar to the LC, chronic exposure to elevated IOP in a primate model induces progressive remodelling, thinning and stiffening of the sclera [128, 138], driven by cellular responses to elevated strain [62].

Since the peripapillary sclera has a major impact on the biomechanics of the LC, its thinning with advanced glaucoma may play a role in the increased susceptibility to damage with advanced glaucoma. Combined with increased peripapillary scleral bowing with age, this may mechanistically contribute to the prevalence of progressive peripapillary atrophy in advanced glaucoma by altering the perfusion from the penetrating branches of the SPCAs [139].

The morphological difference of the ONH load-bearing tissues with progressive glaucoma is also influenced by race. For example, the finding of a thinner peripapillary sclera in African-Americans could contribute to a greater deformability of the ONH and hence damage [15]. This may result in greater strain within the ONH tissues in response to raised IOP [76].

2.6.2.1 Microarchitecture

Posterior bowing of the peripapillary sclera, expansion of the scleral canal and scleral stiffening is marked in non-human primates exposed to chronic IOP elevation [16, 140]. This eventually leads to profound scleral canal wall expansion and excavation of the scleral canal beneath the optic disc margin in advanced glaucoma [1]. Progressive posterior migration of the anterior laminar insertion with advancing glaucoma likely reduces the laminar portion of the scleral canal's resistance to radial expansion and may be a contributing factor to the clinical phenomenon of glaucomatous excavation [86].

2.6.2.2 Cellular Changes

Chronic IOP elevation causes remodelling of the peripapillary scleral collagen structure and a stiffer pressure-strain response that occurs concurrently with optic nerve damage [16].

Increased strain levels and increased frequency of strain fluctuations cause myofibroblast differentiation and increased cytoskeletal changes in scleral fibroblasts [123]. As glaucoma progresses, the collagen structure in the peripapillary sclera overall becomes more uniform and less organised [114, 116, 141]. Animal models have shown an increase in the number and cross-sectional area of collagen fibrils, with a higher number of smaller diameter fibrils compared with larger diameter fibrils [142]. These lead to a sclera which appears to be progressively stiffer with progressing glaucoma [116].

2.7 Changes to Optic Nerve Head Vasculature in Glaucoma

The aged and glaucomatous ONH is more likely to have stiff connective tissues and a compromised blood supply [143, 144]. The biomechanical environment of the ONH also applies to blood vessels in the region, especially those within the laminar beams, and the diffusion properties of the vessel walls.

The SPCAs pass through the peripapillary sclera immediately adjacent to the scleral portion of the neural canal. The sclera thins here to accommodate any expansion of the neural tissues and may impart an IOP-related mechanical stress or strain on the penetrating SPCAs. Thus, the vascular supply to the load-bearing connective tissues occurs through an end- organ capillary bed encase load-bearing tissue. Thus, these branches of the SPCA without the sclera and the capillary beds they supply experience continuous direct strain, which may explain the link between deep ONH circulation to IOP elevation [145].

Imaging modalities such as OCT angiography have shown there is a significant difference in ONH vascular density between glaucoma and normal patients, with a significant correlation between ONH perfusion and glaucomatous damage [146–151]. There is also generalised narrowing of the retinal vessels [149] as well as reduced ONH and peripapillary blood flow dynamics [150–152] in advanced glaucoma, which may also be due to loss of metabolic demand. Currently, no clinical device can reliably image the deeper circulation provided by the SPCA to the load-bearing tissues of the ONH.

There is no direct blood supply to the axons or axon bundles within the LC. However, tensile, compressive or shear strains within laminar beams may also cause occlusion of the capillaries running within each beam [5]. In addition to increased laminar beam stiffness, age- and IOP-related increases in laminar beam thickness, laminar astrocyte basement membrane thickness and laminar ECM stiffening may diminish nutrient diffusion from the laminar capillaries into adjacent axons [5]. Reduced blood flow within the LC has been demonstrated in glaucoma patients compared to normal subjects [153] and those with ocular hypertension [154]. Similar changes have also been seen in the neuroretinal rim [154, 155].

ONH blood flow is tightly autoregulated to meet the functional and metabolic demands of the retina, including RGC. Deficient autoregulation has been reported in both the ONH and retina of glaucomatous eyes, indicating that chronic alterations in perfusion accompany the altered connective tissue architecture and material properties of the ONH [156].

2.8 Conclusion

Glaucomatous remodelling of the ONH is driven by strain within these tissues in response to IOP-related stress. How strain is experienced within the ONH, which drives the cellular reaction, is mediated by the morphology and material properties of these tissue. These biomechanical properties are heavily influenced by the three-dimensional geometry and material properties of the load-bearing tissues of the ONH. The changes in the ONH associated with glaucoma represent complex alterations in the connective tissues, cells and vasculature within the LC and peripapillary sclera. This deleterious remodelling is a critical component in the development of the toxic milieu the RGC axons must pass as they traverse this region.

References

1. Burgoyne CF, Downs JC, Bellezza AJ, Suh J-KF, Hart RT. The optic nerve head as a biomechanical structure: a new paradigm for understanding the role of IOP-related stress and strain in the pathophysiology of glaucomatous optic nerve head damage. Prog Retin Eye Res. 2005;24(1):39–73.
2. Downs JC. Optic nerve head biomechanics in aging and disease. Exp Eye Res. 2015;133:19–29.
3. Downs JC, Roberts MD, Burgoyne CF. Mechanical environment of the optic nerve head in glaucoma. Optom Vis Sci Off Publ Am Acad Optom. 2008;85(6):425–35.

4. Campbell IC, Coudrillier B, Ross Ethier C. Biomechanics of the posterior eye: a critical role in health and disease. J Biomech Eng. 2014;136(2):021005.
5. Burgoyne CF. A biomechanical paradigm for axonal insult within the optic nerve head in aging and glaucoma. Exp Eye Res. 2011;93(2):120–32.
6. Burgoyne CF, Downs JC, Bellezza AJ, Hart RT. Three-dimensional reconstruction of normal and early glaucoma monkey optic nerve head connective tissues. Invest Ophthalmol Vis Sci. 2004;45(12):4388–99.
7. Hoyt WF, Luis O. Visual fiber anatomy in the infrageniculate pathway of the primate. Arch Ophthalmol Chic Ill 1960. 1962;68:94–106.
8. Wolff E, Penmann G. The position occupied by the peripheral retinal fibres in the nerve-fibre layer and at the nerve head. Concil Ophthalmol. Acta. 1951;XVI:625–35.
9. Triviño A, Ramírez JM, Salazar JJ, Ramírez AI, García-Sánchez J. Immunohistochemical study of human optic nerve head astroglia. Vis Res. 1996;36(14):2015–28.
10. Downs JC, Girkin CA. Lamina Cribrosa in Glaucoma. Curr Opin Ophthalmol. 2017;28(2):113–9.
11. Zeimer RC, Ogura Y. The relation between glaucomatous damage and optic nerve head mechanical compliance. Arch Ophthalmol Chic Ill 1960. 1989;107(8):1232–4.
12. Anderson DR. Ultrastructure of human and monkey lamina cribrosa and optic nerve head. Arch Ophthalmol Chic Ill 1960. 1969;82(6):800–14.
13. Sigal IA, Flanagan JG, Tertinegg I, Ethier CR. 3D morphometry of the human optic nerve head. Exp Eye Res. 2010;90(1):70–80.
14. Park SC, Hsu AT, Su D, Simonson JL, Al-Jumayli M, Liu Y, et al. Factors associated with focal lamina cribrosa defects in glaucoma. Invest Ophthalmol Vis Sci. 2013;54(13):8401–7.
15. Girkin CA, Fazio MA, Yang H, Reynaud J, Burgoyne CF, Smith B, et al. Variation in the three-dimensional histomorphometry of the normal human optic nerve head with age and race: lamina cribrosa and peripapillary scleral thickness and position. Invest Ophthalmol Vis Sci. 2017;58(9):3759–69.
16. Girard MJA, Suh J-KF, Bottlang M, Burgoyne CF, Downs JC. Biomechanical changes in the sclera of monkey eyes exposed to chronic IOP elevations. Invest Ophthalmol Vis Sci. 2011;52(8):5656–69.
17. Komai Y, Ushiki T. The three-dimensional organization of collagen fibrils in the human cornea and sclera. Invest Ophthalmol Vis Sci. 1991;32(8):2244–58.
18. Quigley HA, Dorman-Pease ME, Brown AE. Quantitative study of collagen and elastin of the optic nerve head and sclera in human and experimental monkey glaucoma. Curr Eye Res. 1991;10(9):877–88.
19. Gogola A, Jan N-J, Brazile B, Lam P, Lathrop KL, Chan KC, et al. Spatial patterns and age-related changes of the collagen crimp in the human cornea and sclera. Invest Ophthalmol Vis Sci. 2018;59(7):2987–98.
20. Coudrillier B, Tian J, Alexander S, Myers KM, Quigley HA, Nguyen TD. Biomechanics of the human posterior sclera: age- and glaucoma-related changes measured using inflation testing. Invest Ophthalmol Vis Sci. 2012;53(4):1714–28.
21. Quigley HA, Addicks EM. Regional differences in the structure of the lamina cribrosa and their relation to glaucomatous optic nerve damage. Arch Ophthalmol Chic Ill 1960. 1981;99(1):137–43.
22. Nickells RW, Howell GR, Soto I, John SWM. Under pressure: cellular and molecular responses during glaucoma, a common neurodegeneration with axonopathy. Annu Rev Neurosci. 2012;35:153–79.
23. Howell GR, Soto I, Libby RT, John SWM. Intrinsic axonal degeneration pathways are critical for glaucomatous damage. Exp Neurol. 2013;246:54–61.
24. Quigley HA, Hohman RM, Addicks EM, Massof RW, Green WR. Morphologic changes in the lamina cribrosa correlated with neural loss in open-angle glaucoma. Am J Ophthalmol. 1983;95(5):673–91.
25. Radius RL. Anatomy of the optic nerve head and glaucomatous optic neuropathy. Surv Ophthalmol. 1987 Aug;32(1):35–44.
26. Radius RL, Gonzales M. Anatomy of the lamina cribrosa in human eyes. Arch Ophthalmol Chic Ill 1960. 1981;99(12):2159–62.
27. Roberts MD, Liang Y, Sigal IA, Grimm J, Reynaud J, Bellezza A, et al. Correlation between local stress and strain and lamina cribrosa connective tissue volume fraction in normal monkey eyes. Invest Ophthalmol Vis Sci. 2010 Jan;51(1):295–307.
28. Dandona L, Quigley HA, Brown AE, Enger C. Quantitative regional structure of the normal human lamina cribrosa. A racial comparison. Arch Ophthalmol Chic Ill 1960. 1990;108(3):393–8.
29. Dichtl A, Jonas JB, Naumann GO. Course of the optic nerve fibers through the lamina cibrosa in human eyes. Graefes Arch Clin Exp Ophthalmol Albrecht Von Graefes Arch Klin Exp Ophthalmol. 1996;234(9):581–5.
30. Morgan JE, Jeffery G, Foss AJ. Axon deviation in the human lamina cribrosa. Br J Ophthalmol. 1998;82(6):680–3.
31. Fitzgibbon T, Taylor SF. Retinotopy of the human retinal nerve fibre layer and optic nerve head. J Comp Neurol. 1996;375(2):238–51.
32. Downs JC, Burgoyne CF, Grytz R. Mechanical strain and restructuring of the optic nerve head. In: Glaucoma medical diagnosis & therapy. 2nd ed. Elsevier; 2015. p. 67–87.
33. Brazile B, Yang B, Gogola A, Lam P, Voorhees A, Sigal IA. One beam-one vessel is not true: lamina cribrosa vessel and collagen beam networks have distinct topologies. Invest Ophthalmol Vis Sci. 2019;60(9):4275.
34. Wang L, Cioffi GA, Cull G, Dong J, Fortune B. Immunohistologic evidence for retinal glial cell

changes in human glaucoma. Invest Ophthalmol Vis Sci. 2002;43(4):1088–94.
35. Hernandez MR, Igoe F, Neufeld AH. Cell culture of the human lamina cribrosa. Invest Ophthalmol Vis Sci. 1988;29(1):78–89.
36. Varela HJ, Hernandez MR. Astrocyte responses in human optic nerve head with primary open-angle glaucoma. J Glaucoma. 1997;6(5):303–13.
37. Kerr NM, Johnson CS, Green CR, Danesh-Meyer HV. Gap junction protein connexin43 (GJA1) in the human glaucomatous optic nerve head and retina. J Clin Neurosci Off J Neurosurg Soc Aust. 2011;18(1):102–8.
38. Liu B, Neufeld AH. Expression of nitric oxide synthase-2 (NOS-2) in reactive astrocytes of the human glaucomatous optic nerve head. Glia. 2000;30(2):178–86.
39. Nguyen JV, Soto I, Kim K-Y, Bushong EA, Oglesby E, Valiente-Soriano FJ, et al. Myelination transition zone astrocytes are constitutively phagocytic and have synuclein dependent reactivity in glaucoma. Proc Natl Acad Sci U S A. 2011;108(3):1176–81.
40. Kirwan RP, Leonard MO, Murphy M, Clark AF, O'Brien CJ. Transforming growth factor-beta-regulated gene transcription and protein expression in human GFAP-negative lamina cribrosa cells. Glia. 2005;52(4):309–24.
41. Kirwan RP, Felice L, Clark AF, O'Brien CJ, Leonard MO. Hypoxia regulated gene transcription in human optic nerve lamina cribrosa cells in culture. Invest Ophthalmol Vis Sci. 2012;53(4):2243–55.
42. Balaratnasingam C, Morgan WH, Johnstone V, Cringle SJ, Yu D-Y. Heterogeneous distribution of axonal cytoskeleton proteins in the human optic nerve. Invest Ophthalmol Vis Sci. 2009;50(6):2824–38.
43. Lu L, Oswald SJ, Ngu H, Yin FC-P. Mechanical properties of actin stress fibers in living cells. Biophys J. 2008;95(12):6060–71.
44. Morrison JC. Integrins in the optic nerve head: potential roles in glaucomatous optic neuropathy (an American ophthalmological society thesis). Trans Am Ophthalmol Soc. 2006;104:453–77.
45. Wipff P-J, Hinz B. Integrins and the activation of latent transforming growth factor beta1—an intimate relationship. Eur J Cell Biol. 2008;87(8–9):601–15.
46. Baker EL, Zaman MH. The biomechanical integrin. J Biomech. 2010;43(1):38–44.
47. Crawford Downs J, Roberts MD, Sigal IA. Glaucomatous cupping of the lamina cribrosa: a review of the evidence for active progressive remodeling as a mechanism. Exp Eye Res. 2011;93(2):133–40.
48. Downs JC, Blidner RA, Bellezza AJ, Thompson HW, Hart RT, Burgoyne CF. Peripapillary scleral thickness in perfusion-fixed normal monkey eyes. Invest Ophthalmol Vis Sci. 2002;43(7):2229–35.
49. Winkler M, Jester B, Nien-Shy C, Massei S, Minckler DS, Jester JV, et al. High resolution three dimensional reconstruction of the collagenous matrix of the human optic nerve head. Brain Res Bull. 2010;81(2–3):339.
50. Grytz R, Meschke G. Constitutive modeling of crimped collagen fibrils in soft tissues. J Mech Behav Biomed Mater. 2009 Oct 1;2(5):522–33.
51. Girard M, Downs JC, Burgoyne CF, Bottlang M, Suh J-KF. Anisotropic and nonlinear mechanical behavior of monkey posterior sclera under intraocular pressure. Invest Ophthalmol Vis Sci. 2007;48(13):3304.
52. Bellezza AJ, Hart RT, Burgoyne CF. The optic nerve head as a biomechanical structure: initial finite element modeling. Invest Ophthalmol Vis Sci. 2000 Sep;41(10):2991–3000.
53. Sigal IA, Girard M, Burgoyne C, Downs JC. Biomechanical changes of the optic disc. In: Ocular disease: mechanisms and management. 1st ed. London: Elsevier; 2010.
54. Burgoyne CF, Morrison JC. The anatomy and pathophysiology of the optic nerve head in glaucoma. J Glaucoma. 2001;10(5):S16.
55. Fazio MA, Grytz R, Morris JS, Bruno L, Gardiner SK, Girkin CA, et al. Age-related changes in human peripapillary scleral strain. Biomech Model Mechanobiol. 2014 Jun;13(3):551–63.
56. Albon J, Karwatowski WS, Avery N, Easty DL, Duance VC. Changes in the collagenous matrix of the aging human lamina cribrosa. Br J Ophthalmol. 1995;79(4):368–75.
57. Bailey AJ, Paul RG, Knott L. Mechanisms of maturation and ageing of collagen. Mech Ageing Dev. 1998;106(1–2):1–56.
58. Goldbaum MH, Jeng SY, Logemann R, Weinreb RN. The extracellular matrix of the human optic nerve. Arch Ophthalmol Chic Ill 1960. 1989;107(8):1225–31.
59. Albon J, Karwatowski WS, Easty DL, Sims TJ, Duance VC. Age related changes in the non-collagenous components of the extracellular matrix of the human lamina cribrosa. Br J Ophthalmol. 2000;84(3):311–7.
60. Sawaguchi S, Yue BY, Fukuchi T, Iwata K, Kaiya T. Age-related changes of sulfated proteoglycans in the human lamina cribrosa. Curr Eye Res. 1993;12(8):685–92.
61. Morrison JC, Jerdan JA, Dorman ME, Quigley HA. Structural proteins of the neonatal and adult lamina cribrosa. Arch Ophthalmol Chic Ill 1960. 1989;107(8):1220–4.
62. Morrison JC, Dorman-Pease ME, Dunkelberger GR, Quigley HA. Optic nerve head extracellular matrix in primary optic atrophy and experimental glaucoma. Arch Ophthalmol Chic Ill 1960. 1990;108(7):1020–4.
63. Albon J, Purslow PP, Karwatowski WS, Easty DL. Age related compliance of the lamina cribrosa in human eyes. Br J Ophthalmol. 2000;84(3):318–23.
64. Geraghty B, Jones SW, Rama P, Akhtar R, Elsheikh A. Age-related variations in the biomechanical properties of human sclera. J Mech Behav Biomed Mater. 2012;16:181–91.

65. Grytz R, Fazio MA, Libertiaux V, Bruno L, Gardiner S, Girkin CA, et al. Age- and race-related differences in human scleral material properties. Invest Ophthalmol Vis Sci. 2014;55(12):8163–72.
66. Murienne BJ, Chen ML, Quigley HA, Nguyen TD. The contribution of glycosaminoglycans to the mechanical behaviour of the posterior human sclera. J R Soc Interface. 2016;13(119):20160367.
67. Coudrillier B, Pijanka J, Jefferys J, Sorensen T, Quigley HA, Boote C, et al. Collagen structure and mechanical properties of the human sclera: analysis for the effects of age. J Biomech Eng. 2015;137(4):0410061–04100614.
68. Fazio MA, Grytz R, Morris JS, Bruno L, Girkin CA, Downs JC. Human scleral structural stiffness increases more rapidly with age in donors of African descent compared to donors of European descent. Invest Ophthalmol Vis Sci. 2014;55(11):7189–98.
69. Steinhart MR, Cone-Kimball E, Nguyen C, Nguyen TD, Pease ME, Chakravarti S, et al. Susceptibility to glaucoma damage related to age and connective tissue mutations in mice. Exp Eye Res. 2014;119:54–60.
70. Nguyen C, Cone FE, Nguyen TD, Coudrillier B, Pease ME, Steinhart MR, et al. Studies of scleral biomechanical behavior related to susceptibility for retinal ganglion cell loss in experimental mouse glaucoma. Invest Ophthalmol Vis Sci. 2013;54(3):1767–80.
71. Pease ME, Oglesby EN, Cone-Kimball E, Jefferys JL, Steinhart MR, Kim AJ, et al. Scleral permeability varies by mouse strain and is decreased by chronic experimental glaucoma. Invest Ophthalmol Vis Sci. 2014 Apr 21;55(4):2564–73.
72. Anderson OA, Jackson TL, Singh JK, Hussain AA, Marshall J. Human transscleral albumin permeability and the effect of topographical location and donor age. Invest Ophthalmol Vis Sci. 2008;49(9):4041–5.
73. Tun TA, Wang X, Baskaran M, Nongpiur ME, Tham Y-C, Perera SA, et al. Variation of Peripapillary scleral shape with age. Invest Ophthalmol Vis Sci. 2019;60(10):3275–82.
74. Yang H, Downs JC, Bellezza A, Thompson H, Burgoyne CF. 3-D histomorphometry of the normal and early glaucomatous monkey optic nerve head: prelaminar neural tissues and cupping. Invest Ophthalmol Vis Sci. 2007;48(11):5068–84.
75. Burgoyne CF, Downs JC. Premise and prediction-how optic nerve head biomechanics underlies the susceptibility and clinical behavior of the aged optic nerve head. J Glaucoma. 2008;17(4):318–28.
76. Sigal IA, Flanagan JG, Ethier CR. Factors influencing optic nerve head biomechanics. Invest Ophthalmol Vis Sci. 2005;46(11):4189–99.
77. Yang H, Downs JC, Sigal IA, Roberts MD, Thompson H, Burgoyne CF. Deformation of the normal monkey optic nerve head connective tissue after acute IOP elevation within 3-D histomorphometric reconstructions. Invest Ophthalmol Vis Sci. 2009;50(12):5785–99.
78. Roberts MD, Sigal IA, Liang Y, Burgoyne CF, Downs JC. Changes in the biomechanical response of the optic nerve head in early experimental glaucoma. Invest Ophthalmol Vis Sci. 2010;51(11):5675–84.
79. Agoumi Y, Sharpe GP, Hutchison DM, Nicolela MT, Artes PH, Chauhan BC. Laminar and prelaminar tissue displacement during intraocular pressure elevation in glaucoma patients and healthy controls. Ophthalmology. 2011;118(1):52–9.
80. Sigal IA, Flanagan JG, Tertinegg I, Ethier CR. Predicted extension, compression and shearing of optic nerve head tissues. Exp Eye Res. 2007;85(3):312–22.
81. Sigal IA, Flanagan JG, Tertinegg I, Ethier CR. Modeling individual-specific human optic nerve head biomechanics. Part I: IOP-induced deformations and influence of geometry. Biomech Model Mechanobiol. 2009;8(2):85–98.
82. Downs JC. IOP telemetry in the nonhuman primate. Exp Eye Res. 2015;141:91–8.
83. Coleman DJ. Trokel S. direct-recorded intraocular pressure variations in a human subject. Arch Ophthalmol Chic Ill 1960. 1969;82(5):637–40.
84. Turner DC, Edmiston AM, Zohner YE, Byrne KJ, Seigfreid WP, Girkin CA, et al. Transient intraocular pressure fluctuations: source, magnitude, frequency, and associated mechanical energy. Invest Ophthalmol Vis Sci. 2019;60(7):2572–82.
85. Morris HJ, Tang J, Cruz Perez B, Pan X, Hart RT, Weber PA, et al. Correlation between biomechanical responses of posterior sclera and IOP elevations during micro intraocular volume change. Invest Ophthalmol Vis Sci. 2013;54(12):7215–22.
86. Yang H, Williams G, Downs JC, Sigal IA, Roberts MD, Thompson H, et al. Posterior (outward) migration of the lamina cribrosa and early cupping in monkey experimental glaucoma. Invest Ophthalmol Vis Sci. 2011;52(10):7109–21.
87. Downs JC, Yang H, Girkin C, Sakata L, Bellezza A, Thompson H, et al. Three-dimensional histomorphometry of the normal and early glaucomatous monkey optic nerve head: neural canal and subarachnoid space architecture. Invest Ophthalmol Vis Sci. 2007;48(7):3195–208.
88. Jonas JB, Ritch R, Panda-Jonas S. Chapter 2—cerebrospinal fluid pressure in the pathogenesis of glaucoma. In: Bagetta G, Nucci C, editors. Progress in Brain Research [Internet]. Elsevier; 2015 [cited 2020 May 31]. p. 33–47. (New Trends in Basic and Clinical Research of Glaucoma: A Neurodegenerative Disease of the Visual System, Part B; vol. 221). Retrieved from http://www.sciencedirect.com/science/article/pii/S007961231500093X
89. Wang B, Lucy KA, Schuman JS, Sigal IA, Bilonick RA, Kagemann L, et al. Decreased lamina cribrosa beam thickness and pore diameter relative to distance from the central retinal vessel trunk. Invest Ophthalmol Vis Sci. 2016;57(7):3088–92.
90. Downs JC, Roberts MD, Burgoyne CF, Hart RT. Multiscale finite element modeling of the lamina

cribrosa microarchitecture in the eye. Conference of Proceedings Annual International Conference IEEE Engineer Med Biol Soc IEEE Eng Med Biol Soc Annu Conf. 2009;2009:4277–80.
91. Sigal IA, Grimm JL, Jan N-J, Reid K, Minckler DS, Brown DJ. Eye-specific IOP-induced displacements and deformations of human lamina cribrosa. Invest Ophthalmol Vis Sci. 2014;55(1):1–15.
92. Reynaud J, Lockwood H, Gardiner SK, Williams G, Yang H, Burgoyne CF. Lamina cribrosa microarchitecture in monkey early experimental glaucoma: global change. Invest Ophthalmol Vis Sci. 2016;57(7):3451–69.
93. Roberts MD, Grau V, Grimm J, Reynaud J, Bellezza AJ, Burgoyne CF, et al. Remodeling of the connective tissue microarchitecture of the lamina cribrosa in early experimental glaucoma. Invest Ophthalmol Vis Sci. 2009 Feb;50(2):681–90.
94. Jung KI, Jung Y, Park KT, Park CK. Factors affecting plastic lamina cribrosa displacement in glaucoma patients. Invest Ophthalmol Vis Sci. 2014 Nov 4;55(12):7709–15.
95. Grytz R, Sigal IA, Ruberti JW, Meschke G, Downs JC. Lamina cribrosa thickening in early glaucoma predicted by a microstructure motivated growth and remodeling approach. Mech Mater Int J. 2012;44:99–109.
96. Hernandez MR, Andrzejewska WM, Neufeld AH. Changes in the extracellular matrix of the human optic nerve head in primary open-angle glaucoma. Am J Ophthalmol. 1990;109(2):180–8.
97. Quigley HA, Brown A, Dorman-Pease ME. Alterations in elastin of the optic nerve head in human and experimental glaucoma. Br J Ophthalmol. 1991 Sep;75(9):552–7.
98. Hernandez MR. Ultrastructural immunocytochemical analysis of elastin in the human lamina cribrosa. Changes in elastic fibers in primary open-angle glaucoma. Invest Ophthalmol Vis Sci. 1992;33(10):2891–903.
99. Fukuchi T, Sawaguchi S, Hara H, Shirakashi M, Iwata K. Extracellular matrix changes of the optic nerve lamina cribrosa in monkey eyes with experimentally chronic glaucoma. Graefes Arch Clin Exp Ophthalmol Albrecht Von Graefes Arch Klin Exp Ophthalmol. 1992;230(5):421–7.
100. Fukuchi T, Sawaguchi S, Yue BY, Iwata K, Hara H, Kaiya T. Sulfated proteoglycans in the lamina cribrosa of normal monkey eyes and monkey eyes with laser-induced glaucoma. Exp Eye Res. 1994;58(2):231–43.
101. Kirwan RP, Wordinger RJ, Clark AF, O'Brien CJ. Differential global and extra-cellular matrix focused gene expression patterns between normal and glaucomatous human lamina cribrosa cells. Mol Vis. 2009;15:76–88.
102. Rogers R, Dharsee M, Ackloo S, Flanagan JG. Proteomics analyses of activated human optic nerve head lamina cribrosa cells following biomechanical strain. Invest Ophthalmol Vis Sci. 2012;53(7):3806–16.
103. Job R, Raja V, Grierson I, Currie L, O'Reilly S, Pollock N, et al. Cross-linked actin networks (CLANs) are present in lamina cribrosa cells. Br J Ophthalmol. 2010;94(10):1388–92.
104. Ridet JL, Malhotra SK, Privat A, Gage FH. Reactive astrocytes: cellular and molecular cues to biological function. Trends Neurosci. 1997;20(12):570–7.
105. Agapova OA, Ricard CS, Salvador-Silva M, Hernandez MR. Expression of matrix metalloproteinases and tissue inhibitors of metalloproteinases in human optic nerve head astrocytes. Glia. 2001;33(3):205–16.
106. Hernandez MR. The optic nerve head in glaucoma: role of astrocytes in tissue remodeling. Prog Retin Eye Res. 2000;19(3):297–321.
107. Tezel G, Hernandez MR, Wax MB. In vitro evaluation of reactive astrocyte migration, a component of tissue remodeling in glaucomatous optic nerve head. Glia. 2001;34(3):178–89.
108. Sigal IA, Flanagan JG, Tertinegg I, Ethier CR. Finite element modeling of optic nerve head biomechanics. Invest Ophthalmol Vis Sci. 2004;45(12):4378–87.
109. Sigal IA, Flanagan JG, Tertinegg I, Ethier CR. Modeling individual-specific human optic nerve head biomechanics. Part II: influence of material properties. Biomech Model Mechanobiol. 2009;8(2):99–109.
110. Sigal IA, Yang H, Roberts MD, Burgoyne CF, Downs JC. IOP-induced lamina cribrosa displacement and scleral canal expansion: an analysis of factor interactions using parameterized eye-specific models. Invest Ophthalmol Vis Sci. 2011;52(3):1896–907.
111. Downs JC, Suh J-KF, Thomas KA, Bellezza AJ, Hart RT, Burgoyne CF. Viscoelastic material properties of the peripapillary sclera in normal and early-glaucoma monkey eyes. Invest Ophthalmol Vis Sci. 2005;46(2):540–6.
112. Coudrillier B, Boote C, Quigley HA, Nguyen TD. Scleral anisotropy and its effects on the mechanical response of the optic nerve head. Biomech Model Mechanobiol. 2013 Oct;12(5):941–63.
113. Watson PG, Young RD. Scleral structure, organisation and disease. A review. Exp Eye Res. 2004;78(3):609–23.
114. Pijanka JK, Coudrillier B, Ziegler K, Sorensen T, Meek KM, Nguyen TD, et al. Quantitative mapping of collagen fiber orientation in non-glaucoma and glaucoma posterior human sclerae. Invest Ophthalmol Vis Sci. 2012;53(9):5258–70.
115. Danford FL, Yan D, Dreier RA, Cahir TM, Girkin CA, Geest JPV. Differences in the region- and depth-dependent microstructural organization in normal versus glaucomatous human posterior sclerae. Invest Ophthalmol Vis Sci. 2013;54(13):7922–32.
116. Coudrillier B, Pijanka JK, Jefferys JL, Goel A, Quigley HA, Boote C, et al. Glaucoma-related changes in the mechanical properties and collagen

micro-architecture of the human sclera. PLoS One. 2015;10(7):e0131396.
117. Grytz R, Meschke G, Jonas JB. The collagen fibril architecture in the lamina cribrosa and peripapillary sclera predicted by a computational remodeling approach. Biomech Model Mechanobiol. 2011;10(3):371–82.
118. Ma Y, Pavlatos E, Clayson K, Pan X, Kwok S, Sandwisch T, et al. Mechanical deformation of human optic nerve head and peripapillary tissue in response to acute IOP elevation. Invest Ophthalmol Vis Sci. 2019;60(4):913–20.
119. Pavlatos E, Ma Y, Clayson K, Pan X, Liu J. Regional deformation of the optic nerve head and peripapillary sclera during IOP elevation. Invest Ophthalmol Vis Sci. 2018;59(8):3779–88.
120. Yan D, McPheeters S, Johnson G, Utzinger U, Vande Geest JP. Microstructural differences in the human posterior sclera as a function of age and race. Invest Ophthalmol Vis Sci. 2011;52(2):821–9.
121. Cui W, Bryant MR, Sweet PM, McDonnell PJ. Changes in gene expression in response to mechanical strain in human scleral fibroblasts. Exp Eye Res. 2004;78(2):275–84.
122. Shelton L, Rada JS. Effects of cyclic mechanical stretch on extracellular matrix synthesis by human scleral fibroblasts. Exp Eye Res. 2007;84(2):314–22.
123. Qu J, Chen H, Zhu L, Ambalavanan N, Girkin CA, Murphy-Ullrich JE, et al. High-magnitude and/or high-frequency mechanical strain promotes peripapillary scleral myofibroblast differentiation. Invest Ophthalmol Vis Sci. 2015;56(13):7821–30.
124. Oglesby EN, Tezel G, Cone-Kimball E, Steinhart MR, Jefferys J, Pease ME, et al. Scleral fibroblast response to experimental glaucoma in mice. Mol Vis. 2016;22:82–99.
125. Emery JM, Landis D, Paton D, Boniuk M, Craig JM. The lamina cribrosa in normal and glaucomatous human eyes. Trans - Am Acad Ophthalmol Otolaryngol Am Acad Ophthalmol Otolaryngol. 1974;78(2):OP290–7.
126. Stamper RL, Lieberman MF, Drake MV. Becker-Shaffer's diagnosis and therapy of the glaucomas. 8th ed. Elsevier Health Sciences; 2009. p. 580.
127. Yang H, He L, Gardiner SK, Reynaud J, Williams G, Hardin C, et al. Age-related differences in longitudinal structural change by spectral-domain optical coherence tomography in early experimental glaucoma. Invest Ophthalmol Vis Sci. 2014;55(10):6409–20.
128. Hayreh SS, Pe'er J, Zimmerman MB. Morphologic changes in chronic high-pressure experimental glaucoma in rhesus monkeys. J Glaucoma. 1999;8(1):56–71.
129. Quigley HA, Addicks EM, Green WR, Maumenee AE. Optic nerve damage in human glaucoma. II. The site of injury and susceptibility to damage. Arch Ophthalmol Chic Ill 1960. 1981;99(4):635–49.
130. Jonas JB, Königsreuther KA, Naumann GO. Optic disc histomorphometry in normal eyes and eyes with secondary angle-closure glaucoma. I. Intrapapillary region. Graefes Arch Clin Exp Ophthalmol Albrecht Von Graefes Arch Klin Exp Ophthalmol. 1992;230(2):129–33.
131. Jonas JB, Berenshtein E, Holbach L. Anatomic relationship between lamina cribrosa, intraocular space, and cerebrospinal fluid space. Invest Ophthalmol Vis Sci. 2003;44(12):5189–95.
132. Morgan WH, Yu DY, Alder VA, Cringle SJ, Cooper RL, House PH, et al. The correlation between cerebrospinal fluid pressure and retrolaminar tissue pressure. Invest Ophthalmol Vis Sci. 1998;39(8):1419–28.
133. Investigators AGIS. The advanced glaucoma intervention study (AGIS): 12. Baseline risk factors for sustained loss of visual field and visual acuity in patients with advanced glaucoma. Am J Ophthalmol. 2002;134(4):499–512.
134. Hernandez MR, Ye H. Glaucoma: changes in extracellular matrix in the optic nerve head. Ann Med. 1993;25(4):309–15.
135. Jonas JB, Xu L. Optic disk hemorrhages in glaucoma. Am J Ophthalmol. 1994 Jul 15;118(1):1–8.
136. Siegner SW, Netland PA. Optic disc hemorrhages and progression of glaucoma. Ophthalmology. 1996;103(7):1014–24.
137. Johnson EC, Jia L, Cepurna WO, Doser TA, Morrison JC. Global changes in optic nerve head gene expression after exposure to elevated intraocular pressure in a rat glaucoma model. Invest Ophthalmol Vis Sci. 2007;48(7):3161–77.
138. Girard MJA, Suh J-KF, Bottlang M, Burgoyne CF, Downs JC. Scleral biomechanics in the aging monkey eye. Invest Ophthalmol Vis Sci. 2009;50(11):5226–37.
139. Jonas JB. Clinical implications of peripapillary atrophy in glaucoma. Curr Opin Ophthalmol. 2005;16(2):84–8.
140. Yang H, Downs JC, Girkin C, Sakata L, Bellezza A, Thompson H, et al. 3-D histomorphometry of the normal and early glaucomatous monkey optic nerve head: lamina cribrosa and peripapillary scleral position and thickness. Invest Ophthalmol Vis Sci. 2007;48(10):4597–607.
141. Pijanka JK, Kimball EC, Pease ME, Abass A, Sorensen T, Nguyen TD, et al. Changes in scleral collagen organization in murine chronic experimental glaucoma. Invest Ophthalmol Vis Sci. 2014;55(10):6554–64.
142. Cone-Kimball E, Nguyen C, Oglesby EN, Pease ME, Steinhart MR, Quigley HA. Scleral structural alterations associated with chronic experimental intraocular pressure elevation in mice. Mol Vis. 2013;19:2023–39.
143. Grunwald JE, Piltz J, Patel N, Bose S, Riva CE. Effect of aging on retinal macular microcirculation: a blue field simulation study. Invest Ophthalmol Vis Sci. 1993;34(13):3609–13.
144. Harris A, Harris M, Biller J, Garzozi H, Zarfty D, Ciulla TA, et al. Aging affects the retrobulbar circula-

tion differently in women and men Arch Ophthalmol Chic Ill 1960. 2000;118(8):1076–80.
145. Hayreh SS. Blood supply of the optic nerve head and its role in optic atrophy, glaucoma, and oedema of the optic disc. Br J Ophthalmol. 1969;53(11):721–48.
146. Lévêque P-M, Zéboulon P, Brasnu E, Baudouin C, Labbé A. Optic disc vascularization in glaucoma: value of spectral-domain optical coherence tomography angiography. J Ophthalmol. 2016; 2016 [cited 2020 Jun 27]: e6956717. Retrieved from https://www.hindawi.com/journals/joph/2016/6956717/
147. Harris A, Kagemann L, Ehrlich R, Rospigliosi C, Moore D, Siesky B. Measuring and interpreting ocular blood flow and metabolism in glaucoma. Can J Ophthalmol. 2008;43(3):328–36.
148. Hitchings RA, Spaeth GL. Fluorescein angiography in chronic simple and low-tension glaucoma. Br J Ophthalmol. 1977;61(2):126–32.
149. Jonas JB, Nguyen XN, Naumann GO. Parapapillary retinal vessel diameter in normal and glaucoma eyes. I. Morphometric data. Invest Ophthalmol Vis Sci. 1989;30(7):1599–603.
150. Tobe LA, Harris A, Hussain RM, Eckert G, Huck A, Park J, et al. The role of retrobulbar and retinal circulation on optic nerve head and retinal nerve fibre layer structure in patients with open-angle glaucoma over an 18-month period. Br J Ophthalmol. 2015;99(5):609–12.
151. Yokoyama Y, Aizawa N, Chiba N, Omodaka K, Nakamura M, Otomo T, et al. Significant correlations between optic nerve head microcirculation and visual field defects and nerve fiber layer loss in glaucoma patients with myopic glaucomatous disk. Clin Ophthalmol Auckl NZ. 2011;5:1721–7.
152. Piltz-Seymour JR. Laser doppler flowmetry of the optic nerve head in glaucoma. Surv Ophthalmol. 1999;43:S191–8.
153. Nicolela MT, Hnik P, Drance SM. Scanning laser Doppler flowmeter study of retinal and optic disk blood flow in glaucomatous patients. Am J Ophthalmol. 1996;122(6):775–83.
154. Kerr J, Nelson P, O'Brien C. A comparison of ocular blood flow in untreated primary open-angle glaucoma and ocular hypertension. Am J Ophthalmol. 1998;126(1):42–51.
155. Findl O, Rainer G, Dallinger S, Dorner G, Polak K, Kiss B, et al. Assessment of optic disk blood flow in patients with open-angle glaucoma. Am J Ophthalmol. 2000 Nov;130(5):589–96.
156. Grunwald JE, Riva CE, Stone RA, Keates EU, Petrig BL. Retinal autoregulation in open-angle glaucoma. Ophthalmology. 1984;91(12):1690–4.

How to Interpret Optic Disc in Myopes?

3

Vinay Nangia

3.1 Introduction

The optic disc in myopia, associated with increased axial length has different characteristics compared to those found in emmetropes. The changes in the morphometric characteristics of the optic nerve head, are often unpredictable with increase in axial length (AXL).

Many studies have shown an increase in the optic disc size in association with myopic refractive error and increase in AXL [1, 2]. Large discs have been especially associated with high myopia of greater than −8.00 Dioptres (D) compared to those with lesser degrees of myopia or with emmetropia or hypermetropia. Jonas and co-workers found the mean optic disc area to be 6.87 ± 3.99 mm^2, which was much larger than that seen in non-myopic or low myopic eyes (2.69 ± 0.70 mm^2) [3]. It may be important to study not only the degree of myopia but also the relationship with the AXL, to offset the effect of corneal curvature on these measurements. In a clinic-based study in Central India in high myopes, with a mean spherical equivalent of −10.12 ± 2.47 D and a mean AXL of 27.14 ± 1.99 mm the mean disc area was 2.26 ± 0.70 mm^2 (unpublished data from the author). This may indicate that the size of the optic disc may differ in myopes across regions and that not all discs in high myopia may be large. This has implications for understanding the features of optic disc in myopia and glaucoma (Fig. 3.1a, b). In another study, optic disc area was associated with increased AXL ($r = 0.13$, $p < 0.035$). The study included whites and African Americans [4]. This study, however, included all AXLs and had very few subjects over 26 mm.

The optic disc in myopia differs in its morphometry which is influenced by growth of the eye. This effect appears to be largely dependent on the AXL and the associated parapapillary changes that accompany it. In a study which included normal with a range of refractive error from +0.75 D to −12.75 D, the authors found that the ratio of the vertical disc diameter (VDD) to the horizontal disc diameter (HDD) was significantly increased with increasing myopia [5].

In a study on the shape of the optic disc in glaucoma it was determined that the optic disc form did not differ significantly for the low myopes less than −8.0 D with the normal optic disc shape being slightly vertically oval [6]. One of the typical shapes which accompany high myopia is of a vertically or obliquely oval disc with significantly increased vertical diameters. This is generally associated with the presence of temporal parapapillary changes. One of the significant changes found in moderate to high myopia especially when accompanied by peripapillary changes is the presence of a cup which appears to have a shallow appearance. This is considered

V. Nangia (✉)
Glaucoma Service, Suraj Eye Institute, Nagpur, India

S. Pandav et al. (eds.), *The Optic Nerve Head in Health and Disease*,
https://doi.org/10.1007/978-981-33-6838-5_3

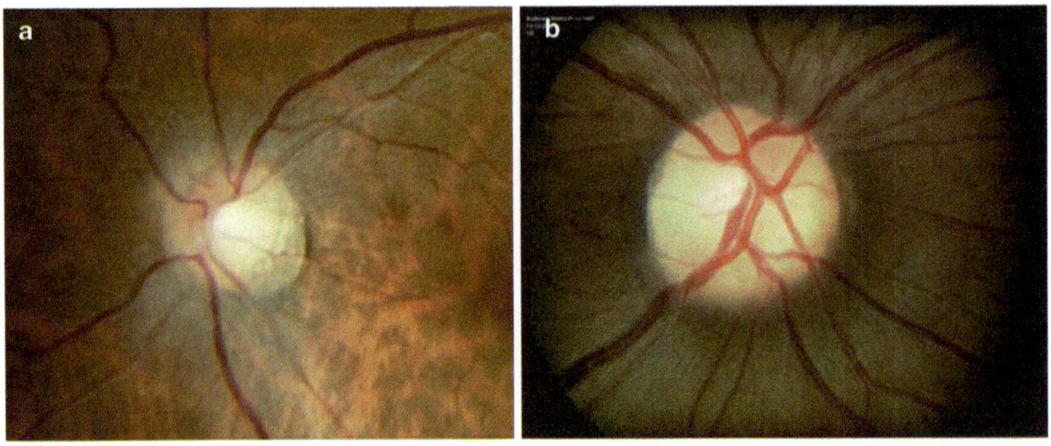

Fig. 3.1 Size of the optic disc in myopia can vary significantly depending on the accompanying parapapillary changes. (**a**) This subject has myopia of −9.5 D, axial length of 26.61 mm, and a disc area of 1.54 mm^2. (**b**) Subject has myopia of −4.50 D, axial length of 23.56 mm, and a disc area of 3.95 mm^2 (Image Courtesy: Central India Myopia Eye Study, Suraj Eye Institute; With Permission)

classical of the optic disc in high myopia. The presence of shallow cupping even in myopic subjects with glaucoma may make it difficult to use the cup depth as a sign of glaucoma in high myopia, contrary to the increased cup depth that may be seen in subjects with emmetropia and low myopia.

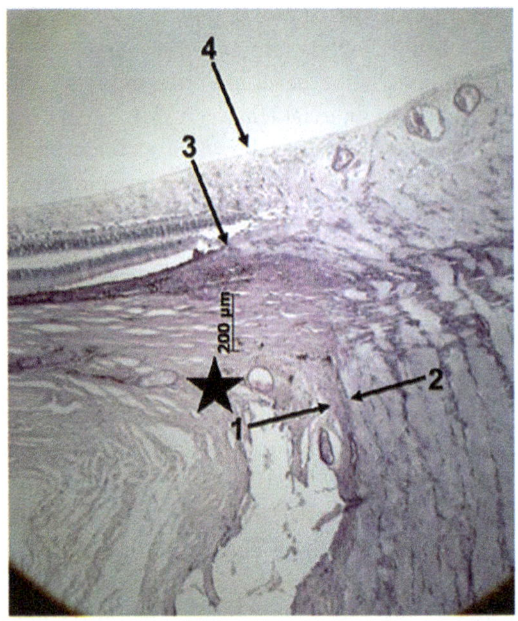

Fig. 3.2 Histopathology of gamma zone. Photomicrograph of the optic nerve head (staining: PAS); Arrows #1 and #2: Pia mater of the optic nerve; Arrow #3: End of Bruch's membrane; Arrow #4: Projection of the outer margin of the pia mater of the optic nerve; Gamma zone: region between Arrows #3 and #4; Black star: Beginning of dura mater of the optic nerve (Courtesy of Jonas JB, et al. PLoS One 7(10): e47237. With Permission)

3.2 Parapapillary Changes in Myopia

Parapapillary changes in myopia have been called parapapillary atrophy and were indistinguishable from the parapapillary changes seen in non-myopic and non-high myopic subjects clinically (beta, β zone). The parapapillary area was called "gamma, γ zone" by Jonas and colleagues in 2012 [7], defined as the distance between the end of Bruch's membrane and the outer margin of the optic nerve, which is covered by the pia mater. The gamma zone is known to be associated significantly with increasing AXL and this space is largely bridged below the nerve fibers by the scleral lamina also called the scleral flange, which separates it from the subarachnoid space, which is enlarged in such eyes and lies below the gamma zone (Fig. 3.2) [7]. This has been shown also not to be related to the presence or progression of glaucoma [8]. Gamma zone is seen clinically but best defined using enhanced depth imaging using SDOCT or swept source OCT. It was found in 101 (51.27%) of 197 myopes (range −1 D onwards). The mean axial length in the high myopia group defined as myopia more than −6 D was 26.58±1.98 mm. The prevalence of gamma zone in this group was 73.86% (65/88 eyes) more than in the moderate and low myopia group. Further, the extent of the gamma zone was significantly correlated with increasing axial length ($p < 0.001$; $r = 0.559$) and with decreasing visual acuity ($p = 0.043$; $r = 0.244$) (unpublished data from author). The identification of gamma zone is considerably important because it is associated with changes in the shape of the optic nerve and that may have implications in recognition of glaucomatous damage in such eyes (Fig. 3.3a–d).

3.3 Glaucoma and Myopia

Myopia is an important risk factor for glaucoma and several studies have come to a similar conclusion [9, 10]. A study showed that at a given intraocular pressure (IOP) in primary open angle glaucoma (POAG), optic nerve damage may be more pronounced in highly myopic eyes with

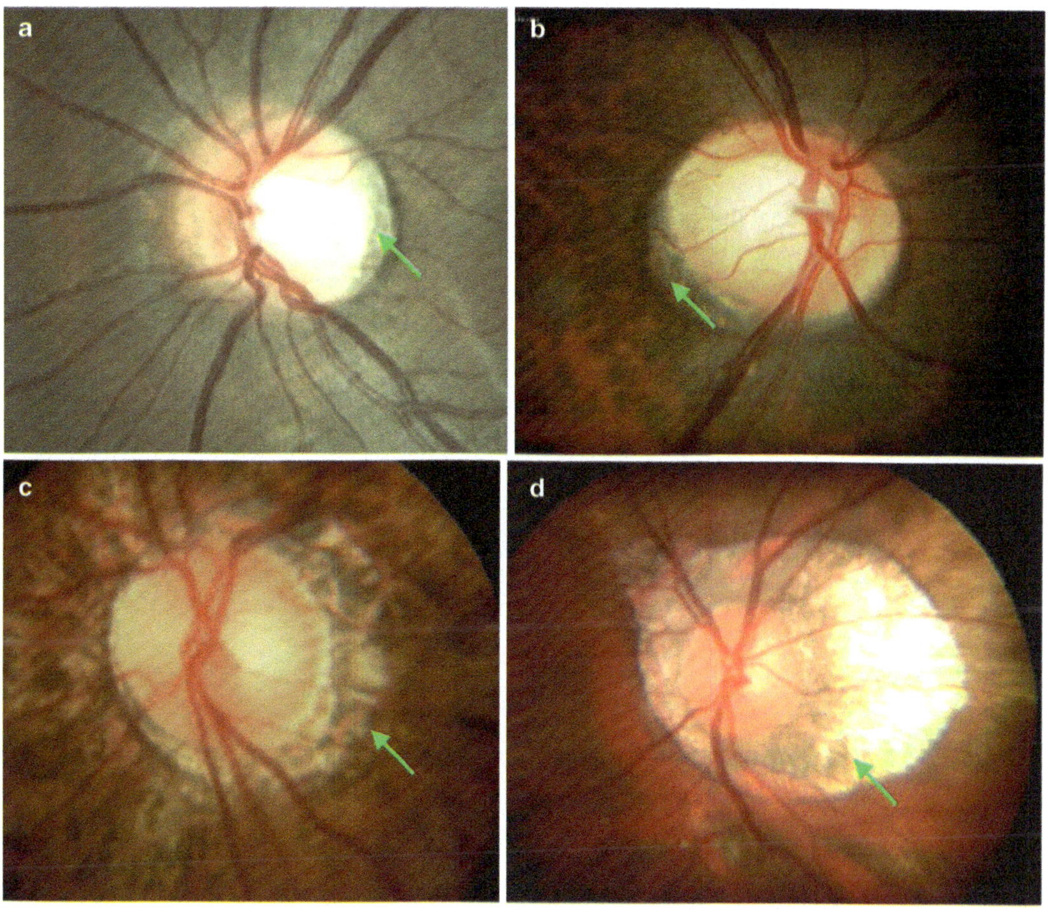

Fig. 3.3 (**a–d**) Gamma zone (space between the margin of the optic disc and the Bruchs membrane opening). (**a**) Subject with gamma zone (green arrows) with a refractive error of −6.5 DSph and +0.50 DCyl and axial length of 24.24 mm. (**b**) Subject with refraction of −10.25 DSph. and axial length of 27.39 mm. C. Subject has refractive error of −22.00 DSph and +4.00 DCyl with an axial length of 31.30 mm. (**d**) Subject has a refractive error of −19.75 DSph. and an axial length of 35.35 mm. The appearance of the gamma zone varies between subjects and should be distinguished from a beta zone (Courtesy of Central India Myopia Eye Study, Suraj Eye Institute; With Permission)

large optic discs than in non-highly myopic eyes, suggesting a greater susceptibility of the high myopic eyes to glaucomatous damage [11]. The presence of myopia (>−4 D) is also considered to be a significant risk factor for visual field loss in subjects with POAG [12]. In the Tajimi Study, besides the IOP, myopia and age were identified as significant risk factors for having POAG [13]. In a study to determine the influence of large megalodiscs (>3.79 mm^2), multivariate analysis showed glaucoma prevalence in these myopes was 3.2 times higher ($p < 0.001$) than in normal sized discs or small discs (<1.51 mm^2) [14]. In this model, however, AXL was not found to be associated with glaucoma prevalence. In low and moderate myopes, the appearance of the optic disc in glaucoma may be very similar to that which has been described in POAG. In high myopes however, because of the structural changes in the optic disc tissue, the presence of parapapillary area, the inability to identify the beta zone clinically as separate from the gamma zone, the thinning of the lamina cribrosa [15], the shallow cup, the vertically oval shape of the disc with an increase in vertical disc diameters, the possible role of optic disc size and sometimes irregular or generalized pallor of the optic disc, a normal IOP, and the difficulty in assessment of visual fields especially in association with myopic macular degeneration and similar challenges in assessing the retinal nerve fiber layer (RNFL) clinically because of the tessellation, poor visibility, and relative thinning that already exists in high myopia and sometimes, even in moderate myopia and difficulty also in assessing the RNFL with the SDOCT because of the migration of Bruch's membrane temporally and the change in the vascular landmarks, there may be difficulty in diagnosing glaucoma at a relatively early stage and sometimes the diagnosis of even moderate severity of glaucoma may be an important goal to prevent further loss (Fig. 3.4a, b).

3.4 Pallor of Optic Disc in Myopia

Pallor of the optic disc in myopia is known to occur in high myopia and also in association with glaucoma. This type of significant pallor is different in a subject with high myopia and glaucoma,

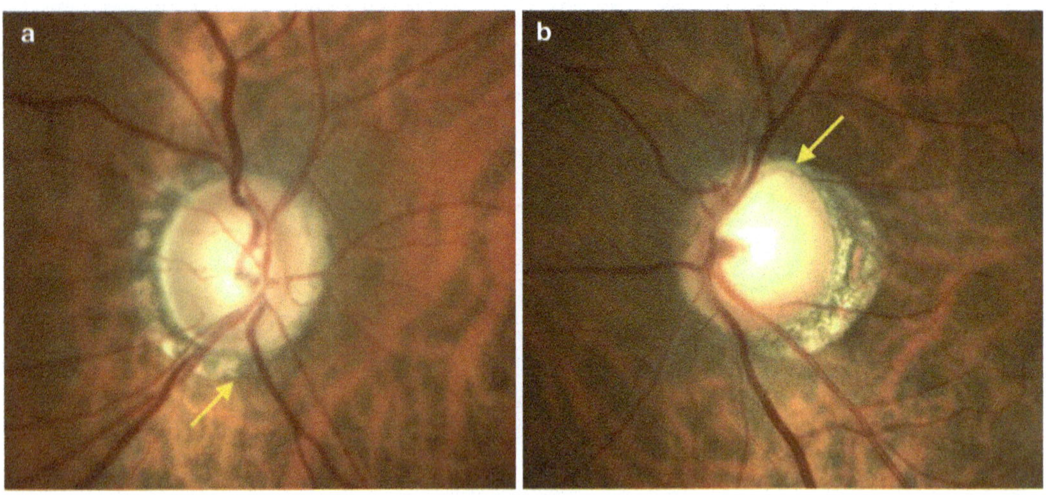

Fig. 3.4 (**a** and **b**) Glaucoma in myopia. (**a**) 79 years of age male patient has a refractive error of −3.25 DS and +3.00 DC. The axial length is 25.56 mm. (**b**) A 61 years of age male pseudophakic subject with an axial length of 26.62 mm. It is important in these subjects to differentiate beta zone and gamma zone since patients of glaucoma may have a beta zone and those with increased axial length are likely to have a gamma zone (yellow arrow shows NRR loss)

when the entire disc may appear pale. Sometimes a shallow cup may be visible and at times, the disc is pale without the classical cupping that one would typically expect in glaucoma. Generalized or patchy pallor in the absence of glaucoma may be associated with reduced vascular flow due to the structural changes associated with the increased axial length, the associated distortion of the parapapillary area due to the separation of the Bruch's membrane leading to compromised posterior ciliary and choroidal circulation that supplies the optic disc tissue. Pallor as a finding may be important especially in the presence of normal IOP to distinguish it from glaucoma. Normal IOP in a patient of myopia with glaucoma and the presence of pallor which may or may not be associated due to glaucomatous damage may present a clinical challenge in the assessment, management, and follow-up of such patients (Fig. 3.5a, b).

3.5 Tilt of the Optic Disc

The tilt of the optic disc has been described based on the disc ovality [16], raised margin of the optic disc [17] and the classical tilted disc [18]. It has also been defined by the levels of the Bruch's membrane opening (BMO) on two sides of the horizontal and/or vertical meridians of the optic disc [19].

Disc ovality is a concept that involves measurement of the longest and shortest diameter of the optic disc. A ratio of minimum to maximum disc diameter of ≤0.8 is considered as a significant disc tilt [16]. Likewise a ratio of ≥1.33 for the longest versus the shortest diameter is also considered as a disc tilt. The prevalence of optic disc tilt was 40.2% in a young myopic population [16]. Myopia was found in 66.2% of eyes with tilted discs compared to 12.4% of eyes with normal discs [20] (Fig. 3.6a, b). High disc ovality ratio has also been found to be associated with older age, higher time spent indoors, greater increase in myopia, and larger beta parapapillary zone in school children in Beijing.

Optic disc tilt was also diagnosed based on the greater height of one margin of the optic disc above the opposite margin [17]. This is possible using stereo viewing or also when using the horizontal and/or vertical sections of the optic disc using the SDOCT (Fig. 3.7a, b).

The authors in this study on adolescent children from Singapore found a significant association with refractive error, higher axial length, and the presence of beta parapapillary changes.

The optic disc tilt has also been calculated based on the BMO. The BMO margin on the nasal side is often higher than the BMO margin on the temporal side. The angle of difference between the two sides may be calculated using the SDOCT sections and this would be an indi-

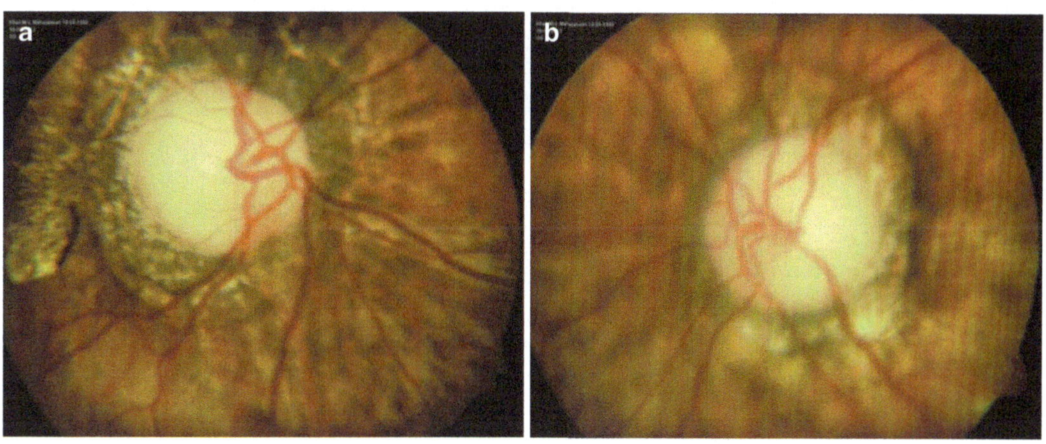

Fig. 3.5 (**a** and **b**) Pallor of optic disc in myopia. This 33 year old female had a refractive error of −18 D in BE. (**a**) RE Axial length is 28.95 mm and (**b**) LE AXL is 28.54 mm

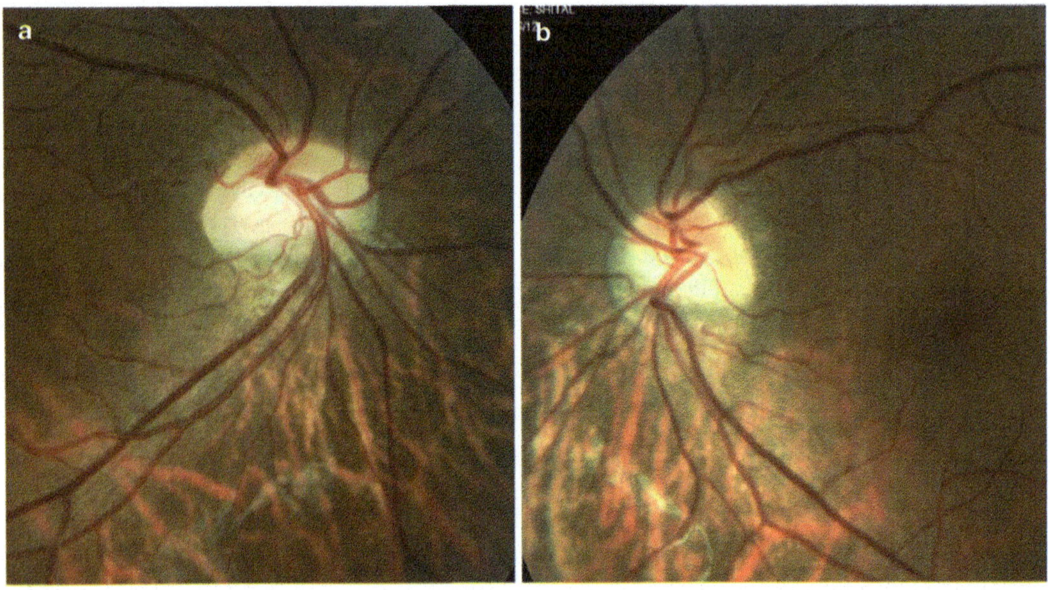

Fig. 3.6 (**a** and **b**) Classical tilted disc. (**a**) RE subject with refractive error of −0.50 Dsph and −0.50 Dcyl, axial length 23.65 mm. Tilt index (disc ovality ratio) of 1.60 and torsion angle of 80 deg. (**b**) LE same subject as in (**a**), with a refractive error of −0.50 Dsph and −1.00 Dcyl. Axial length 23.90 mm. Tilt index 1.60, torsion angle of 90°

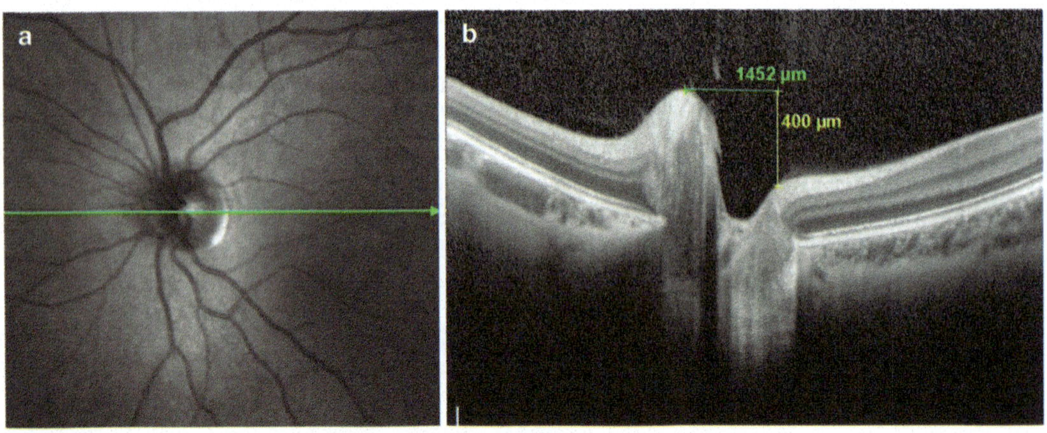

Fig. 3.7 (**a** and **b**) Showing the relatively elevated nasal disc margin relative to the temporal disc margin by 400 microns (**b**, arrows)

cation of the optic disc tilt, often also called rotation of the disc [18, 21]. The tilt forms a part of several changes that occur in the myopic optic disc and the course of the vessels originating from the papillae. The authors found that horizontal tilt was associated with high myopia, greater AXL, and thicker temporal RNFL.

The classical tilted optic disc was described as a congenital tilted optic disc and was long considered to be due to the entry of the optic nerve into the eye at an angle, thus resulting in one margin being more prominent and the corresponding opposite margin being less prominent [20, 21]. Several terms have been used to describe discs with a tilt, such as Fuchs's coloboma, congenital crescents, conus, dysversion of the optic nerve head (ONH), and situs inversus. Associated with such a typical tilted disc is a rotation (i.e. torsion) of the disc around the sagittal axis. There is currently no proof to suggest that there is indeed a congenital actual tilt and/or rotation of the optic nerve, especially since the tilt of the optic nerve has been documented to evolve over a period of time in subjects with myopia under observation over several years. The most frequent orientation of the tilted optic nerve is inferonasal, and this is accompanied by a pseudo-rotation of the superior pole of the optic disc and elevation of the supero-temporal NRR [22]. Dorrel in his earlier observations described three features of the tilted disc, the crescent, presence of depression of one side of the disc, and the oblique direction of the retinal vessels as they entered the eye [21]. Young and associates also described the hypo-pigmentation of the inferonasal fundus, myopic astigmatism, and static visual field depression and/or defects [23].

In the Beijing Eye Study, the presence of the tilted disc as defined here was found in 31 eyes of 23 patients out of 4324 subjects. They were associated with myopia, astigmatism, lower BCVA, small optic discs, and visual field defects [24]. In the Blue Mountains Eye Study, the prevalence was 1.6% out of 3583 participants. The prevalence of the tilted disc increased with increase in astigmatism. Myopia was present in 66.2% of eyes with tilted discs and features of pallor, tessellation, situs inversus, beta parapapillary atrophy, visual field defects, and staphyloma were associated [19].

In another unpublished data by the author and Shaikh C on 104 eyes of 52 subjects with classical tilted optic disc, the mean myopia was −7.05 ± 3.63 D, mean AXL was 25.80 ± 1.50 mm, the mean disc ovality ratio was 1.28 ± 0.21, the mean torsion was 44.64 ± 33.29° and Parapapillary atrophy was detected in 102/104 eyes.

The challenge of the classical tilt of the optic disc lies in being able to clinically assess the optic disc. With the change in the morphometric character of the optic disc, the appearance of a rotation of the poles, abnormal appearance of the superior origin of blood vessels, the appearance of inferior or inferonasal pallor and slope of the NRR—where one would expect the inferior NRR—and the changes in visual field findings and RNFL thickness, all become barriers to diagnosing early and moderate glaucoma. These patients should therefore be followed up even more carefully, in order to detect glaucoma at an early stage (Fig. 3.8a, b).

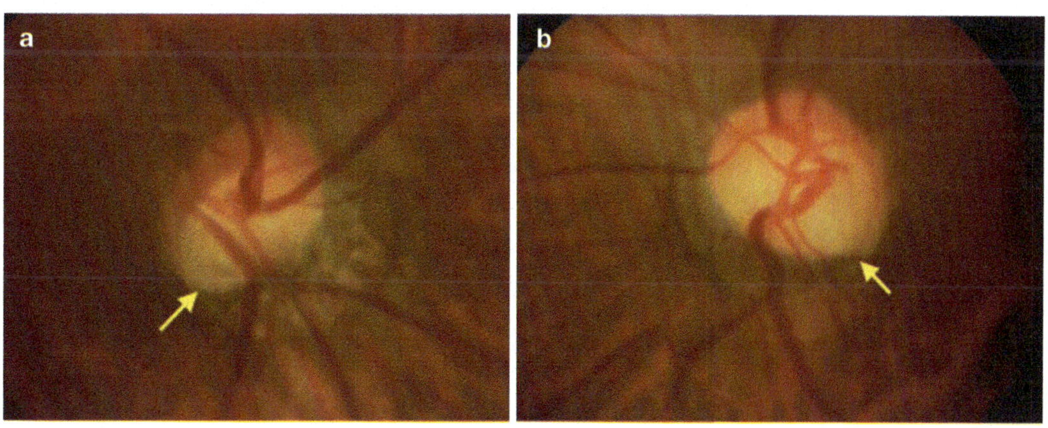

Fig. 3.8 (**a** and **b**) Showing glaucoma in tilted disc female 47 year. (**a**) RE Refractive error of −9.00 D, (**b**) LE Sph. Equ. −7.00 D, IOP BE 14 mmHg, CCT RE 502 u, LE 510 u. Disc shows significant cupping, which is hard to differentiate from a tilted disc that does not have glaucoma. Yellow arrows show loss of inferotemporal NRR

Acknowledgements I would like to acknowledge my team at the Suraj Eye Institute that has worked with me over several years particularly on studying the optic disc: Dr. Karishma Bhate, Dr. Shubhra Agarwal, Dr. Krishna Bhojwani, Dr. Priyanka Pardhi, Dr. Chandini Shaikh, Dr. Swati Mishra, Dr. Rajesh Gupta, Dr. Anshu Khare, Dr. Hemangi Rathi, Dr. Deepti Jain, Dr. Sarang Lambat, and Dr. Prabhat Nangia.

References

1. Nangia V, Matin A, Bhojwani K, Kulkarni M, et al. Optic disc size in a population-based study: the Central India eye and medical study. Acta Ophthalmol. 2008;86(1):103–4.
2. Jonas JB, Dichtl A. Optic disc morphology in myopic primary open angle glaucoma. Graefes Arch Clin Exp Ophthalmol. 1997;235:627–33.
3. Jonas JB, Gusek GC, Naumann GOH. Optic disc morphometry in high myopia. Graefes Arch Clin Exp Ophthalmol. 1988;226:587–90.
4. Oliveira C, Harizman N, Girkin CA, Xie A, et al. Axial length and optic disc size in normal eyes. Br J Ophthalmol. 2007;91:37–9.
5. Hyung SM, Kim DM, Hong C, Youn D. Optic disc of the myopic eye: relationship between refractive error and morphometric characteristics. Korean J Ophthalmol. 1992;6:32–5.
6. Jonas JB, Papastathopoulos KI. Optic disc shape in glaucoma. Graefes Arch Clin Exp Ophthalmol. 1996;234:167–73.
7. Jonas JB, Jonas SB, Jonas RA, Holbach L, Dai Y, et al. Parapapillary atrophy: histological Gama zone and delta zone. PLoS One. 2012;7(10):e47237.
8. Yi D, Jost JB, Huang H, Wang M, Sun X. Microstructure of parapapillary atrophy beta zone and gamma zone. Invest Ophthalmol and Vis Sci. 2013;54(3):2013–7.
9. Marcus MW, de Vries MM, Montolio JGF, Jansonius MN. Myopia as a risk factor for open angle glaucoma: a systematic review and meta-analysis. Ophthalmology. 2011;118:1989–94.
10. Xu L, Wang Y, Wang S, et al. High myopia and glaucoma susceptibility. The Beijing eye study. Ophthalmology. 2007;114:216–20.
11. Jonas JB, Budde WM. Optic nerve damage in highly myopic eyes with chronic open angle glaucoma. Eur J Ophthalmol. 2005;15(1):41–7.
12. Chihara E, Liu X, Dong J, et al. Severe myopia is a risk factor for progressive visual field loss in primary open angle glaucoma. Ophthalmologica. 1997;211:66–71.
13. Suzuki Y, Iwase A, Araie M, et al. Risk factors for open angle glaucoma in a Japanese population. The Tajimi study. Ophthalmology. 2006;113:1613–7.
14. Nagaoka N, Jonas JB, Morohoshi K, Moriyama M, Shimada N, Yoshida T, et al. Glaucomatous-type optic discs in high myopia. PLoS One. 2015;10(10):e0138825.
15. Jonas JB. Role of cerebrospinal fluid pressure in the pathogenesis of glaucoma. Acta Ophthalmol. 2011;89:505–14.
16. Tay E, Seah S, Chan SP, et al. Optic disc ovality as an index of tilt and its relationship to myopia and perimetry. Am J Ophthalmol. 2005;139:247–52.
17. Samarawickrama C, Mitchell P, Tong L, et al. Myopia-related optic disc and retinal changes in adolescent children from Singapore. Ophthalmology. 2011;118:2050–7.
18. Hwang HY, Yoo C, Kim YY. Myopic optic disc tilt and the characteristics of the peripapillary retinal nerve fiber layer thickness measured by spectral domain optical coherence tomography. J Glaucoma. 2012;21:260–5.
19. Vongphanit MP, Wang JJ. Population prevalence of tilted optic disc and the relationship of this sign to refractive error. Am J Ophthalmol. 2002;133:679–85.
20. Witmer MT, Margo CE, Drucker M. Tilted optic disks. Surv Ophthalmol. 2010;55(5):403–28.
21. Dorrel D. The tilted disc. Br J Ophthalmol. 1978;62:16–20.
22. Apple DJ, Rabb MF, Walsh PM. Congenital anomalies of the optic disk. Surv Ophthalmol. 1982;27:3–41.
23. Young SE, Walsh FB, Knox DL. The tilted disc syndrome. Am J Ophthalmol. 1976;82(1):16–23.
24. You QS, Xu L, Jonas JB. Tilted optic discs. The Beijing eye study. Eye. 2008;22:728–9.

4 What Are the Key Clinical Skills and Investigative Techniques for Disc Evaluation?

Sushma Tejwani and Parin Mehta

Optic nerve head (ONH) evaluation plays a key role in the diagnosis and assessment of glaucoma and effective clinical evaluation is a technical skill that requires acquisition and practice. Stereo-photographs allow review of the nerve without the technical difficulty, are an excellent record, but are hard to follow and cannot (practically) be performed at every visit. The physical examination findings of the ONH should be documented each visit, with a drawing (preferably with imaging) for comparison with future examinations [1].

4.1 Clinical Examination of the Optic Nerve

A magnified stereoscopic optic disc examination using +60, +78, or +90 dioptre (D) lens with slit lamp bio-microscopy is the ideal technique and is the single most important clinical skill that is mandatory for ONH assessment for glaucoma [2].

The red-free light source from the slit lamp helps identify the retinal nerve fibre layer (RNFL) defects as well, although the specialized photography systems are ideal for the same [3]. The direct ophthalmoscope provides a magnified image, but does not give a stereoscopic view and hence is not the ideal way to assess; however, indirect ophthalmoscope provides a low magnification that makes it unsuitable for documenting subtle signs.

For the systematic evaluation and documentation of the ONH the clinical examination can be divided into following components.

4.1.1 Description of the ONH

The ONH description should address its size, shape, tilt, or any deviation in morphology from normal, some of which has already been addressed in Chap. 1.

4.1.1.1 Size

Disc size varies according to ethnicity, e.g. Caucasians have smaller disc, followed by Mexicans, Asians, and then Africans. The average area of disc in whites ranges from 2.1 to 2.8 mm^2 [4]. Estimation of disc size can be done on slit lamp with the slit lamp graticule by adjusting the height of the slit to the edges of the optic size while examining with +60 D lens [5]. The multiplication factor used for different lenses is 1.26 with Goldman contact lens, 1.5 with Volk superfields lens, 1.15 with +78D, and 1.41 for +90 D lens. Thus, it is important to have an accurate assessment of the size, as the smaller cup may be abnormal for a smaller disc and a larger cup may be normal for a larger disc (Fig. 4.1).

S. Tejwani (✉) · P. Mehta
Glaucoma Service, Narayana Nethralaya-2, Bangalore, India
e-mail: sushma@narayananethralaya.com

S. Pandav et al. (eds.), *The Optic Nerve Head in Health and Disease*,
https://doi.org/10.1007/978-981-33-6838-5_4

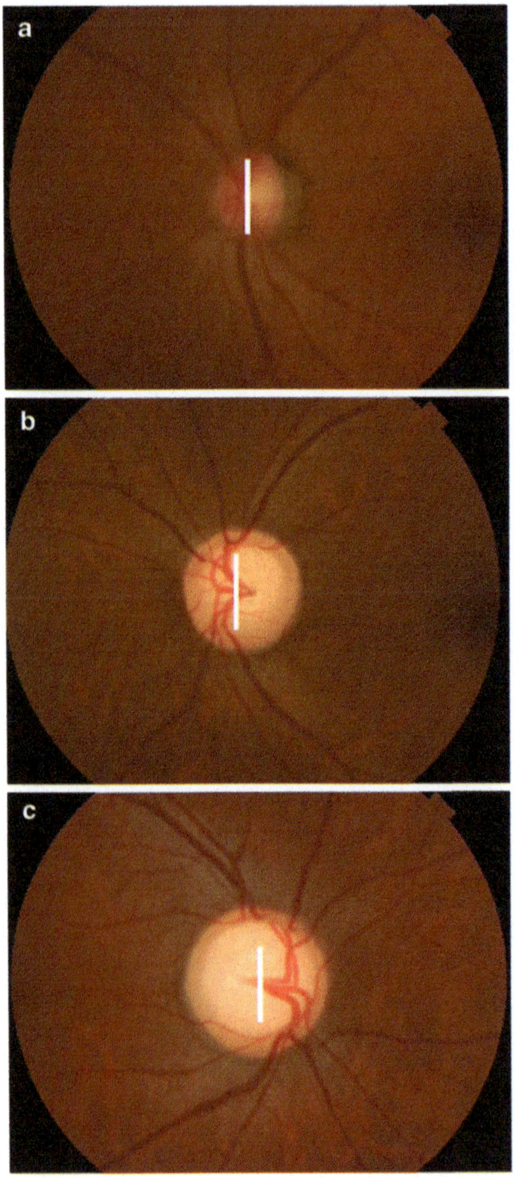

Fig. 4.1 Different sizes of the ONH. Comparison with the same sized vertical bar indicates the difference between (**a**) small disc, (**b**) medium disc, and (**c**) large disc

4.1.1.2 Shape

The shape of the ONH is usually vertically oval, so that vertical diameter being 7–10% larger than horizontal [5]. If there is a disparity, the shape may actually be horizontally oval, round, oblique, slit like, and may influence the configuration of the neuro-retinal rim (NRR) as well.

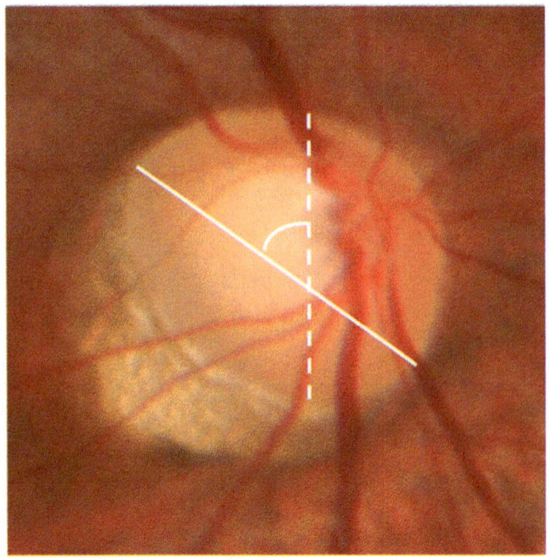

Fig. 4.2 Hashed line is the expected vertical axis of a normal disc. The solid line in this image shows a 45° tilt

4.1.1.3 Tilt

The tilt in the vertical axis of the disc may be a sign of myopia (Fig. 4.2) and may actually be protective for progression [6]. An elongated optic disc is known to be associated with higher astigmatism or amblyopia [7].

4.1.2 Cup-to-Disc Ratio

Cup-to-disc ratio (CDR) is a well-established index of glaucoma damage severity to the optic nerve head. Conventionally concern about glaucomatous damage to the nerve starts at about 0.7 (vertical CDR) but this has been criticized over many years as being independent of disc size. When the underlying scleral canal size is considered, then the range of normality varies, with smaller nerves potentially being glaucomatous at CDR greater than or equal to 0.6, and with very large that number increases to 0.8.

> CD ratio is meaningful only in relation to the disc size, whether small, medium, or large, and normal shape of the disc. On its own, it may not mean anything.

Cup is a potentially empty space in the centre of the ONH after all the ganglion cell axons have been circumferentially distributed in the space bounded by the scleral canal. This circumferential arrangement forms the NRR. Hence, CDR alone is fallacious and is only a surrogate measure for estimation of glaucomatous damage in conjunction with the disc size. Given the same disc size, asymmetry between the two eyes of >0.2 (Fig. 4.3) is a strong predictor of glaucoma, as is progression over time [3].

Rim–disc ratio (RDR) is a new concept that helps overcome some of the shortcomings of the cup:disc ratio system. RDR is used by the disc damage likelihood scale (DDLS), which has been discussed in detail in Chap. 8.

In order to identify the inner dimensions of the NRR, or the outer margins of the cup, we must identify a change in the contour and/or the colour. Clues about the junction of the rim with the cup can be taken from the bending of blood vessels as they follow the contour (Fig. 4.4). Not all vessels follow the contour of the rim faithfully and some may traverse the rim without deviation (known as overpass vessels). Accurate identification of the inner margin of the NRR is vital to determining glaucoma damage and must be practised.

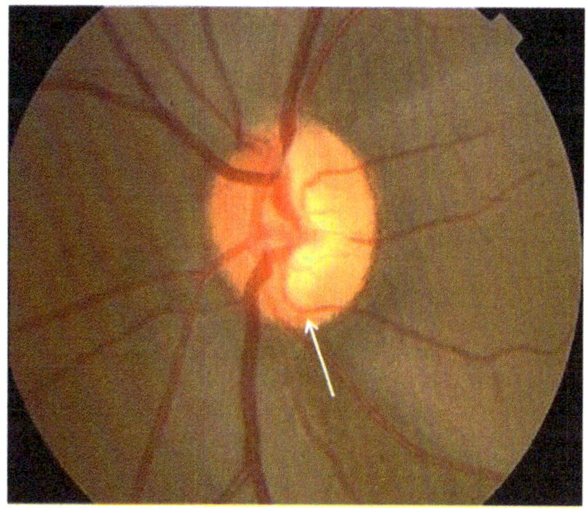

Fig. 4.4 Cupping can be judged by observing bending of vessels at cup and rim junction (white arrow)

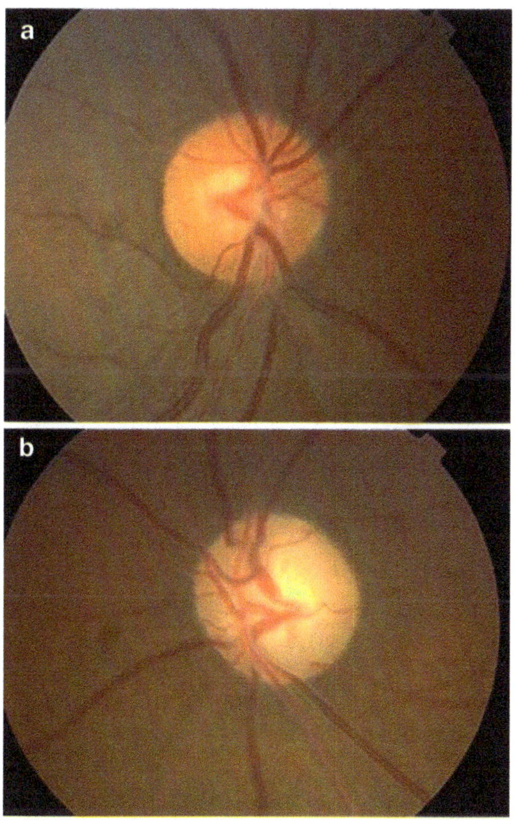

Fig. 4.3 Cup–disc ratio asymmetry: (**a**) right eye and (**b**) left eye (glaucomatous)

4.1.3 Neuroretinal Rim (NRR)

NRR consists of the area occupied by retinal ganglion cells (RGCs) in cross-section and loss of this tissue is an unequivocal feature of disease. Loss of the NRR is required in glaucoma. The size of NRR correlates with disc size—larger nerves have a larger NRR and hence more axons. The area of NRR reported for Caucasians is 1.97 ± 0.5 mm^2, and the Indians eye has much higher (2.29 ± 0.39 mm^2) [8, 9]. The NRR follows a particular pattern, that is inferior rim is thicker than superior, then nasal, temporal being the thinnest [9] and this is known as ISNT rule seen in 80% of the normal ONHs.

The first change that is observed in NRR with glaucoma is the change in contour, that is backward bowing or saucerisation of a segment or whole of NRR (Fig. 4.5) subsequently the sloping, shelving, and excavation happens leading to change in the NRR width and breach of the ISNT rule. Additionally, the localized loss of NRR can

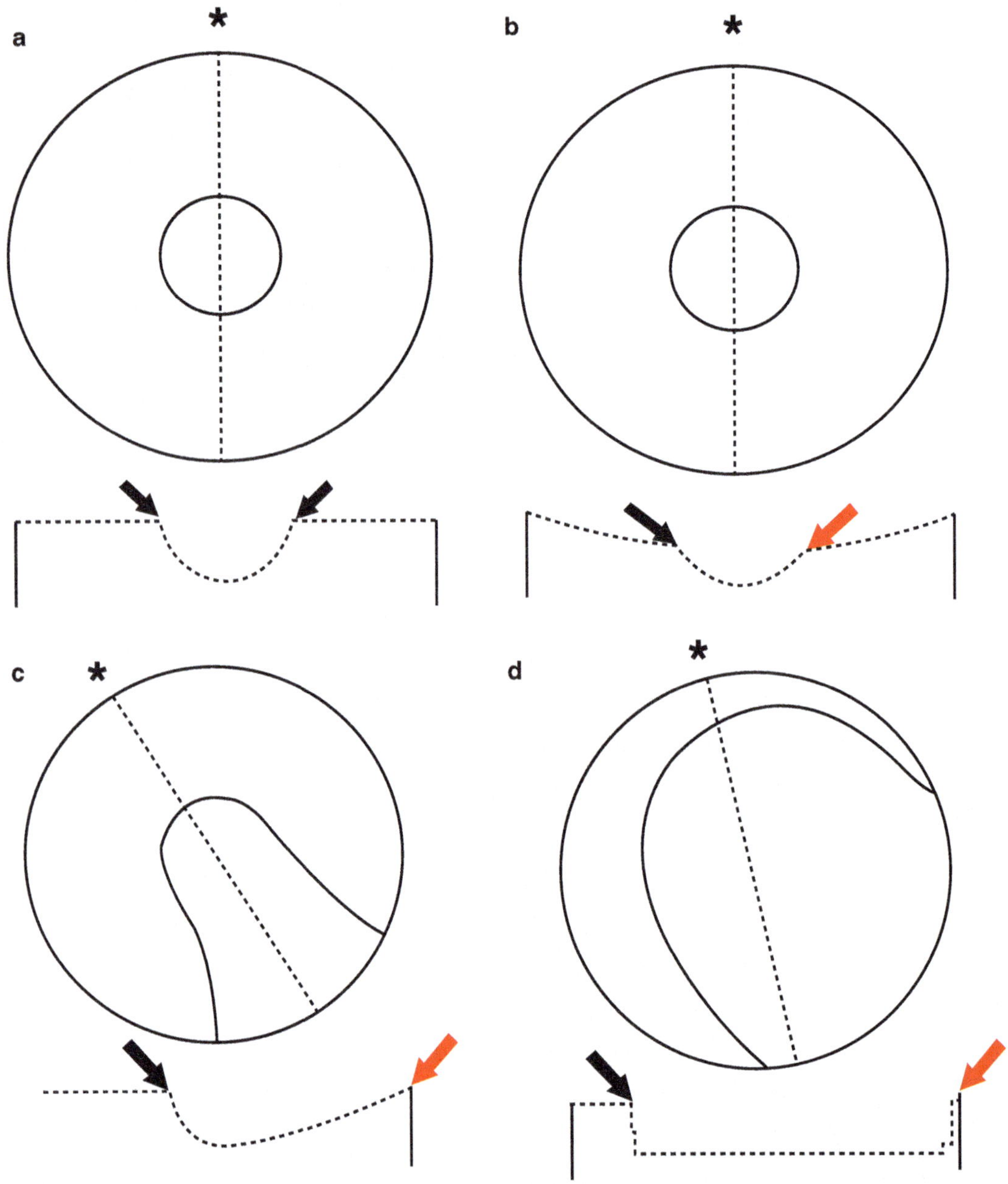

Fig. 4.5 Schematic diagram showing progressive changes in contour of neuroretinal rim demonstrated by horizontal sections at the bottom of each diagram starting from (**a**) normal, (**b**) saucerization, (**c**) shelving, and (**d**) excavation

happen leading to absence of rim in a segment forming a notch (Fig. 4.6). The loss is usually seen first in the inferotemporal or superotemporal disc region; hence, these should be examined carefully. Presence of a notch, pallor, or thinning of superior or inferior NRR are strong indicators of glaucoma. Pallor is more marked in non-glaucomatous optic neuropathy rather than glaucoma (Fig. 4.7). Pallor in excess of cupping can occur in multiple scenarios, such as, if there is sudden acute rise intraocular pressure in angle closure crisis or secondary glaucoma [10], or potentially other non-glaucomatous causes of cupping, such as autosomal dominant optic

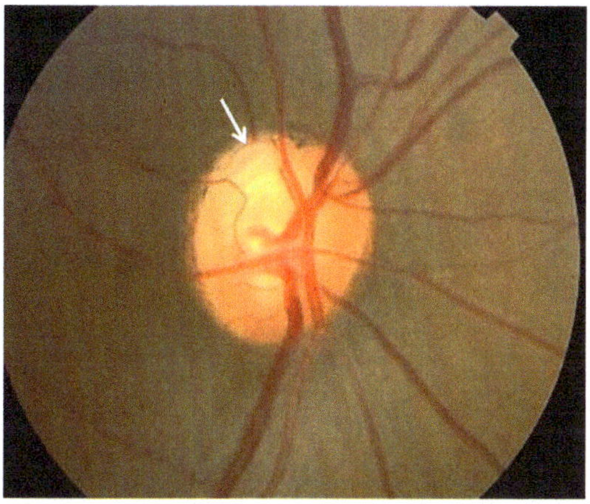

Fig. 4.6 Localized rim loss showing absence of neuroretinal rim in that area forming a superior notch (white arrow)

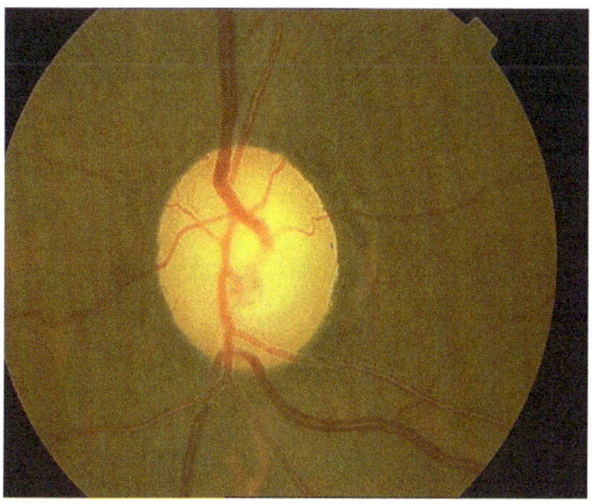

Fig. 4.7 Optic disc pallor seen in anterior ischemic optic neuropathy (AION) which mimics glaucoma

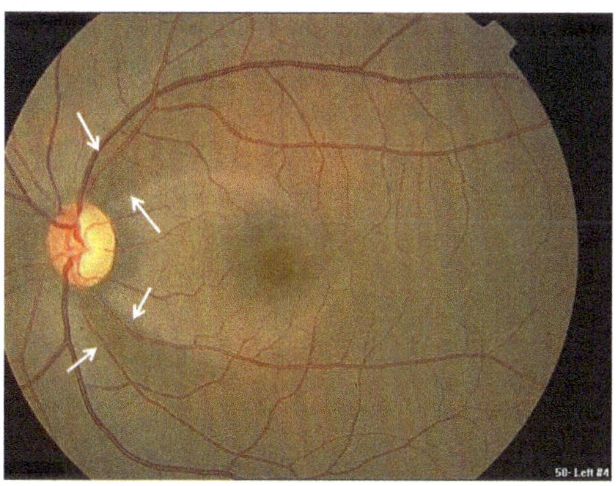

Fig. 4.8 Typical wedge-shaped nerve fibre layer defects seen superiorly and inferiorly (white arrows)

atrophy, methanol toxicity, and some forms of vascular insult (some of these conditions are addressed in Chap. 9).

4.1.4 Retinal Nerve Fibre Layer (RNFL) Evaluation

Dilated disc evaluation with slit lamp biomicroscopy using +78D lens with red-free light along with red-free photographs is the most useful way to examine RNFL.

Normal RNFL when seen from superior to inferior area appears to have bright, dark, bright pattern with fine striations that are less than retinal vessels in width. Bright correlates with superior and inferior arcuate regions and dark with the macula corresponding with the thickness of physiological RNFL distribution. The deviation from this pattern is suggestive of RNFL loss. Diffuse loss may occur for reasons other than glaucoma. When RNFL loss is extensive and diffuse it may be hard to detect clinically—look for baring of vessels and a lack of fine striations on reflected light. A localized RNFL (Fig. 4.8) loss appears as a wedge-shaped defect that begins at the margin of the disc and enlarges as it moves towards periphery [11]. This localized RNFL defect is very specific for glaucoma and is highly suggestive of early glaucoma. Although RNFL defects may be identified by examination they cannot be quantified except with cross-sectional imaging [5].

4.1.4.1 Disc Haemorrhage.

Isolated disc haemorrhage along the RNFL (Fig. 4.9), or a NRR notch, usually in the superotemporal and inferotemporal quadrant, in the absence of other retinal haemorrhages is a specific sign of glaucoma [3, 5]. These are seen in 4–7% of glaucoma patients but do occur in normal eyes. A recent study found that over half of isolated disc haemorrhages referred for assessment of glaucoma were found not to have the disease. Disc haemorrhages are seen in all types of glaucoma, from ocular hypertension to advanced primary open-angle glaucoma and from normal tension glaucoma to high-tension

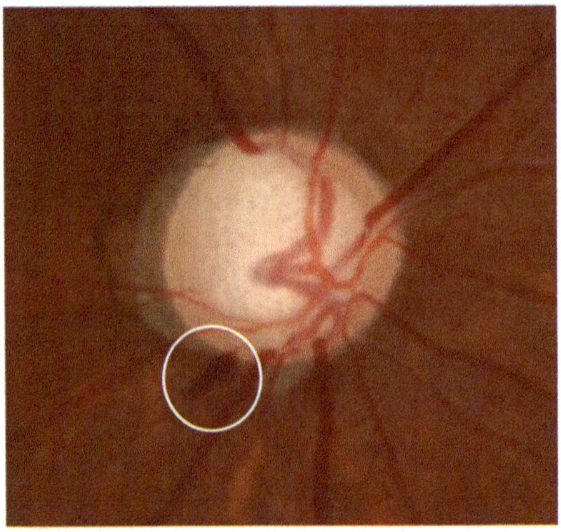

Fig. 4.9 Isolated disc haemorrhage (white circle), a classical sign of glaucoma progression

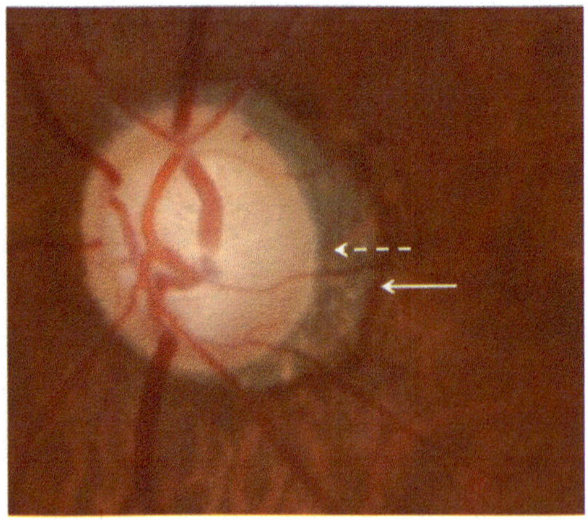

Fig. 4.10 Peripapillary chorioretinal atrophy with peripheral alpha zone (solid arrow) and central beta zone (hashed arrow)

glaucomas. They last for few weeks and then may or may not translate into RNFL defects [4]. In a patient on treatment, the appearance of disc hemorrhage may be a sign of the disease progression. An extra attention is needed to detect disc haemorrhage, even in the Ocular Hypertension Treatment Study (OHTS), only 17% of disc haemorrhages identified on photographs were spotted on clinical examination [12]. These are addressed in detail in Chaps. 5 and 7.

> Localized RNFL defects and isolated disc hemorrhages are very specific and objective signs of early glaucoma and should be carefully looked for during optic disc evaluation.

4.1.5 Peripapillary Chorioretinal Atrophy (PPCRA)

PPCRA consists of beta zone and alpha zone and is also seen in age-related changes, myopia, oblique entry disc in addition to glaucoma. Beta zone is closer to the optic nerve and consists of retinal pigment epithelial (RPE) and choroidal atrophy, whereas alpha zone is peripheral to the disc and has only RPE atrophy (Fig. 4.10). Beta zone correlates more with glaucoma and has been reported to be associated with location of disc haemorrhages [13]. This has been addressed in detail in Chap. 3.

4.1.6 'Glaucoma-Like Discs'

This is a false positive and needs to be differentiated from the true positive. There are many reasons for this and they will be reviewed later in this book. It is important to differentiate the changes in the disc due to reasons other than glaucoma, as there are certain common signs that can overlap. For instance, many myopic changes in the optic nerve like oblique entry, peripapillary atrophy, sloping rims can be seen in myopia and can be considered as glaucoma or vice versa.

> All myopes should be carefully evaluated for glaucoma with high index of suspicion as the disc changes may overlap and affect the estimation.

Hence it is important to carefully evaluate the contour of the vessel and its change at the NRR margin to understand the shape of NRR and CDR. Certain other conditions like optic disc pit

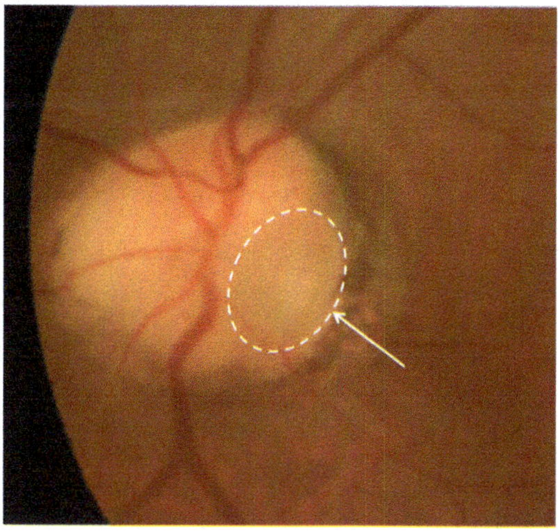

Fig. 4.11 Optic disc pit (hashed circle) mimicking glaucomatous disc

(Fig. 4.11) resolved arteritic anterior ischemic optic neuropathy (AAION), leutic or Kjer's dominant optic atrophy, methanol poisoning may give the false impression of glaucoma due to increased cupping or pallor. Therefore, the appearance of the ONH in conjunction with other clinical symptoms and sign can help differentiate these from glaucoma.

This is addressed in detail in a subsequent chapter.

4.1.7 Overall Impression of the Disc

Based on the above mentioned features the ONH should be described in a way that an overall impression of being normal, suspect, or glaucoma can be made. If there are specific and objective signs of glaucoma such as RNFL defect, disc haemorrhage, or notch, the diagnosis of glaucoma is certain; however, subjective signs like sloping of the rim, increased CDR, diffuse loss of RNFL can qualify a disc to be having suspicion and may require further evaluation. ONH that is ambiguous and cannot be resolved by the clinician to normal or diseased needs to be 'risk managed'. They need photos and imaging and need review at set time in the future—depending upon the rest of the risk profile of the patient.

4.2 Imaging the ONH

Clinical evaluation of the ONH does involve some subjectivity, leading to high rates of intra-observer as well as inter-observer variability. The recent advances in imaging instruments are an objective means of achieving reproducible information aiding the clinician in the early diagnosis [14].

The automated imaging technologies used so far include:

1. Optical coherence tomography (OCT).
2. Confocal scanning laser ophthalmoscopy (CSLO).
3. Scanning laser polarimetry (SLP).

Each of these has their own fundamental method of acquiring and processing images, despite providing similar information, however, they are not interchangeable. We shall describe interpretation of OCT in detail.

4.2.1 Optical Coherence Tomography (OCT)

Over the last two decades, OCT has evolved as the most commonly used techniques for ONH and peripapillary retinal imaging in glaucoma [15].

All forms of OCT use the principle of low coherence interferometry to acquire high-resolution images of ocular structures. A near-infrared (840-nm) light beam is projected by a superluminescent diode into a beam splitter which in turn creates a reference and a measurement beam. The measurement beam is directed onto the subject's eye, and based on the distance, thickness, and reflectivity of intraocular tissues, it is reflected back. The reference beam is reflected from the reference mirror. The pattern of interference (Michelson principle) created by difference in echo propagation of the two beams is measured by a photosensitive detector (Fig. 4.12). This information is used to create bi-dimensional images of the different layers at a given point.

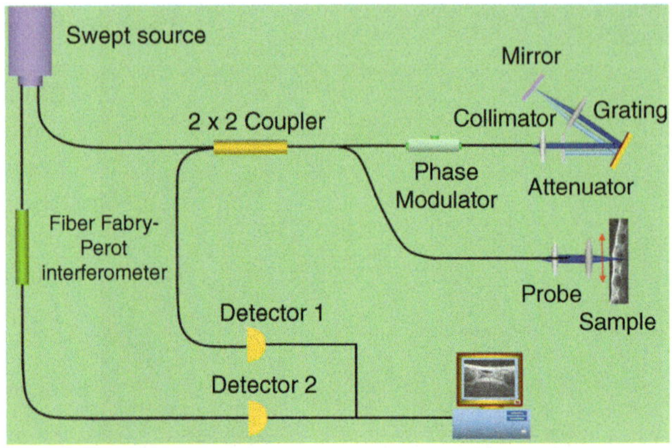

Fig. 4.12 Image acquisition by OCT using Michelson interferometer principle

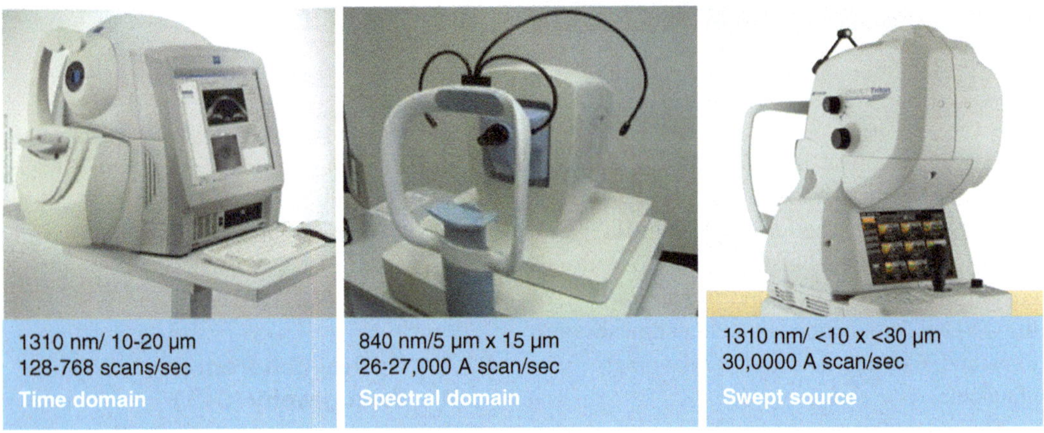

Fig. 4.13 Three generations of OCT machines: Carl Zeiss Meditec (Cirrus), Optovue (RTVue), and Topcon Medical Systems (Triton)

4.2.1.1 Types of OCT

There are three generations of OCT: time domain (TD), spectral domain (SD), and swept source (SS) OCT. Axial resolution (depth) varies from 2 to 7 microns. The speed of scanning has drastically improved allowing for a more detailed sampling of the area of interest, as we have moved from TD to SD and SSOCT (Fig. 4.13).

Nowadays all OCT devices have spectral domain technology, which has a significantly higher resolution and shorter image acquisition time. Time domain OCT and spectral domain OCT have a different operating principle; time domain OCT was associated with the delay in the reflection time of light, while the actual variable in spectral domain OCT is the change in the optic frequency.

In a spectral domain OCT, the ONH is scanned with a 6 × 6 mm cube consisting of serial B scans that take 30,000–40,000 A mode scans. A 3.46 mm circle centred at optic disc is identified automatically using 3D software enabling the analysis of peripapillary RNFL. The standard OCT acquires 3D images of the ONH region which enables accurate and reproducible measurements of parameters like disc and rim area, CDR, cup volume, and others.

The acquired data is then compared with the normative database of the machine. Table 4.1 gives the normative database for the different machines including GDx and HRT. Based on the patient's ethnicity one can determine the validity of statistical comparisons for a particular machine.

Table 4.1 Normative database details of three different types of OCT, HRT 3, and GDX

Model	Carl Zeiss Meditec (Cirrus)	Topcon Medical Systems (Triton)	Heidelberg Engineering (Spectralis)	Optovue (RTVue)	HRT3	GDx
No. of subjects	284	182	201	80	>1000	540
Ages (years)	19–84	19–84	18–78	18–84	18–80	18–80
Gender (M/F)	133 M 149 F	Disc: 54 M/92 F Macula: 112 F/61 M	111 M 90 F	N/A	N/A	N/A
Ethnicity	43% Caucasian24% Asian18% African American12% Hispanic1% Indian6% mixed ethnicity	64% Caucasian21% African American15% Hispanic	Caucasian	33% Caucasian22% Asian20% African American12% Hispanics12% Indian1% other	>700 Caucasian >200 African-American >100 Indian (southeast Asian) Hispanics and Asians are in process	Asian African-American Caucasian Hispanic
Anatomy evaluated	RNFL thickness ONH parameters GCL + IPL thicknessmacula	Optic disc macula	RNFL thickness	RNFL thickness ganglion cell complex macular thickness	RNFL thickness Optic nerve parameters	RNFL thickness Optic nerve parameters

Most of the SDOCT machines have high precision quality and eye trackers which allows minimal deviation of data [16]. However diagnostic accuracy of TDOCT versus SDOCT [17, 18] and SDOCT versus SSOCT [19] is statistically similar for early or pre-perimetric glaucoma. Parameters used for diagnosing glaucoma as well as for evaluating risk in glaucoma suspects include peripapillary RNFL, ganglion cells, ONH, and macular parameters. Although there are many SDOCT brands in the world, the most commonly used SD-OCTs are the Spectralis (Heidelberg Engineering, Dossenheim, Germany), the Cirrus (Carl Zeiss Meditec, Dublin, CA), Triton (Topcon Inc.), and the RTVue (Optovue Inc., Fremont, CA). Each OCT machine has different glaucoma scan patterns, proprietary software segmentation algorithms, and display outputs (Fig. 4.14).

4.2.1.2 Components of the Printouts and their Interpretation

Although each machine provides slightly different printouts as reports, but their components and the interpretation remain the same. We shall describe each component in detail by taking different sections of the report.

4.2.1.2.1 Fundus Image and Scan Quality

The fundus image in OCT is created by superimposing the image obtained through scanning laser ophthalmoscopy (SLO) and OCT. This image appears on the upper section of the RNFL analysis screen and shows where the scan is centred, an ideal centring of the scan should be equidistant from the centre of the disc. This section determines the quality of the scan, a well centred and equally illuminated image represents a good quality scan (Fig. 4.15a). The scan quality is documented by machine on the top panel of the report [20]. One must remember that the normative database varies with age, ethnicity, and machine.

All OCT algorithms attempt to identify the internal limiting membrane as the upper boundary of the RNFL. The OCT software-related artefacts include algorithm failure and the

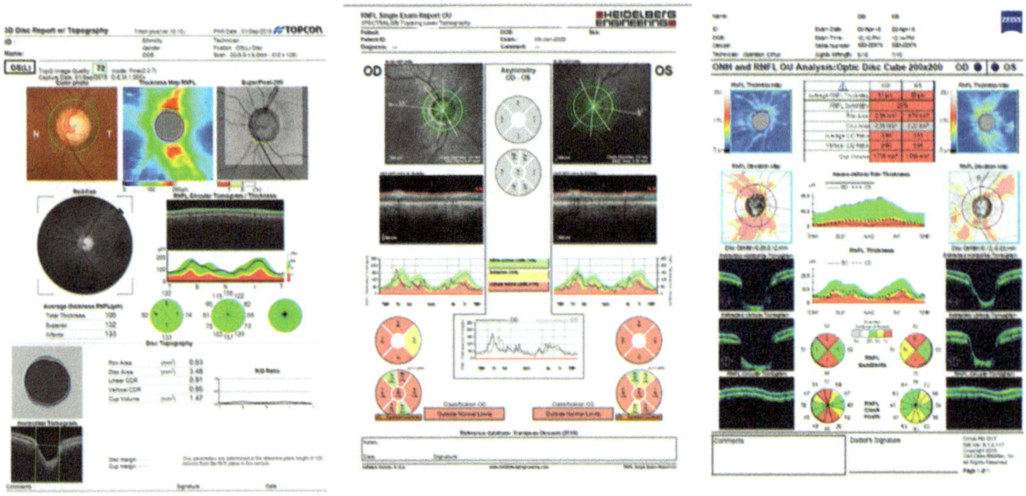

Fig. 4.14 Standard OCT printouts of Triton (Topcon medical systems), Spectralis (Heidelberg Engineering), and Cirrus (Carl Zeiss Meditec)

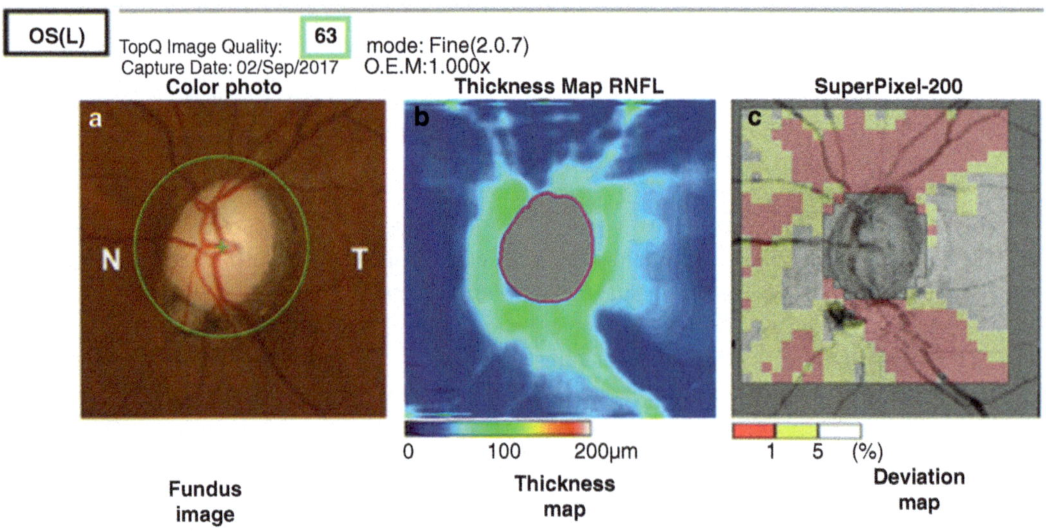

Fig. 4.15 (**a**) Upper section of OCT printout depicting image quality in green box along with fundus image and centration circle, (**b**) thickness map, and (**c**) deviation or superpixel map

misidentification of the anterior–posterior retinal boundaries. This is commonly seen in eyes with prominent posterior hyaloid, marked peripapillary atrophy, high myopia, or with significant media opacities (dry eye, corneal opacities, cataract, and vitreous opacities).

Focal media opacities, such as floater, posterior vitreous detachment and haemorrhage, can cause a focal loss of signal strength giving a false appearance of focal RNFL drop out that can artificially create segmental areas of thinning or lower the average RNFL thickness.

If the scan is decentred inferiorly, it measures the RNFL at a distance further away from the ONH and will show lower values, this will give a false impression of nerve fibre loss and glaucoma.

> The image quality and centration are important parameters to be checked before paying attention to numerical details and statistical comparisons in an imaging printout.

4.2.1.2.2 RNFL Thickness Map

The RNFL thickness map is calculated based on all the data of the scanned 6 × 6 cube. Similar to a topographic map, a colour scale is used for show variation in the RNFL thickness (Fig. 4.15b). The colder colours (blue, green) represent thinned areas, while hotter colours (red, yellow) represent thick areas. The map excludes the optic disc displayed in dark blue.

4.2.1.2.3 The Deviation Map

The patient's RNFL thickness is compared with the normative data through the deviation map. Deviation map or superpixel images gives the colour coding for comparison of RNFL thickness with normative database. The probability of being abnormal is represented by the colour code, cooler colours signify near normal, whereas hotter colours indicate more abnormal values (Fig. 4.15c).

4.2.1.2.4 Average Thickness Values and TSNIT Profile

The calculation of RNFL thickness is then displayed in a numerical chart and plotted as a graph known as TSNIT profile. In this chart, the average thickness of each point across the calculation is demonstrated for both eyes (Fig. 4.16a).

For the graph, RNFL thickness profile is charted temporally, superiorly, nasally, inferiorly, and temporally again, in that order, beginning from around the optic disc is represented by black line. This is superimposed on age matched normative data (colour bands), where band green band indicates that 95% of the normal population. Yellow band depicts the 5% of normal population and the red band indicates 1% of normal population, so part of the line falling in red zone suggests that less than 1% chance of being normal at that point for the given patient.

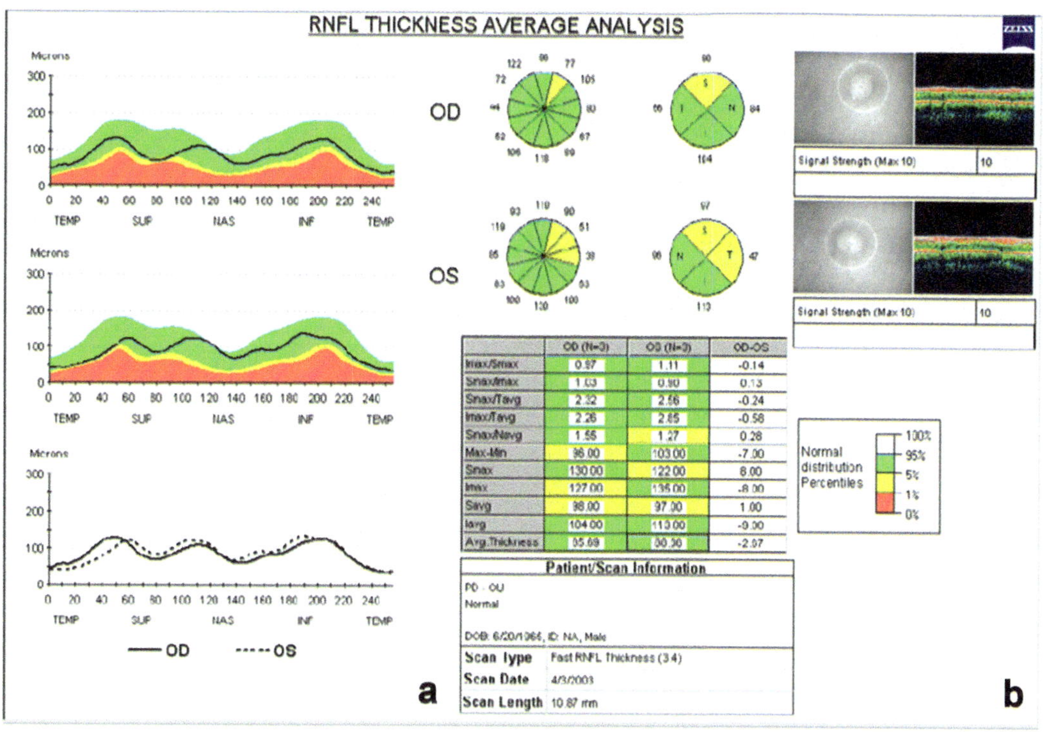

Fig. 4.16 (**a**) Average RNFL thickness and TSNIT profile for right eye, left eye, and inter-eye asymmetry and (**b**) sector wise and quadrant wise thickness profile along with tabular form with inter-eye differences

4.2.1.2.5 Mean Thickness in Quadrants

Normal distribution percentiles for the RNFL (Fig. 4.16b) are represented in sectoral clock hours and quadrants thickness, these are useful in identifying changes overtime. The table represents colour coded percentile distribution of right eye, left eye, and asymmetry, the last row showing the average thickness. Various ratios like inferior maximum thickness/superior maximum thickness for each eye are given in numerical value in a box that is colour coded.

The statistical comparisons with colour codes give a visual impression of the quadrants/clock hours having abnormality and its quantification in comparison to the age-related normative database of the machine, however, needs to be substantiated clinically.

Inter-eye symmetry graph is the superimposition of the two eyes and it gives comparative study between the two eyes, asymmetry being suggestive of glaucoma.

4.2.1.2.6 ONH Parameters and Analysis Results

For the optic nerve head analysis, the radial and the horizontal scan detects the anterior surface of the RNFL and the RPE (Fig. 4.17). Individual radial scan analysis is seen on the left side of large scan image (top) for each of the radial line scans and shows the red shaded area as ***rim area*** above the cup line to anterior surface of disc.

The average of the ***nerve bundle widths at the disc*** is determined on each side, which appears as a straight yellow line from each disc reference point to the nearest point on the anterior surface.

The straight, light blue line between the two disc reference points indicated by a light blue

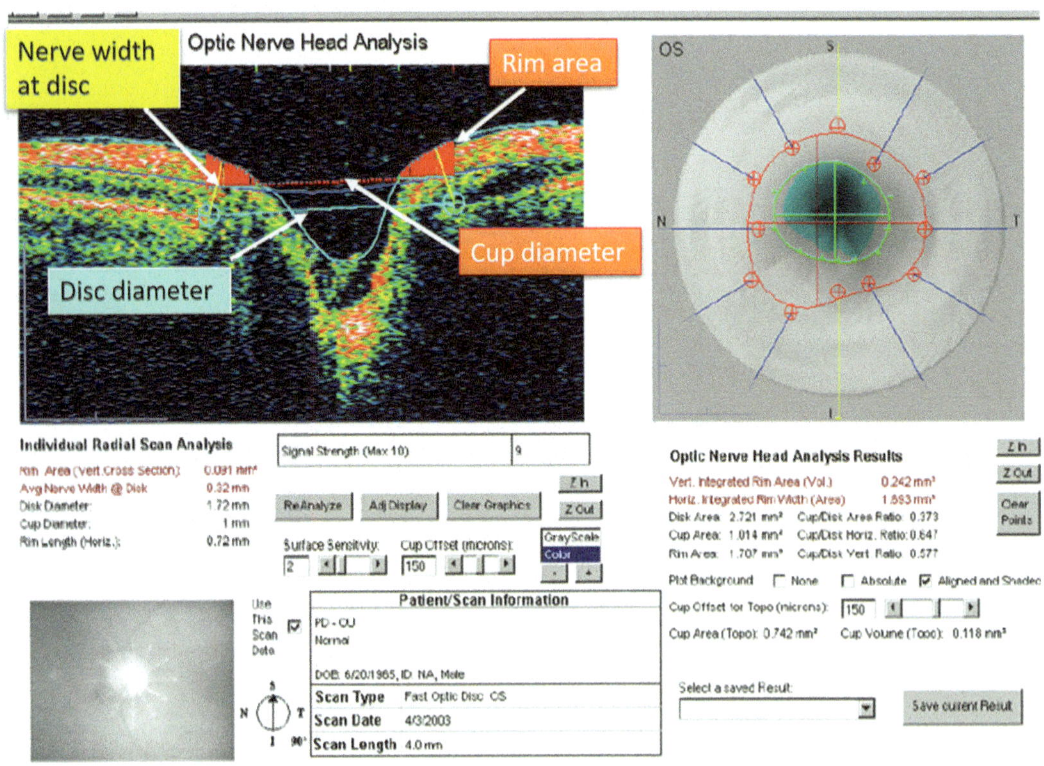

Fig. 4.17 Optic nerve head parameters based on horizontal tomogram showing various landmarks for calculation. The grey box shows disc line and cup line for various measurements

cross inside a circle corresponds with ***disc diameter***.

The disc reference points correspond to the top and inner edges of the RPE, and this line is known as the disc line.

Cup diameter is the dashed, straight red line. This line extends into the rim in light blue, where it represents the posterior boundary of the rim.

Rim length (Horizontal) is the disc diameter minus the cup diameter. ***Optic nerve head analysis results*** are represented in the composite image on the right (top) in the same figure that outlines the disc in red and the cup in green (Fig. 4.17). It shows the longest vertical and horizontal lines across the disc and cup in red and green, respectively.

The nasal (N), inferior(I), temporal(T), and superior(S) quadrants are indicated, it shows the disc reference points with a red cross inside a circle and the cup edges with small green crosses. The following parameters are calculated through this:

- ***Vertical integrated rim area (volume)***: Estimate of the total volume of RNFL tissue in the rim calculated by multiplying the average of the individual rim areas to the disc circumference.
- ***Horizontal integrated rim width (area)***: Estimate of the total rim area calculated by multiplying the average of the individual nerve widths to the disc circumference.
- ***Disc area***: The area bounded by the red outline of the disc.
- ***Cup area***: The area bounded by the green outline of the cup.
- ***Rim area***: Disc area minus cup area.
- ***Cup/disc area ratio.***
- ***Cup/disc horizontal ratio.***
- ***Cup/disc vertical ratio.***

4.2.1.2.7 Posterior Pole Analysis

SDOCT has enabled the measurement of the ganglion cell complex (GCC) comprising of NFL, ganglion cell layer, and inner plexiform layer, loss of which signifies glaucoma. It has been shown that the loss of ganglion cells precedes the visual pathway lesions and RNFL thinning [21]. Another advantage of the GCC thickness analysis is the macula's inclusion of the 50% of the ganglion cells in the retina. 12 vertical lines and 1 horizontal line with a length of 7 mm are scanned in this protocol. The point of focus is 1 mm temporal to fovea, and each line is 0.5 mm width apart so that maximum number of ganglion cells is included.

The GCC scan data is displayed as a thickness map. The ***thickness map*** is colour coded where the thicker areas are represented with hotter colours (yellow, orange) and thinner areas with cooler colours (blue, green) (Fig. 4.18). The GCC map for a normal eye shows a bright circular band around the macula representing a healthy GCC. The centre of the macula has no GCs and hence is thinner and appears black.

The ***deviation or superpixel map*** shows the % loss from normal as determined by the normative database and the hotter colour indicates more abnormality. Lower part of print out in Fig. 4.18 shows superior–inferior average GCC thickness and asymmetry. Focal loss volume (FLV) is the most sensitive parameter for glaucoma and gives a numerical value to the loss of GCC in terms of volume and is expressed as a percentage [22].

Progression software in OCT allows to understand the trend of RNFL loss and also demonstrates the change over a period of time in different parameters (Fig. 4.19). This helps in quantification of anatomical progression in a given patient and helps the clinician to intervene early.

4.2.2 Scanning Laser Polarimetry

SLP is a technique developed on the principle of birefringence, which is an optical property of a structure that changes the polarization of light passing through it. This phase shift is known as retardation and is a quantifiable property which is correspondent to the thickness of the RNFL [23]. The SLP developed commercially is glaucoma diagnostics or GDx (Carl Zeiss Meditec.) measures this retardation per pixel and is displayed as a map of the scanned area. It uses a corneal compensator to account for the variability in the bire-

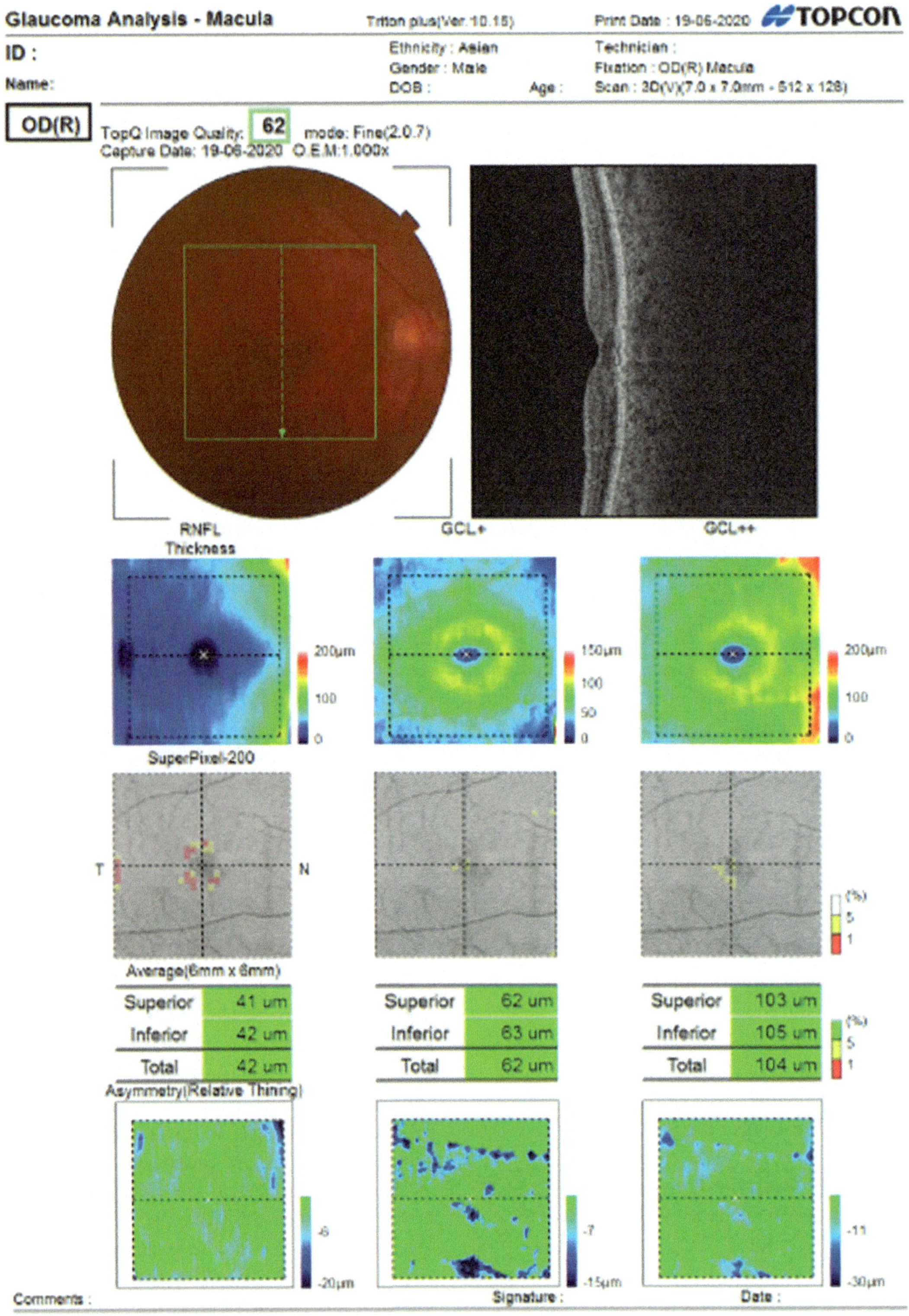

Fig. 4.18 Ganglion cell complex (GCC) analysis showing thickness map, deviation map, and sectoral deviation

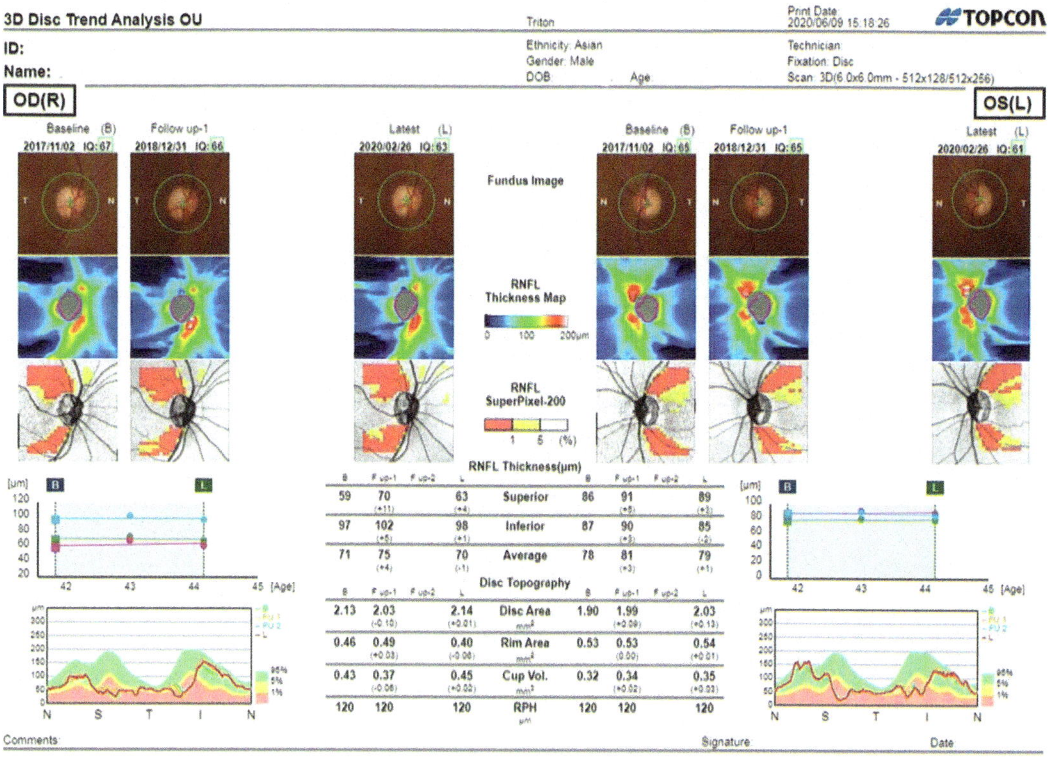

Fig. 4.19 Progression report deviation map, average RNFL thickness changes and their profiles over a period of time

fringence of the cornea to avoid erroneous retardation maps.

4.2.2.1 Standard GDx VCC (Variable Corneal Compensation) Printout

It consists of ONH and peripapillary images which are divided into three parts: the fundus image, RNFL map, and deviation map (Fig. 4.20). The quality of this image determines the focus, centration of scan, and even illumination. The RNFL map is acquired as an image centred at the optic nerve, giving thickness analysis of the surrounding 20 degrees. This analysis is represented as a colour code with the thicker RNFL in the inferior and superior regions shown as bright red and yellow, while the relatively thinner regions in nasal and temporal areas are represented as blue. The third part of the report, deviation map, relays information if the RNFL thickness points are within statistical limits of normality. If not, then the deviations are flagged. If the RNFL has any variation, it is reported as less than 5%, 2%, 1%, or 0.5% chance of being normal.

A similar colour coding is used to indicate if the various thickness parameters like TSNIT average, inferior average, superior average are within statistical limits of normality or not. Nerve fibre indicator (NFI) classifier is a part of the GDx-Pro that ranges 0–100, with a higher number being suggestive of damage and is the best GDx parameter at differentiating ocular healthy and glaucoma eyes [24]. NFI value of less than 30 has a low likelihood of glaucoma, between 30 and 50 is suspect and greater than 50 has a high likelihood of glaucoma. GDx also provides a trend and event analyses known as glaucoma progression analysis (GPA) which documents any statistically significant change in different parameters over the course of the disease.

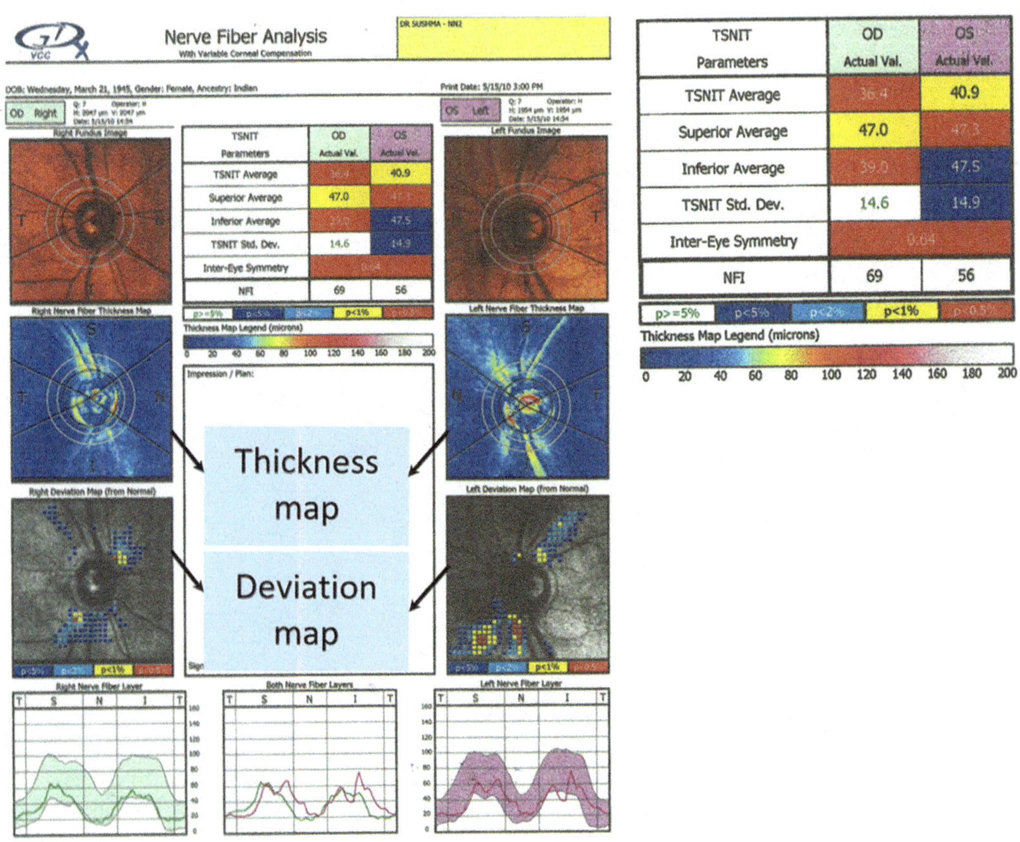

Fig. 4.20 GDx standard printout

4.2.3 Heidelberg Retina Tomography (HRT)

Confocal scanning laser ophthalmoscope (CSLO) technology utilizes diode laser to perform rapid scans of the retina at different heights for commercially available HRT. Using spot illumination principle, it captures confocal slices at x and y axis in multiple z axis planes within 2 seconds and then creates a three-dimensional picture of retinal height between the retinal surface and lamina cribrosa, which may range from 0.5 to 4 mm.

4.2.3.1 Standard HRT Printout

The HRT II and III provide comprehensive software for stereometric analysis of the different images. It measures the optic disc parameters by manually placing a contour line centred at the ONH. The reference plane is placed 50 microns posterior to the mean retinal height along a 5° arc at the temporal sector. It gives in detailed information about the cup, neuroretinal rim, and RNFL and also provides comparison of the two eyes.

The cupping is represented by the linear CDR and cup shape measure, the NRR by rim area and rim volume, and the RNFL by height variation contour and mean RNFL thickness. These parameters are classified as within normal limits (green check), borderline (yellow exclamation), and outside normal limits (red check) (Fig. 4.21a).

In addition to descriptive stereometric measurements, the results from the Moorfields regression analysis (MRA) classification technique also

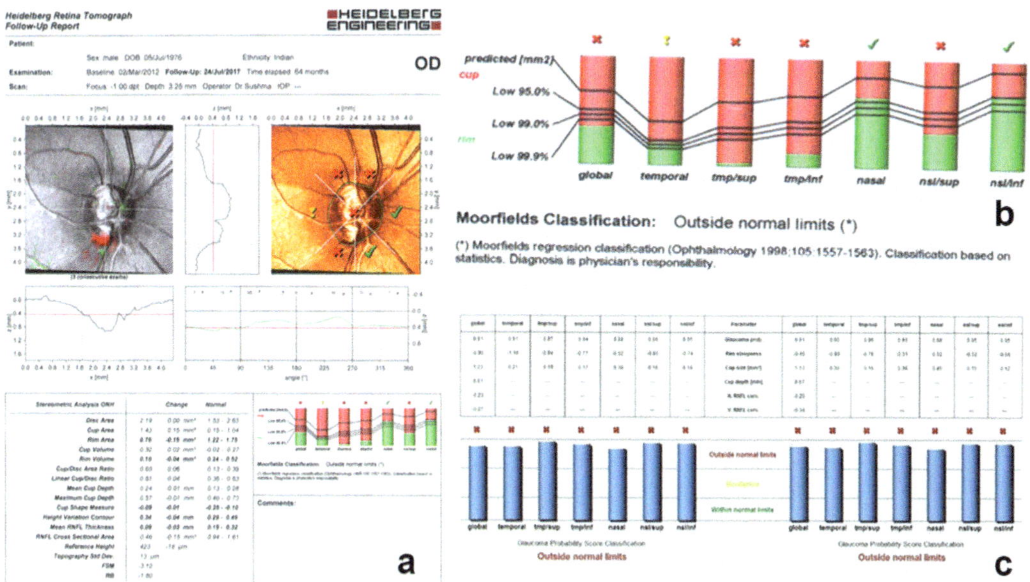

Fig. 4.21 (**a**) Standard HRT report with Moorfields regression analysis and glaucoma probability score, (**b**) Moorfields regression analysis, and (**c**) glaucoma probability score

are provided on the 'OU Report' (Fig. 4.21b). The MRA compares global and local rim area measurements (reference plane dependent) to a normative database and is based on the concept of positive correlation between rim area and disc size. It has been proven to be significant predictor of progression to glaucoma in previous ocular hypertensive eyes [25].

The latest HRT III, however, gives the analysis without the need of operator-based contour delineation. The Glaucoma Probability Score (GPS) uses a geometric model to describe the shape of the optic disc (globally and locally) based on the cup size, cup depth, rim steepness, horizontal and vertical RNFL curvature (Fig. 4.21c).

A relevance vector machine classifier interprets this information and reports the results in terms of probability of the eye being glaucomatous.

Progression software shows the trend analysis with a change in parameters over time and is called topographic change analysis or TCA (Fig. 4.22).

> Sophisticated data points and colourful printouts provided by imaging techniques should not bias our clinical judgement. The decisions for glaucoma management should be taken on the basis of clinical evaluation supported by investigative techniques and not vice versa.

Imaging techniques have revolutionized the glaucoma management in the past two decades; however, it is important to understand strengths and limitations (Table 4.2) of these techniques.

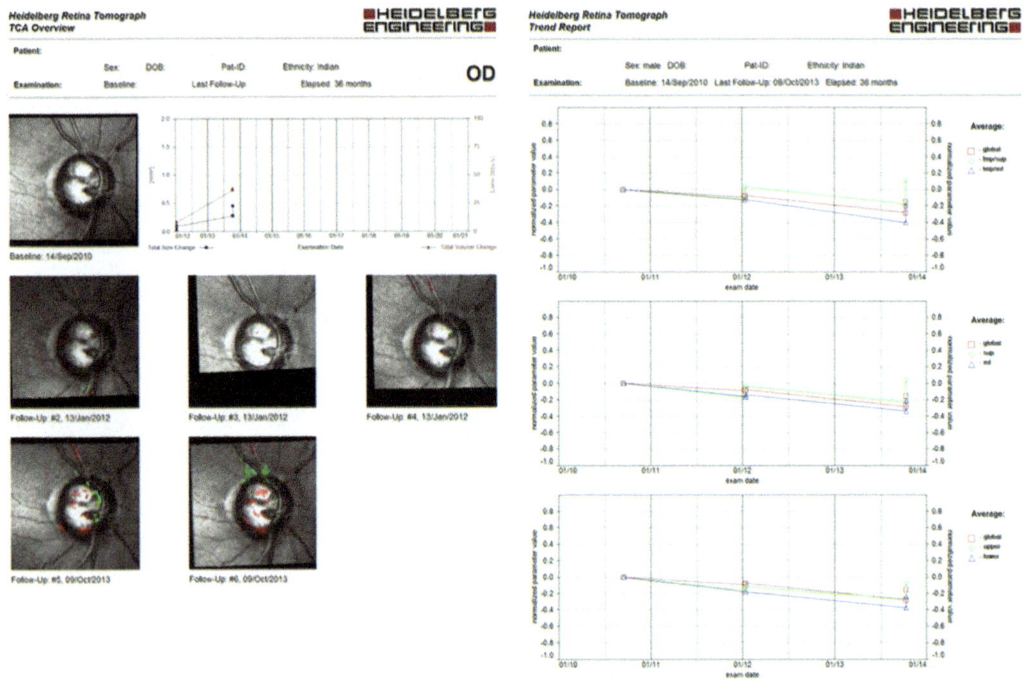

Fig. 4.22 Topographic change analysis with trend report for HRT III

Table 4.2 Limitations and strengths of imaging techniques for glaucoma: OCT, HRT, and GDx

	Strengths	Limitations
OCT	• High sensitivity and specificity for detecting structural damage • Can detect pre-perimetric glaucoma • Can analyse ONH, macula, and RNFL along with statistical comparisons. • Patient friendly reporting.	• Limited normative database • Limited capability of detecting longitudinal progression • Measurements are affected by myopia and axial length changes
GDx	• Simple and rapid imaging technique • Does not require pupil dilation	• Eyes with large peripapillary atrophy cannot be imaged reliably • Corneal surgery may affect corneal compensation • Macular pathologies may hamper evaluation as GDx relies on intact Henle's layer
HRT III	• Real-time quality control during image acquisition • Sophisticated analysis software for glaucoma detection and progression • Large race-specific normative database	• Measurements rely on a reference plane based on the placement of a user-defined contour line • Stereometric analysis can be influenced by moderate changes in IOP

References

1. Weinreb RN, Crowston JG, editors. Glaucoma surgery: open angle glaucoma. World glaucoma association consensus series - 2. Amsterdam: Kugler publications; 2005.
2. Anderson RL, de Los Angeles Ramos Cadena M, Schuman JS. Glaucoma diagnosis: from the artisanal to the defined. Ophthalmol Glaucoma. 2018;1(1):3–14.
3. Hogan B, Trew C, Annoh R, et al. Positive predictive value of optic disc haemorrhages for open angle glaucoma [published online ahead of print, 2019 Nov

26]. Eye (London). 2019; https://doi.org/10.1038/s41433-019-0711-9.
4. Jonas JB, Dichtl A. Advances in the assessment of optic disc changes in early glaucoma. Curr Op Ophthalmol. 1995;6(2):61–6.
5. Jonas JB, Budde WM, Panda-Jonas S. Ophthalmoscopic evaluation of the optic nerve head. Surv Ophthalmol. 1999;43(4):293–320.
6. Lee JE, Sung KR, Lee JY, Park JM. Implications of optic disc tilt in the progression of primary open-angle glaucoma. Invest Ophthalmol Vis Sci. 2015;56(11):6925–31.
7. Jonas JB, Kling F, Gründler AE. Optic disc shape, corneal astigmatism, and amblyopia. Ophthalmology. 1997;104(11):1934–7.
8. Jonas JB, Gusek GC, Naumann GO. Optic disc, cup and neuroretinal rim size, configuration and correlations in normal eyes. Invest Ophthalmol Vis Sci. 1988;29(7):1151–8.
9. Arvind H, George R, Raju P, Ramesh SV, Mani B, Kannan P, Vijaya L. Neural rim characteristics of healthy south Indians: the Chennai glaucoma study. Invest Ophthalmol Vis Sci. 2008;49(8):3457–64.
10. Hitchings RA. The optic disc in glaucoma, III: diffuse optic disc pallor with raised intraocular pressure. Brit J Ophthalmol. 1978;62(10):670–5.
11. Sanfilippo PG, Cardini A, Hewitt AW, Crowston JG, Mackey DA. Optic disc morphology—rethinking shape. Prog Retin Eye Res. 2009;28(4):227–48.
12. Budenz DL, et al. Detection and prognostic significance of optic disc hemorrhages during the ocular hypertension treatment study. Ophthalmology. 2006;113:21372143.
13. Geijssen HC, Greve EL. Disc haemorrhages and peripapillary atrophy. Invest Ophthalmol Vis Sci. 1999;32:1017.
14. Greaney MJ, Hoffman DC, Garway-Heath DF, Nakla M, Coleman AL, Caprioli J. Comparison of optic nerve imaging methods to distinguish normal eyes from those with glaucoma. Invest Ophthalmol Vis Sci. 2002;43(1):140–5.
15. Huang D, Swanson EA, Lin CP, Schuman JS, Stinson WG, Chang W, et al. Optical coherence tomography. Science. 1991;254(5035):1178–81.
16. Hwang YH, Kim YY, Kim HK, Sohn YH. Ability of cirrus high-definition spectral-domain optical coherence tomography clock-hour, deviation, and thickness maps in detecting photographic retinal nerve fiber layer abnormalities. Ophthalmology. 2013;120(7):1380–7.
17. Jeoung JW, Kim TW, Weinreb RN, Kim SH, Park KH, Kim DM. Diagnostic ability of spectral-domain versus time-domain optical coherence tomography in preperimetric glaucoma. J Glaucoma. 2014;23(5):299–306.
18. Sung KR, Kim JS, Wollstein G, Folio L, Kook MS, Schuman JS, et al. Imaging of the retinal nerve fibre layer with SDOCT for glaucoma diagnosis. Brit J Ophthalmol. 2011;95(7):909–14.
19. Lee WJ, Oh S, Kim YK, Jeoung JW, Park KH. Comparison of glaucoma-diagnostic ability between wide-field swept-source OCT retinal nerve fiber layer maps and spectral-domain OCT. Eye. 2018;32(9):1483–92.
20. Huang Y, Gangaputra S, Lee KE, Narkar AR, Klein R, Klein BE, et al. Signal quality assessment of retinal optical coherence tomography images. Invest Ophthalmol Vis Sci. 2012;53(4):2133–41.
21. Hood DC, Raza AS, de Moraes CG, Liebmann JM, Ritch R. Glaucomatous damage of the macula. Prog Retinal Eye Res. 2013;32:1–21.
22. Arintawati P, Sone T, Akita T, Tanaka J, Kiuchi Y. The applicability of ganglion cell complex parameters determined from SD-OCT images to detect glaucomatous eyes. J Glaucoma. 2013;22(9):713–8.
23. Xu L, Chen PP, Chen YY, Takahashi Y, Wang L, Mills RP. Quantitative nerve fiber layer measurement using scanning laser polarimetry and modulation parameters in the detection of glaucoma. J Glaucoma. 1998;7(4):270–7.
24. Reus NJ, Lemij HG. Diagnostic accuracy of the GDx VCC for glaucoma. Ophthalmology. 2004;111(10):1860–5.
25. Weinreb RN, Zangwill LM, Jain S, Becerra LM, Dirkes K, Piltz-Seymour JR, et al. Predicting the onset of glaucoma: the confocal scanning laser ophthalmoscopy ancillary study to the ocular hypertension treatment study. Ophthalmology. 2010;117(9):1674–83.

How to Reduce Error in Optic Nerve Head Examination

5

Craig Ross, George Kong, Keith R. Martin, and Michael A. Coote

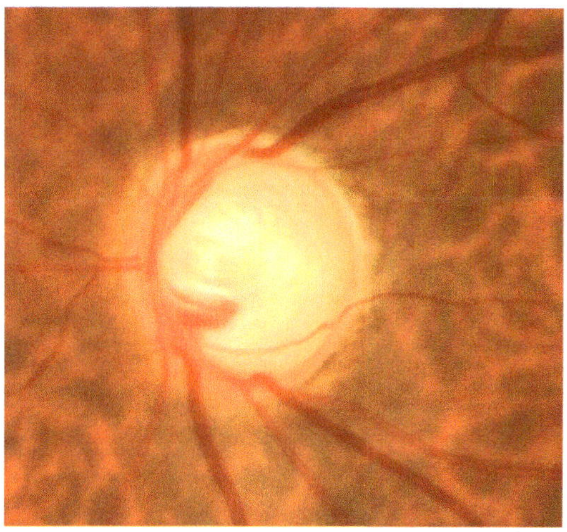

This is the end. How did we get here?

C. Ross
Centre for Eye Research Australia, East Melbourne, VIC, Australia

G. Kong
Centre for Eye Research Australia, East Melbourne, VIC, Australia

University of Melbourne, Parkville, VIC, Australia

Royal Victorian Eye and Ear Hospital, Melbourne, East Melbourne, VIC, Australia

K. R. Martin
Director, Centre for Eye Research Australia, University of Melbourne, Melbourne, Australia

M. A. Coote (✉)
Centre for Eye Research Australia, East Melbourne, VIC, Australia

Royal Victorian Eye and Ear Hospital, Melbourne, East Melbourne, VIC, Australia

University of Melbourne and Latrobe University, Melbourne, Australia

S. Pandav et al. (eds.), *The Optic Nerve Head in Health and Disease*, https://doi.org/10.1007/978-981-33-6838-5_5

5.1 Introduction

The skills required to examine the optic nerve head (ONH, or optic disc) for signs of glaucoma are predominantly possessed by ophthalmologists and optometrists. Glaucoma is the leading cause of irreversible blindness worldwide and early diagnosis is key to the prevention of visual loss [1–4] as errors in the performance of this task can lead to glaucoma treatment being delayed. Although the diagnosis of glaucoma often requires more than the ONH examination findings alone, ONH assessment is important for detection of glaucoma, assessment of severity, and monitoring for disease progression [5–15]. Effective examination of the ONH is a skill; one that must be learnt and practised, and which is performed imperfectly by many eyecare practitioners [16–30].

Population prevalence studies have revealed that approximately half of glaucoma is undiagnosed [31–37], a disappointing statistic that cannot be attributed solely to poor access to eyecare services. The Melbourne Visual Impairment Project (VIP) study found that 45% of glaucoma patients who had been seen by an eyecare professional in the preceding 12 months were not diagnosed at those visits [35–37]. The case study below is an example of this missed opportunity.

Case Study

A 62-year-old university professor with −5.00 dioptres of myopia was unhappy with his multifocal spectacles and made multiple attendances to optometrists. His intraocular pressure (IOP) of 22–24 mmHg demonstrated ocular hypertension, however corrected to within normal IOP limits due to his central corneal thickness (CCT) of 590 μm. Optic disc photographs are seen below in Fig. 5.1. Over 2 years and multiple eyecare appointments, this patient's glaucoma was missed.

The diagnosis was finally made after automated perimetry was performed and his symptoms were revealed to be inferior visual field loss, not his multifocals (see Fig. 5.1). This case of delayed diagnosis rests on the disc exam, irrespective of the issue of IOP calibration. The initial eyecare professionals failed to appreciate the loss of superior rims in both discs, although worse in the right. The discs are both medium-large, tilted temporally, with minimal but potentially confusing PPA.

Loss of both inferior fields is a significant handicap to this patient; however, his field loss has since stabilised with treatment.

Intraocular pressure is an unreliable indicator of glaucoma because it is normal in up to half of patients at the time of diagnosis [32–35]. Other patients with elevated IOP may not have glaucoma [12]. Central to the diagnosis of glaucoma is damage to the ONH. There may be tests that can aid in the detection and measurement of the ONH damage, such as perimetry, ocular coherence tomography (OCT), and electroretinography, but these do not replace the central role of clinical examination and evaluation [14, 15, 38–40]. The 'disc exam' should form part of any eye examination, where it may detect previously undiagnosed glaucoma or (less commonly) other diseases that affect the optic nerve.

The diagnosis of glaucoma requires the findings of the ONH examination to be considered in context, but the assessment of the nerve needs to occur in isolation. Objective assessment of the ONH should occur independent of other clinical features: an ONH exam can be normal in the context of elevated IOP, or glaucomatous with low IOP. In this regard we can conceive of the ONH examination as one of the 'controls' we put in place to address the risk of undiagnosed glaucoma. As such it should be thought of as a separate step in the risk management of missing preventable causes of visual loss.

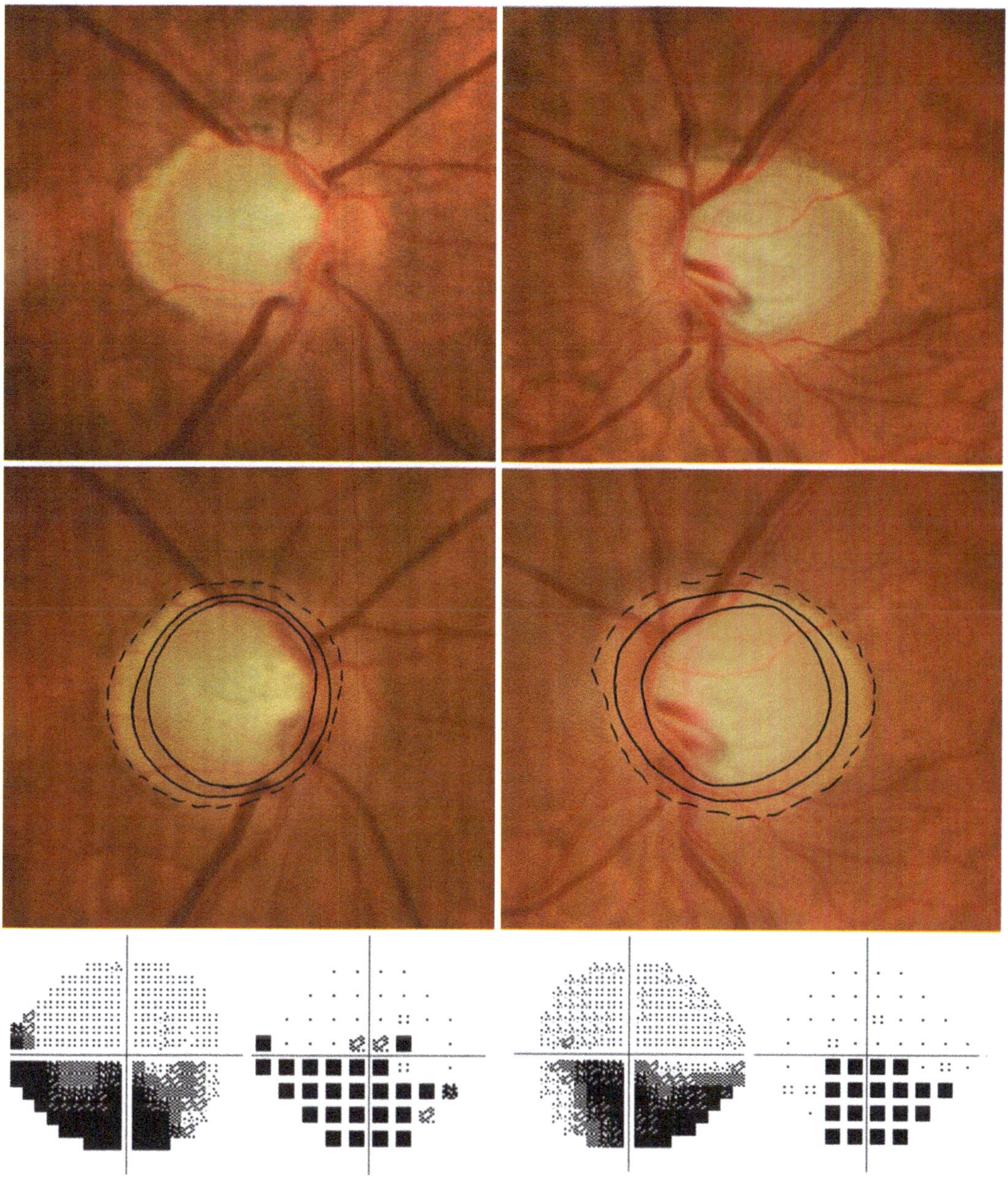

Fig. 5.1 Disc photos (top); annotated disc photos (middle) demonstrating inner and outer margins of neuroretinal rim, NRR (solid line) and PPA (dashed line); perimetry (bottom)

Would you rate this disc differently if you knew the IOP was 14, or if it was 24?

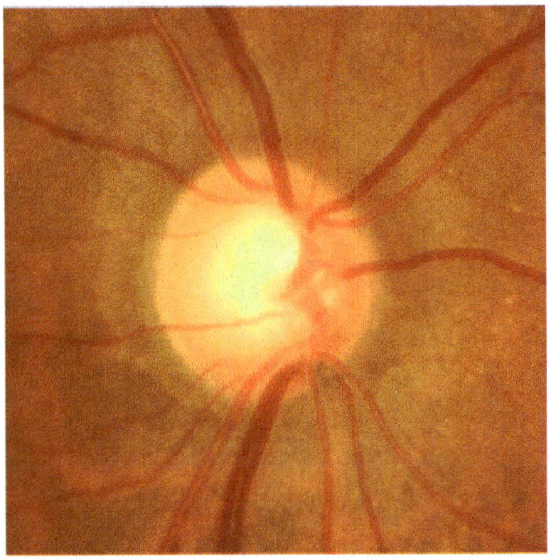

The answer is the same irrespective of the IOP. The disc has a regular shape and orientation with medium canal size, moderate cup depth, intact NRR, and around 0.7 Vertical CDR (cup to disc ratio). There are no disc haemorrhages or retinal nerve fibre layer defects. This nerve is consistent with normality and the IOP is not relevant to that assessment.

Despite the fact that recognisable changes in the ONH may be the only clue to alert the examining eyecare professional, reliable identification of glaucomatous nerve features is not universal—either in a formal testing environment (such as the GONE Project) or in the community [16–19, 37]. This chapter explores the process of examining the disc for glaucoma, where errors may occur, and strategies to avoid them.

5.2 Why Is Disc Examination Difficult?

The ONH in all its measurable dimensions is a hypervariable structure: there is a wide spectrum of 'normality,' much of which overlaps with disease [41–51]. This can make it challenging to identify subtle signs of glaucomatous optic neuropathy (GON). An eye with glaucoma may not have typical or suggestive ONH findings, whereas a healthy eye might have a disc appearance emulating some features of glaucoma [41–51]. A 'glaucoma appearing' ONH can nevertheless go on to develop glaucoma. Progression of glaucoma leads to changes in disc appearance [6–11, 14, 50], although the starting appearance may not be known for sure.

Change over time usually signifies pathology [49, 50], but when longitudinal information is not available variations from normal must be detected, and their likelihood of resulting from change be estimated. In effect, the examiner is trying to imagine the ONH as it would have been had it not suffered loss of structure due to glaucoma—or conversely trying to assess whether the features of the ONH could merely be the result of normal variation.

Progression of glaucomatous disc changes with insufficient treatment

The following cases are examples of progression in disc changes with inadequately treated glaucoma. The first line of photos (untouched image left; then with significant boundaries labelled right) is from before progression occurred, and the second line is after progression. Figures 5.2, 5.3 and 5.4 show progression in early, moderate and advanced disease, respectively.

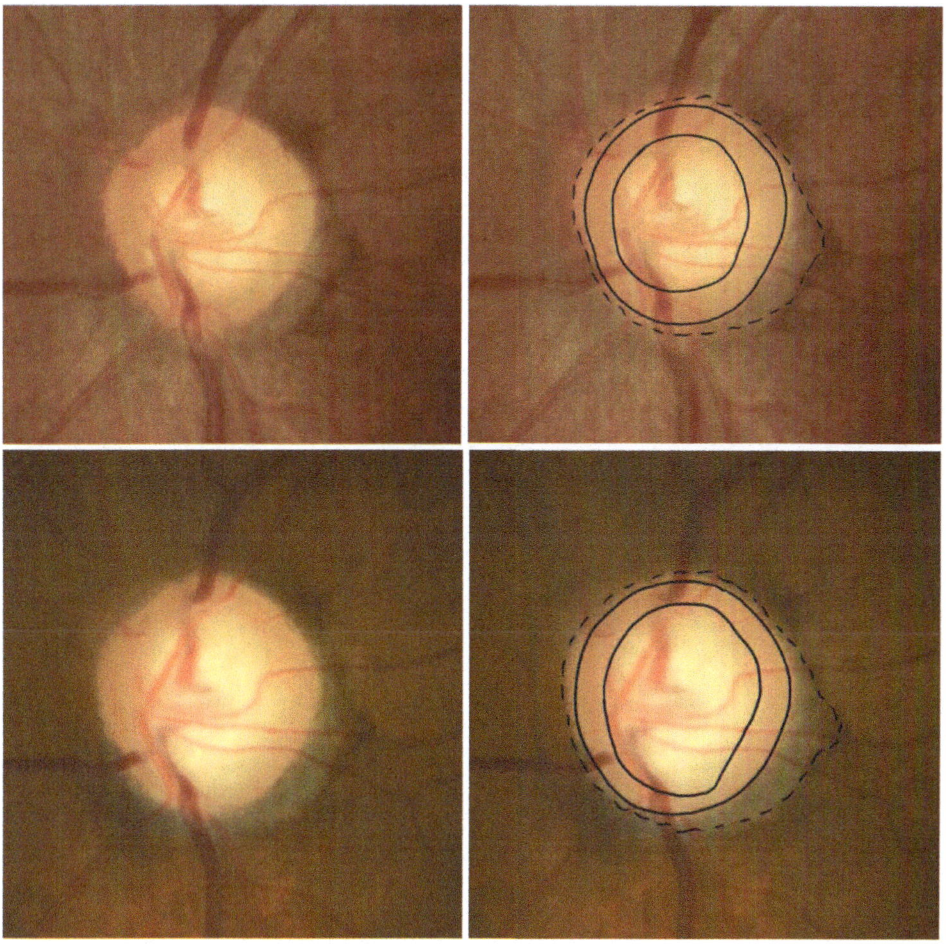

Fig. 5.2 Progression in early disease. A medium to large regular disc with equivocal disc changes of glaucoma, with progression after a prolonged period of steroid-induced high pressure. Disc photographs document an increasing vertical CDR (0.7 to 0.8+) with some early notching superiorly and inferiorly. There is modest increase in the PPA and some increase in the 'nasalisation' of the vessels with loss of the nasal rim

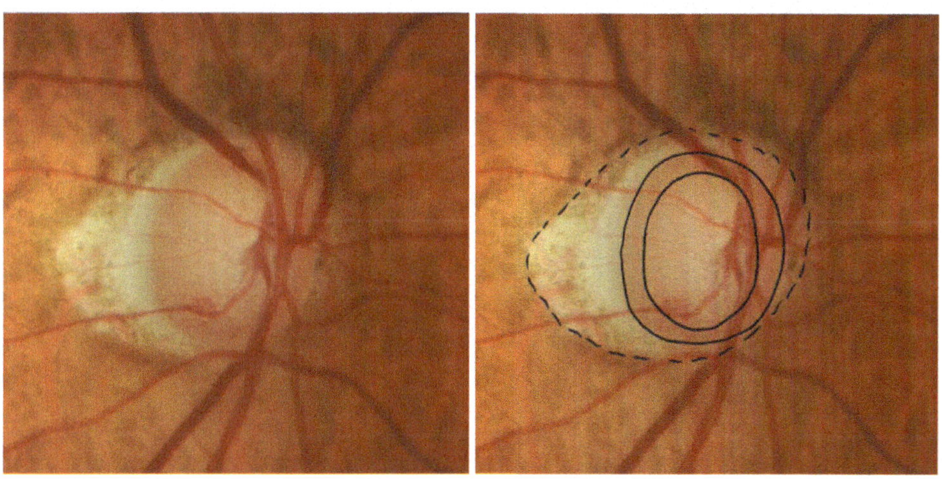

Fig. 5.3 Progression in moderate disease. A medium-sized disc, ovoid vertically with some temporal tilting, worsened as a result of poor compliance and follow-up. The disc has advanced from 0.8 to 0.95 CDR with relatively even expansion of the cup. There is more prominence of the lamina structures and obvious vascular narrowing

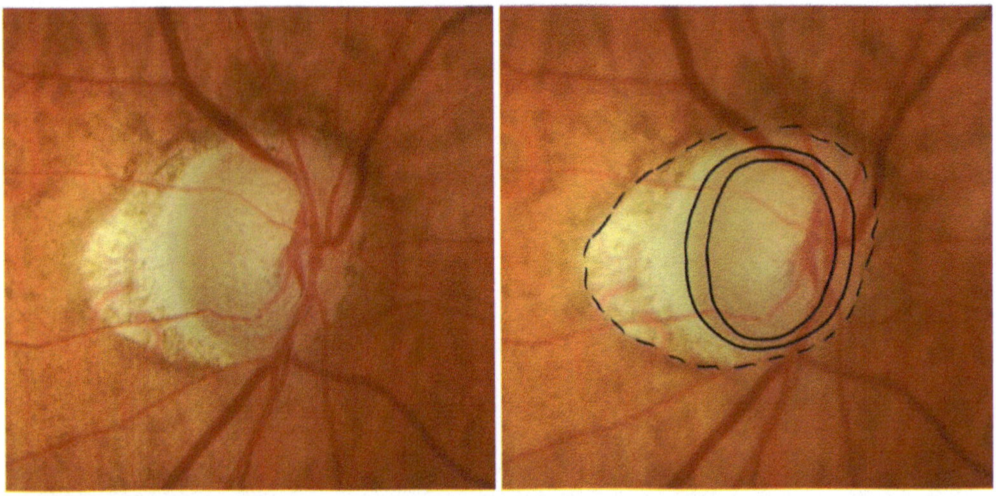

Fig. 5.3 (continued)

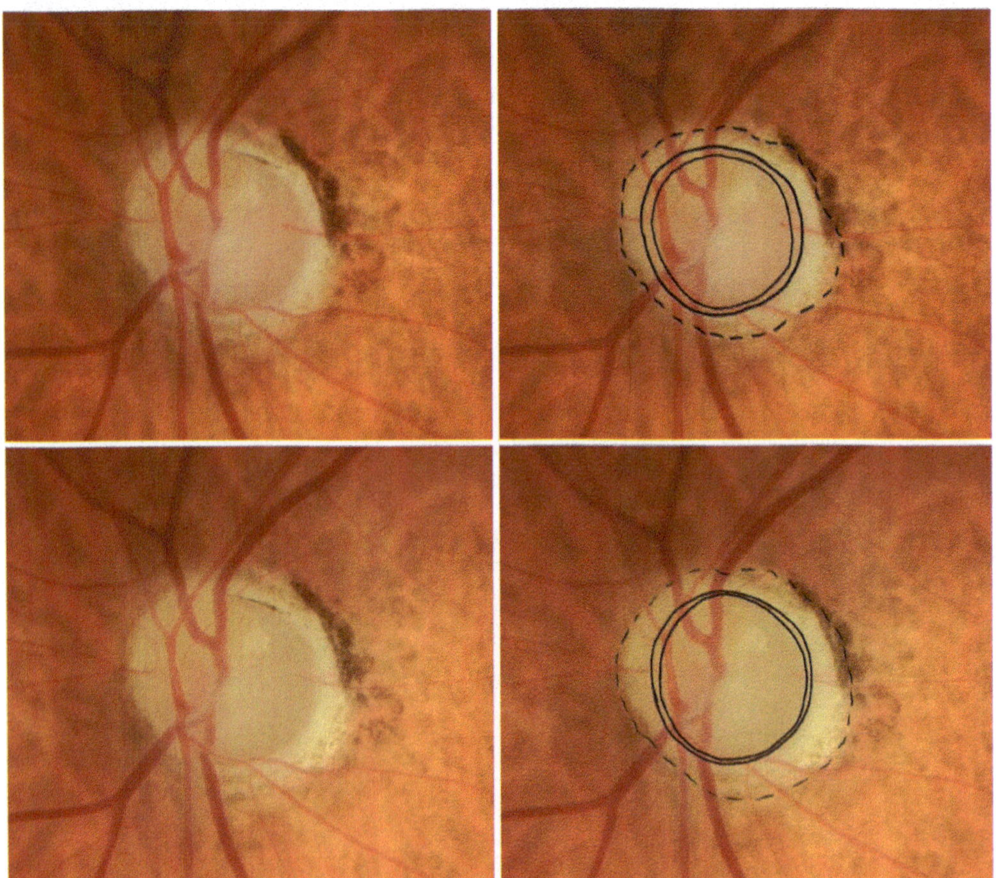

Fig. 5.4 Progression in advanced disease. A medium-sized disc, regular in shape with moderate PPA. Progression occurred because of prolonged overseas travel without monitoring. The disc has advanced from 0.9+ CDR. Although there is discernible increase in CDR, the most prominent feature is arteriolar narrowing and pallor of the nerve head. There is modest increase in the PPA

In essence, glaucomatous ONH examination is the estimation of the neural volume along with any other acquired changes, but in the context of the pre-existing underlying structure. Identifying glaucomatous changes in the regular medium-size disc that are easily visible is (usually) reasonably straightforward. But we know from testing and teaching these skills that where the underlying ONH structure is unexpected and not clearly identified, disc assessment reduces in accuracy [16–19].

In examining the ONH we need to be aware of certain configurations that heighten concern about glaucoma: the tilted nerve, larger diameter nerves with their larger cups, and nerve heads with deeper cups all will appear more like glaucoma. Conversely, there are features that make the discernment of glaucomatous changes difficult, such as small discs, shallow cups and irregular shapes. Indeed, there are structural variations of the nerve—such as extreme tilting, colobomas and highly myopic discs—that make accurate identification of the neural loss very challenging.

To add to this, neuronal loss does not occur at the same pace and in the same pattern in all eyes [49, 50, 52]. There are a number of recognisable patterns of axonal loss at the ONH in glaucoma—some relate to the underlying structure of the nerve (and probably accompanying weaknesses) and some may relate to variations in the pathogenesis of ONH damage in different eyes [41–51]. Historically these differences were interpreted as relating to different mechanisms of disease and glaucoma was, for a time, divided into subgroups based on ONH appearance [53, 54]. Various systems included terms such as 'focal ischaemic' or 'senile sclerotic' discs, or 'concentric cupping'—although these classifications are no longer commonly employed, they remind us of the variation of disease appearance that confronts the examiner looking for evidence of glaucoma. Optic nerve heads which have suffered acute rises in IOP do not tend to develop much 'cupping'—but nonetheless develop axonal loss, loss of visual field and (eventually) pallor [55].

Given the importance and difficulty of this skill, how does an eyecare practitioner learn and perfect it? Perhaps the first step is to acknowledge the difficulties of discerning glaucomatous changes in many discs, as evidenced by the demonstrated failing of eyecare professionals at testing and in identifying disease (undiagnosed glaucoma in spite of eyecare) [16–27, 37].

All skills benefit from a systematic approach to acquisition, but complex ones more so. Examining the ONH accurately is a complex skill. Anders Ericsson coined the term 'directed learning.' Over many years of research in the field of education he propagated the idea that 10,000 hours of practice was required to become truly proficient at a complex skill [56], although he is also sure that skills can be mastered in a much shorter time—but only by better learning techniques. By this Ericsson meant that the more precise the student was in defining the learning objective, the more quickly and effectively they could learn—this is 'directed learning.'

In 2010, we developed an online tool for testing and teaching the skill of optic nerve examination—the GONE Project (found at *www.gone-project.com*) [16]. Eyecare professionals, from glaucoma sub-specialists to optometrists and medical students, have taken the test more than 35,000 times. From this came a wealth of information about how skill-level and level of training affects outcome, as well as what sort of errors were made and whether skill and experience seemed to improve them. Not all experts (glaucoma specialists) got 100% on the test, but they did perform better than trainees and non-glaucoma trained eyecare professionals [16–19]. Training works, but it must be directed and involve feedback. Sometimes this is hard in busy clinics, which is one reason we have kept the GONE Project website open.

But the main aim of this is not to do well on a test; it is that we become competent and effective clinicians. We all should be striving to get better, and as such we should submit ourselves to assessment and relentlessly pursue an understanding of the errors we make in this process.

What follows is a method of ONH examination that has been developed from a deep understanding of the likely errors made by students and clinicians. It is a method aimed at first identifying the structure of the nerve ('the outside') and then the neural elements (in effect 'the inside'). It is not intended to be learned rote, but as an aid to understanding, and to direct learning if there are areas that need improvement. This method was adopted by the World Glaucoma Association (WGA) in 2017 [57].

5.3 The World Glaucoma Association Method of Disc Examination

Disc examination is optimally performed using slit lamp biomicroscopy with pharmacological mydriasis and a fundus lens, where the illumination, magnification, and stereopsis for ONH examination is ideal [57–60]. Examination via an undilated pupil, or with direct or indirect ophthalmoscopy, is possible but at some cost to image detail. Disc photography is widely employed in sub-speciality practice, and experts appear to perform equivalently at disc assessment using monoscopic versus stereoscopic images [61]. Slit lamp examination is still recommended as part of a comprehensive eye exam.

The examination of the ONH is intended to identify the health of the optic nerve end-on as it exits the eye, using the evaluation of the cross-sectional volume as a proxy for axonal mass. The classical features of an ONH with glaucoma are secondary to the loss of ganglion cell axons and their associated astroglia, combined with posterior bowing of the lamina cribrosa [6, 7, 41–45]. This creates the classic 'cupping' with deepening and widening of the cup and hence increase in the cup to disc ratio (CDR) [41–43, 62]. Although this process produces 'classic' or 'typical' glaucoma changes, there are many variations which do not produce such stereotypical appearance—yet are glaucoma nonetheless and will result in loss of vision if not detected and treated [41–51].

The most effective control we can put around the risk of missing glaucomatous changes in the ONH is to approach the examination with the understanding that it is entirely possible to miss important features of glaucoma. This can be either because they are disguised by the underlying structure or because they are variations on the 'classic.' Learning to approach the ONH examination with a systematic approach based upon known errors from the GONE Project should reduce the risk that you will make the same errors and allow you to learn from others [16–19, 63, 64].

The WGA method proposes three stages to ONH assessment [57], followed by synthesis of findings:

1. Determine the outside margins of the neuroretinal rim (the Scleral Canal);
2. Determine the inside margins of the neuroretinal rim (the 'Cup'); then
3. Look for confirmatory findings (disc haemorrhages and loss of Retinal Nerve Fibre Layer).

5.3.1 'Outside' Features

There are four features of the external scleral canal (or scleral ring) to identify (Fig. 5.5). Begin by looking for any peripapillary atrophy (PPA). PPA can blend seamlessly into retinal pigment epithelial changes, or be clearly demarcated. The inner limit of PPA along the scleral rim can be treacherous in disguising the disc and **neuroretinal rim** (NRR) margins. β-zone PPA is associated with glaucoma and increasing PPA over time can indicate disease progression [65–67].

Identify the margins of the scleral ring, which will reveal the **disc size**. The optics of the eye and the fundus lens may influence the apparent disc size to an inexperienced observer; a combination

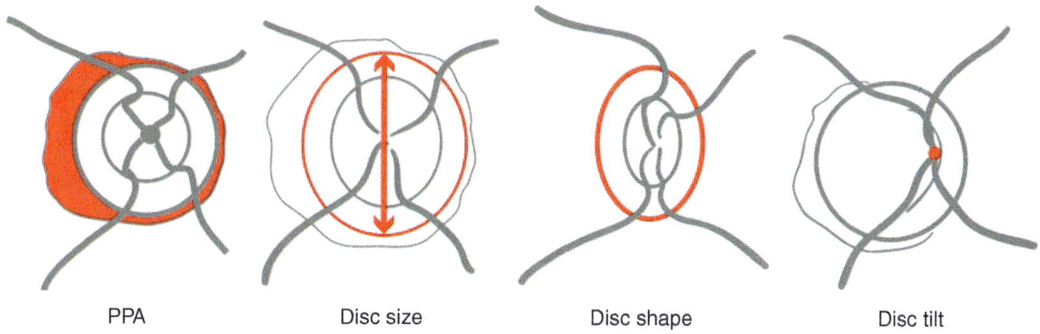

Fig. 5.5 Four 'outside' features of the disc [57]

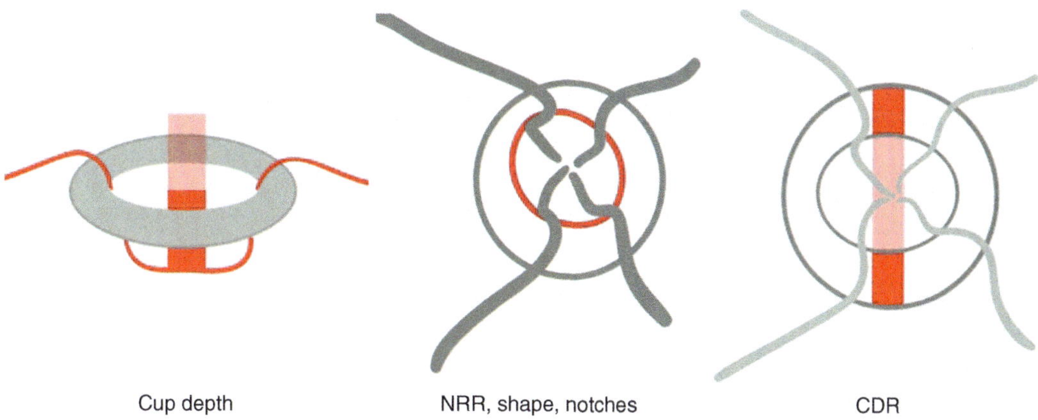

Fig. 5.6 'Inside' features of the disc [57]

of experience and consistency in equipment and technique will assist here. There is a large natural variation in disc size, with correlation to race and very significant refractive error [33, 68–71].

Along with the disc size, the margin of the scleral ring will reveal the **disc shape**. Susceptibility to glaucoma is independent of disc size and shape [44, 68].

It is important to consider the ONH orientation to determine whether any **disc tilt** is present. Tilt can alter the observed perspective of the ONH such that it hides or mimics the appearance of NRR loss. Disc tilt can be associated with visual field defects in the absence of glaucoma [72].

5.3.2 'Inside' Features

There are several features of the internal cup margin to assess (Fig. 5.6). First, assess the **disc colour** and the **depth of the cup**. The depth of the cup is closely correlated to the accuracy of glaucoma diagnosis: in general, deep cups tend to be over-called and shallow cups under-called [18]. In other words, we need to be aware of our biases—a prominent cup can suggest glaucoma, and the absence of a defined cup can suggest the disc is not affected by glaucoma. Cup depth may be influenced by IOP [73, 74]. Inexperienced practitioners show more uncertainty grading cup depth than for other features of the disc [16].

The depth of the cup is an important finding to identify, as noted in Figs. 5.7, 5.8 and 5.9.

Next, assess the contour of the NRR, considering its symmetry, consistency and whether any notches or focal areas of thinning are present. These are typical features of the glaucomatous ONH. The typical disc is vertically oval in shape with a horizontally oval cup, resulting in NRR thickness being greatest inferiorly and superiorly [41–44]. The 'ISNT rule' states that the neuroretinal rim of the average healthy ONH follows a pattern from thickest to thinnest NRR in the order: inferior (I) > superior (S) > nasal (N) and temporal (T) cardinal meridians [75]. ISNT and related rules of thumb are not sensitive or specific enough to guarantee discrimination between the glaucomatous and non-glaucomatous ONH, particularly for tilted or non-vertically ovoid discs [75–77]. For shallow cups, assessment of the NRR may rely on subtle cues related to blood vessel course.

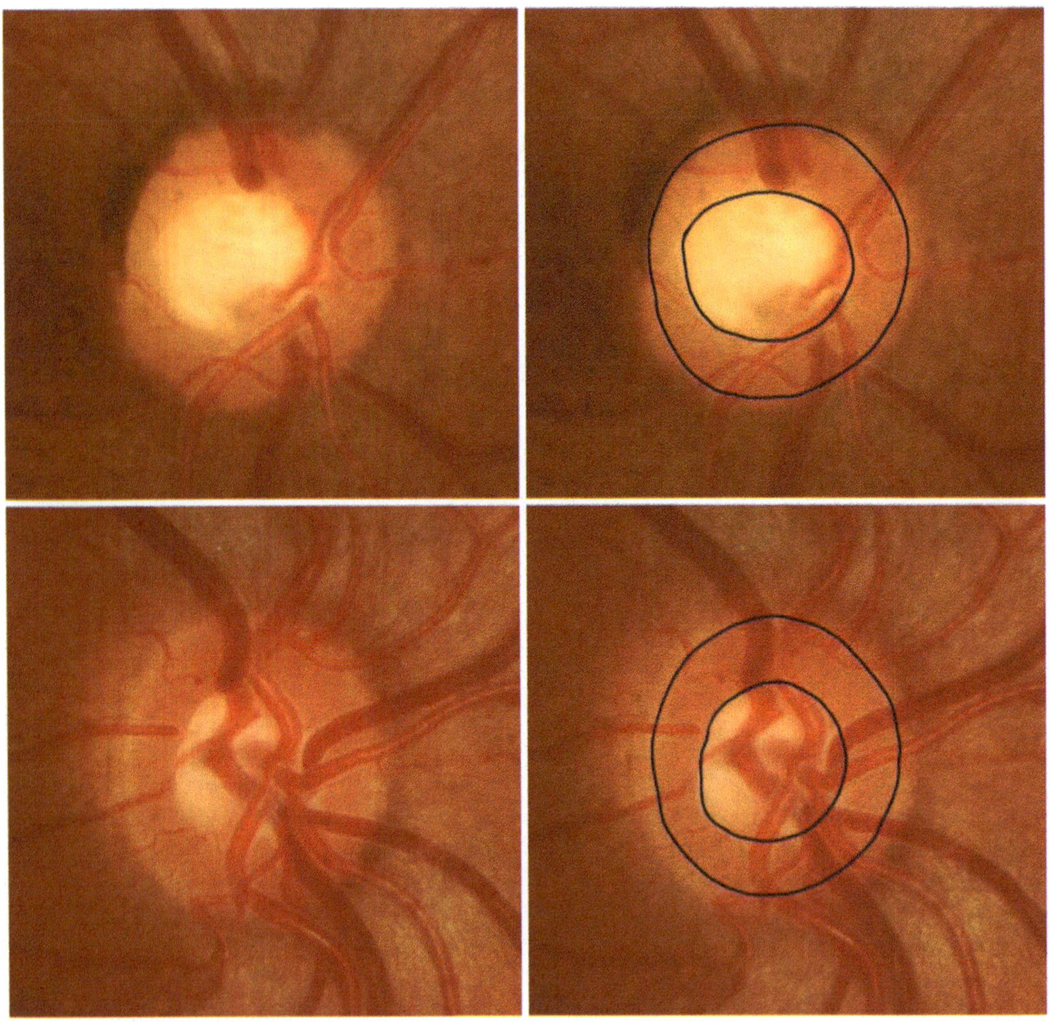

Fig. 5.7 Deep cups: neither of these discs has glaucoma

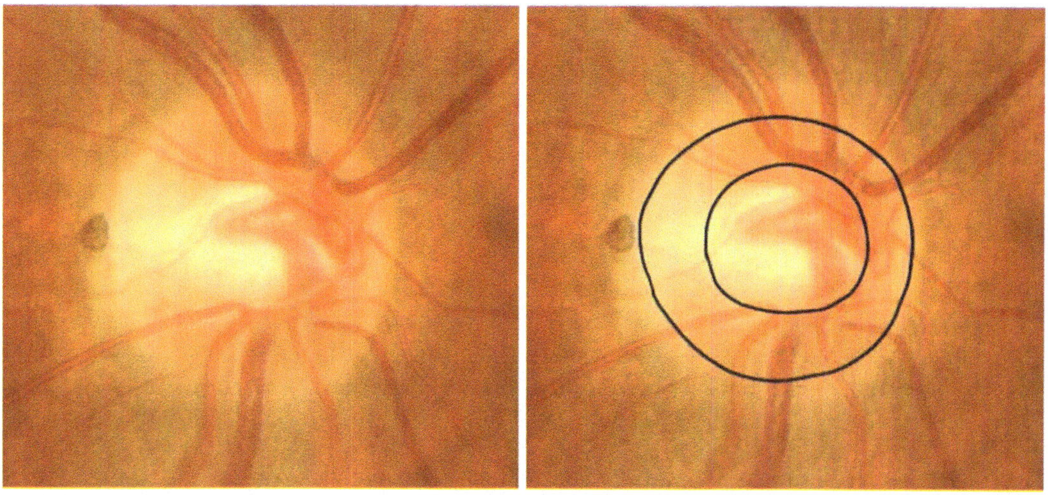

Fig. 5.8 Moderate cup depth

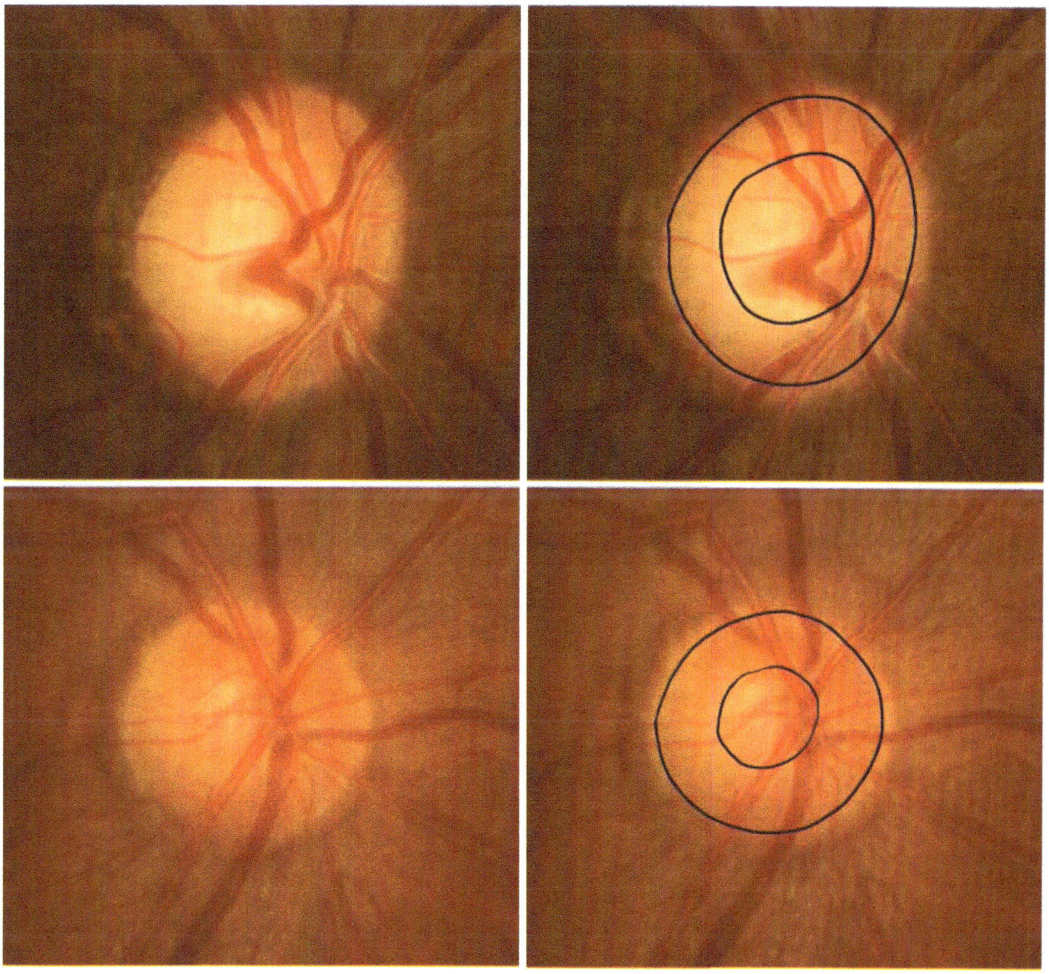

Fig. 5.9 Examples of discs with shallow cups. As the depth of the cup reduces, the definition of the internal rim margin becomes less clear

Consider the external and internal margins of the NRR together to determine the vertical **cup to disc ratio (CDR)**. The CDR is important but is not a reliable measure of NRR loss when considered in isolation; it is highly dependent on disc size [62, 68, 69]. A large disc with a CDR of 0.7 may be normal, however a small disc with the same CDR might have a significantly higher likelihood of glaucoma. The larger disc has more circumferential space for axons to pass through. The compliance of the lamina cribrosa, as influenced by age, can impact the appearance of the ONH, with younger patients demonstrating an exaggerated cup [78]. In spite of all these variations and caveats, experienced observers, when tested, can reliably and accurately estimate the CDR [18, 21, 24].

5.3.3 Additional or Confirmatory Findings

Finally, look for the additional signs of disc haemorrhages or retinal nerve fibre layer (RNFL) loss (Fig. 5.10). Haemorrhage(s) at the disc margin are an important finding and can be overlooked (Fig. 5.11). Disc haemorrhages are related to glaucoma and to progression (and their location with NRR loss) [79–84]. Importantly, they are not pathognomonic, but when associated with other disc features suggest possible worsening or glaucoma [79–84]. Missing a disc haemorrhage may reduce the risk assessment of the eye [18].

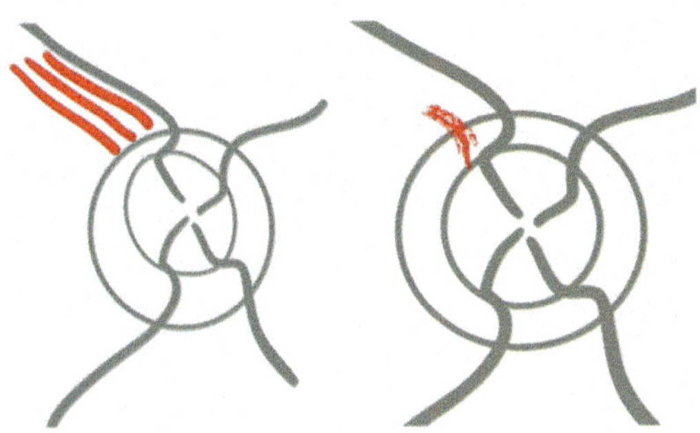

Fig. 5.10 Additional features, RNFL defects and disc haemorrhages [57]

RNFL loss can be challenging for less experienced clinicians to detect, particularly given ageing patients demonstrate a degree of age-related loss [85]. The advent of OCT has greatly assisted clinicians in the quantification of the RNFL and its monitoring over time [15, 28–30]. Although some studies have found imaging algorithms comparable to disc photograph assessment, there remain false positives and negatives and OCT does not replace the role of clinical examination [15, 28–30].

5.3.4 Synthesis

Finally, the clinician should consider all of these findings in making an overall disc assessment based on the systematic examination. It is important to remember that the disc exam forms an independent input into the overall risk estimate for the patient. Carefully consider any asymmetry across the horizontal midline and also between the eyes, although be mindful that many things can cause asymmetry including different size discs, tilt and other pathologies [45, 46, 86, 87].

Eyecare professionals need to look longitudinally at disc changes, and historically this has been greatly facilitated by disc photography. However, shared care is common in glaucoma—between ophthalmologists and optometrists, as well as within hospital glaucoma units. It is therefore imperative that we are not only consistent in our own findings (the intra-observer agreement of our disc assessments), but also that we reliably agree with colleagues (interobserver agreement). In fact, one impetus to the creation of the GONE Project was the observation that cup to disc ratios of some patients would fluctuate over time in clinic notes. Consistent and reliable disc assessment is a key requirement for the detection of ONH changes.

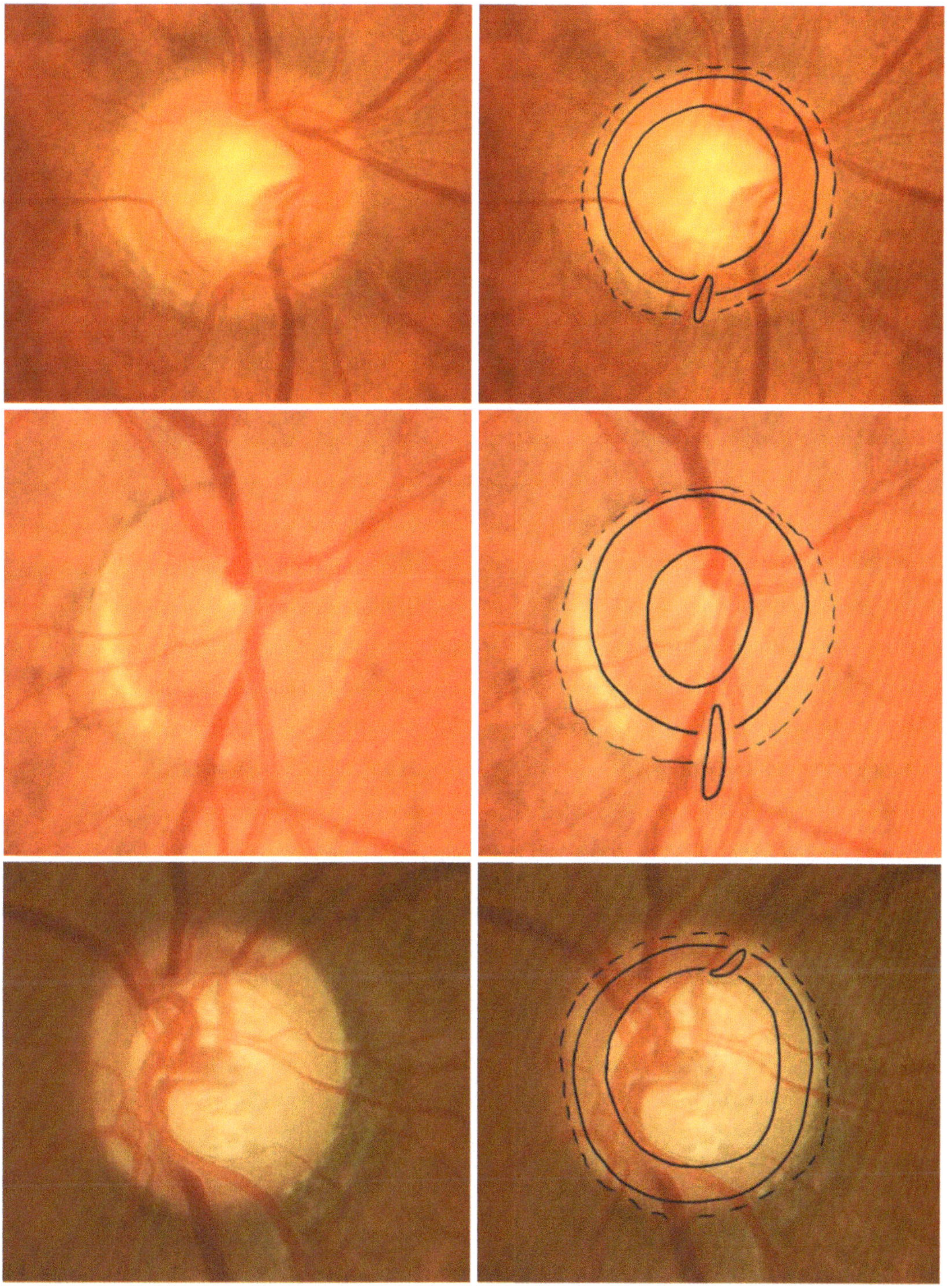

Fig. 5.11 Disc haemorrhages may be easily overlooked

5.4 How Often Are Errors Made?

There is ample evidence that eyecare professionals frequently miss the signs of glaucoma when examining the disc or arrive at an inappropriately high or low likelihood of glaucoma [16–27]. Whilst much focus is directed towards under-diagnosis and under-treatment, over-treatment of glaucoma also has costs to patients and to the healthcare system [88, 89].

Errors made in disc examination can occur at any of the three stages of systematic disc assessment:

1. Missing a sign altogether, for example not identifying a structure of the ONH correctly. These may be called ***errors of not seeing***.
2. After correctly identifying a feature of the ONH, under-estimating or over-estimating the risk conferred by that single feature, for example the diagnostic utility of the presence of a disc haemorrhage. These are ***errors of understanding***.
3. In considering the disc as a whole, an ***error in synthesis*** in calculating the total risk of glaucoma. For example, an error in estimation of NRR loss in a large disc, where disc size influences neural volume.

Table 5.1 ONH features associated with incorrect estimation of glaucoma risk by ophthalmology trainees in the GONE Project

ONH features	Glaucoma risk under-estimated	Glaucoma risk over-estimated
'Outside' disc features	Disc is horizontally ovoid (odds 9.8)	Large discs (odds 2.7)
		Horizontal disc tilt (odds 10.4)
'Inside' disc features	Missed neuroretinal rim loss (odds 4.4)	Cup depth reported to be deeper than it actually is (odds 2.2)
	CDR reported to be smaller than it actually is (odds 2.9)	CDR reported to be larger than it actually is (odds 4.8)
Confirmatory findings	Missed haemorrhage (odds 6.7)	Haemorrhage reported when not present (odds 2.0)
	Missed RNFL loss (odds 11.1)	RNFL loss reported when it was intact (odds 9.0)

*With the odds ratio that trainees would make an error in overall risk assessment—all odds statistically significant to $p \leq 0.05$ [18]

The GONE Project asked participants to grade individual disc features and then to apportion each disc an overall risk estimate for glaucoma [16]. Results showed that ophthalmology trainees and general ophthalmologists under-estimated glaucoma likelihood in more than 20% of discs, and in more than 40% when several individual disc features were incorrectly assessed [18]. When compared to glaucoma specialists, these clinicians were twice as likely to under-estimate the risk than they were to over-estimate it [16]. Inter-observer agreement for both individual disc features and overall glaucoma likelihood was higher among glaucoma specialists, but not unanimous [16]. This is a reminder that disc examination is a challenging skill, but that experience can result in improved consistency of assessment.

Through extensive analysis of the findings of many hundreds of participants in the GONE Project, a number of identifiable ONH features were found to be more likely to be associated with errors in assessment of the ONH overall (see Table 5.1) [18].

From this data it can be seen that accurate assessment of the CDR is important, with incorrect assessment a common cause of both under- and over-estimation of risk [18]. It should be noted that assessment of CDR is a compound skill, requiring the accurate detection of both the 'outside' and 'inside' margins to resolve it. Discs with a CDR of 0.6–0.8 were less consistently assessed by trainees than discs with a CDR under 0.6 or 0.9 and over [18]. This correlation between experience and better interobserver agreement in CDR assessment has also been demonstrated in other studies [21, 24].

The GONE Project also studied, via gaze tracking, the patterns of disc analysis by trainees and glaucoma experts [17]. Whilst trainees did not have ordered patterns of gaze when viewing a disc, experts demonstrated a systematic approach (Fig. 5.12) [17]. Experts spent less time overall

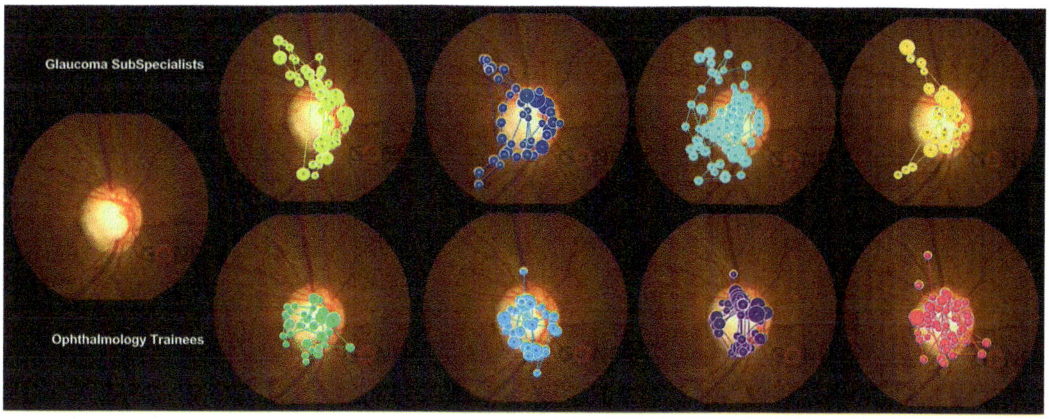

Fig. 5.12 Contrasting gaze patterns of glaucoma subspecialists and ophthalmology trainees in the GONE Project. Experts displayed systematic gaze patterns focusing on the areas with the greatest likelihood of pathology. Trainee viewing behaviour was constricted and lacking a methodical approach (*Reproduced from O'Neill et al. [17])

examining a disc, but more time assessing areas with the greatest likelihood of diagnostic utility: the superior and inferior rim and RNFL [17]. Experts adapted their gaze behaviour to disc morphology, unlike the more scattershot approach of trainees [17].

These insights suggest that eyecare practitioners can aim to reduce error through education about subtle signs at the ONH, awareness of common pitfalls and through learning a systematic technique to disc examination such as the WGA method.

5.5 The Story of a Disc Haemorrhage: How One ONH Reveals Why Errors Are Made

In the GONE Project three images were shown of the same disc. The images were taken 3 months apart and when no change in IOP occurred (Fig. 5.13a). The images show a significant disc haemorrhage (Image 1), a resolving disc haemorrhage (Image 2) and no haemorrhage (Image 3).

Results indicated that experts identified the superior rim thinning whether or not the disc haemorrhage was present. This was not true for less experienced observers, where the presence of the disc haemorrhage appeared to act as a flag drawing attention to the rim loss—which was frequently missed without it. For the image with the resolving haemorrhage (Image 2), observers who detected the haemorrhage also noted the rim thinning, while those who missed the haemorrhage tended to miss the rim loss.

When eye tracking was applied to Image 3 (no haemorrhage), the gaze patterns highlighted why these errors were made by less experienced observers (Fig. 5.13b).

Trainees spent time in un-focused attention with a scattershot gaze pattern, and therefore unsurprisingly often missed the clue of the superior rim loss. Experts focused on relevant areas, noticed the rim loss, directed their attention to the corresponding area inferiorly (to look for rim loss there) and also assessed the RNFL. In other words, the viewing behaviour of expert observers was systematic and therefore less prone to error. Clinicians should learn and practise a careful and methodical approach to ONH examination—such as the WGA method—to reduce the chance of missing key clues to glaucoma.

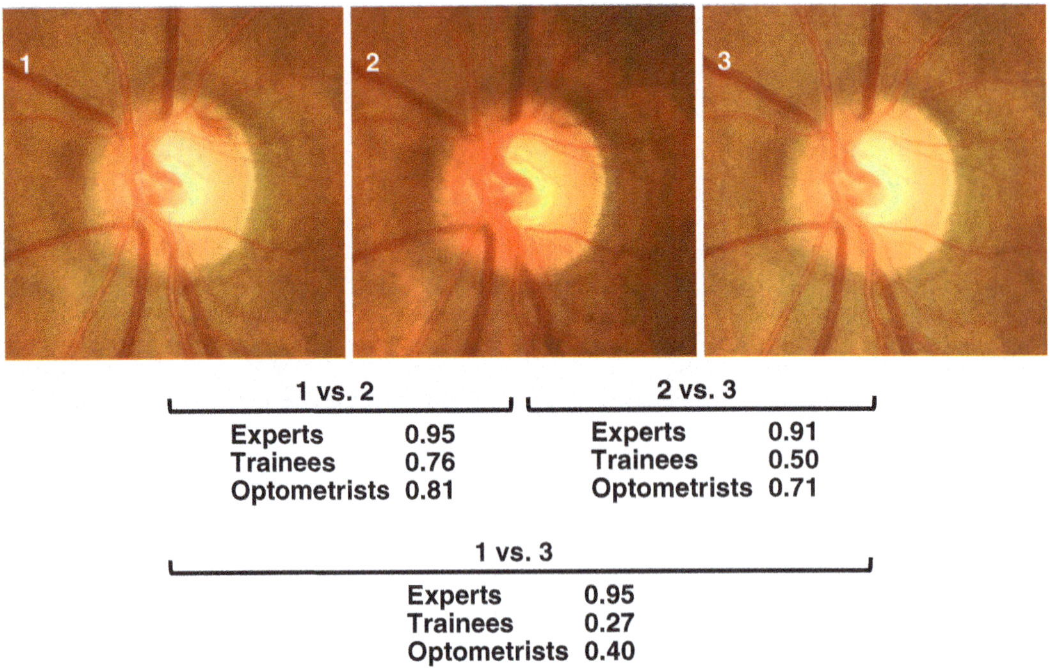

Fig. 5.13 (**a**) An ONH at different points in time. Shown with a disc haemorrhage (Image 1), resolving haemorrhage (Image 2) and no haemorrhage (Image 3). Below, comparison in observer agreement for pairs of images as κ (weighted kappa), where a value of 1 would indicate complete agreement and 0 representing only chance agreement. Note that when experts (Glaucoma Sub-Specialists) are tested, the agreement between the three images is very high (>0.9). But when ophthalmology trainees and optometrists were tested there was poor agreement, particularly between images 1 and 3 (<0.4)

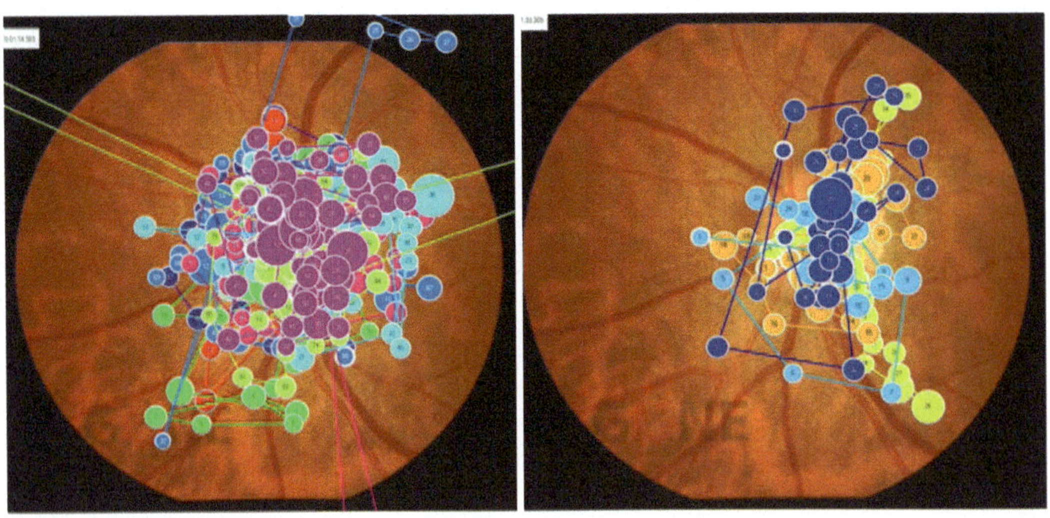

Fig. 5.13 (**b**) Eye tracking of observers presented with Image 3 (without the disc haemorrhage). Trainees (left) compared to experts (right). Different colours represent the gaze patterns of individual observers

5.6 Eight Most Discriminatory Discs from the GONE Project

Clinicians who participated in the GONE Project were asked to provide an overall assessment of the likelihood of each disc being glaucomatous. The following discs represent the greatest difference in assessment between more-experienced and less-experienced observers. Each disc is shown as a plain photograph (left) and with significant boundaries highlighted (right).

5.6.1 Over-Estimation of Glaucoma Risk

With these discs, observers assessed an overly high likelihood of glaucoma. More trained and experienced clinicians tended to perform significantly better on assessment of these images'. These discs were universally larger, with deeper cups (Fig. 5.14a, 5.14b, 5.14c). Note that there are no focal areas of thinning and there is minimal PPA.

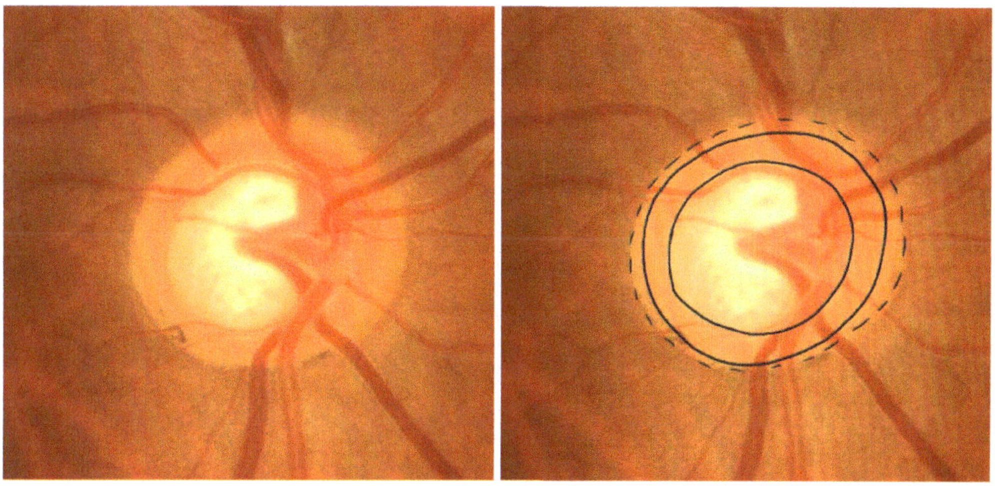

Fig. 5.14 (**a**) This image shows a large, regularly shaped nerve with a clearly demarcated NRR. The circum-linear vessel which demarcates the superior rim has not been bared—this suggests that the vessel and the rim developed together and thus the rim has not retracted. There are no focal defects in the NRR. Larger discs have a larger CDR and can lead to an over-assessment of risk [18]

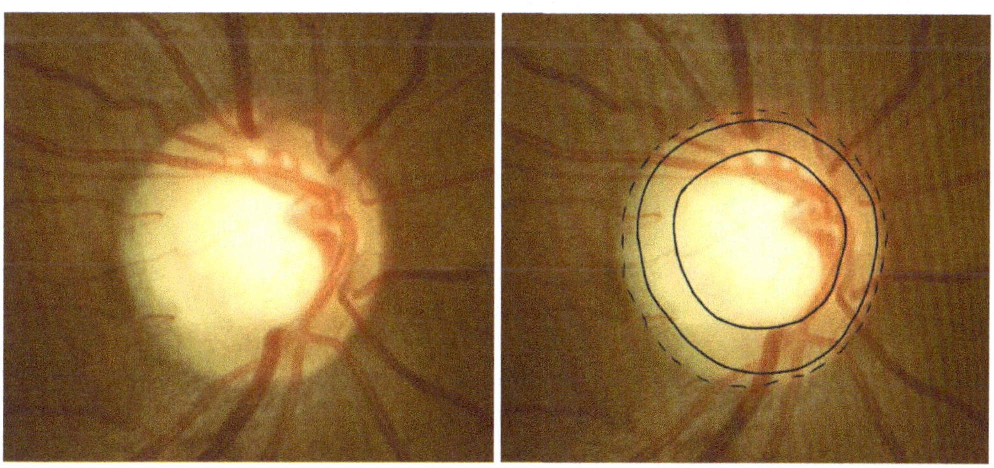

Fig. 5.14 (**b**) This is a large nerve and thus the CDR is approaching 0.8. This should trigger the clinician to have a closer look at this nerve. It is temporally tilted so the temporal margin is not clearly demarcated. There is some asymmetry in the vessel distribution due to some anti-clockwise rotation, but there are no focal areas of loss and the RNFL is intact in all quadrants

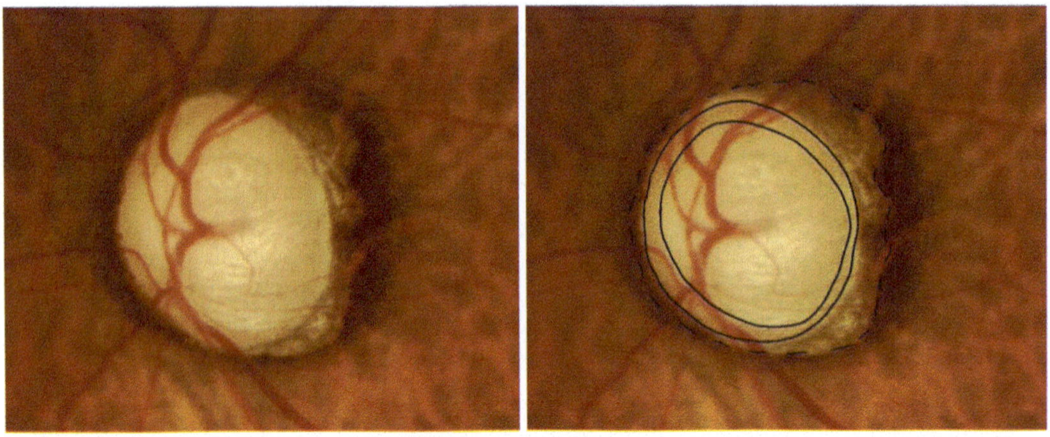

Fig. 5.14 (c) This is a macrodisc in a high myope who also has glaucoma. This disc was thought to be worse than it is, at 0.99 CDR with extensive visual field defects. In fact, there is discernible rim throughout the full extent and there is only mild overall depression and enlargement of the blind spot on perimetry. The assessment of many observers here was incorrect on the severity of glaucomatous changes, not on their presence

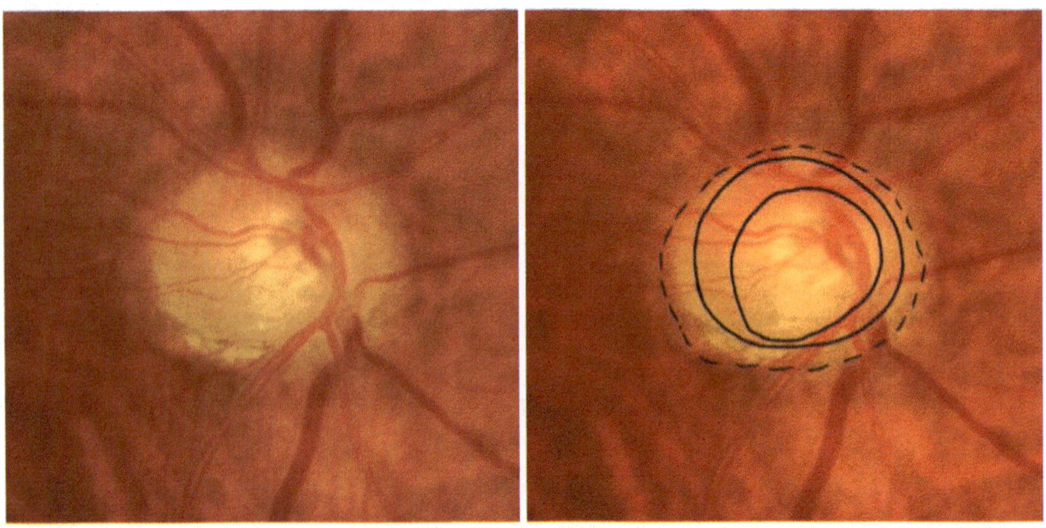

Fig. 5.15 (a) This small-medium disc has an almost full-thickness rim loss inferiorly. There is little PPA and the branch arteriole does not follow the contour of the rim at this point ('overpass cupping'). There is a small amount of temporal tilting which increases the difficulty of recognising the rim margin. Note the small patch of quite marked PPA next to the area of rim loss, which may have helped to disguise the area of loss

5.6.2 Under-Estimation of Glaucoma Risk

For these discs the clinician under-appreciated the signs of glaucoma. There are a variety of underlying reasons for these errors as shown in Figs. 5.15a, 5.15b, 5.15c, 5.15d and 5.15e.

5.7 Difficult Discs

5.7.1 The Tilted Disc

Figure 5.16a shows an optic disc with marked vertical and slightly nasal tilting with subtle peripapillary changes. Figure 5.16b shows a very

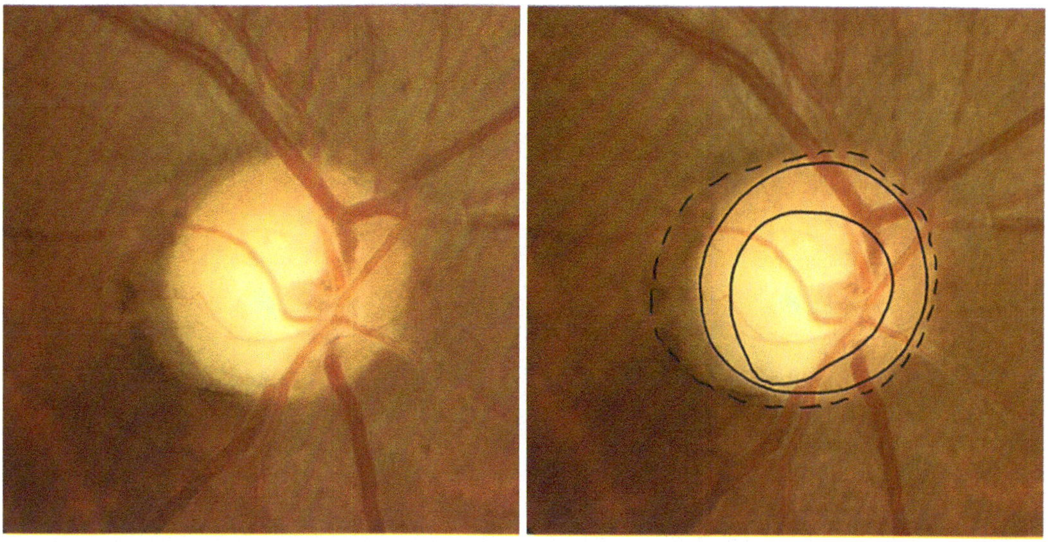

Fig. 5.15 (**b**) This disc is regular in shape and only mildly temporally tilted. Smooth shallow cupping removes one of the triggers to identifying the rim margin ('the inside'). Once again, the inferior arteriole skirts around the margin of the defect and so the contour of this vessel is not revealing. There is a cilioretinal arterial branch at 6 o'clock which serves to distract. There is marked RNFL loss associated with the inferotemporal rim defect

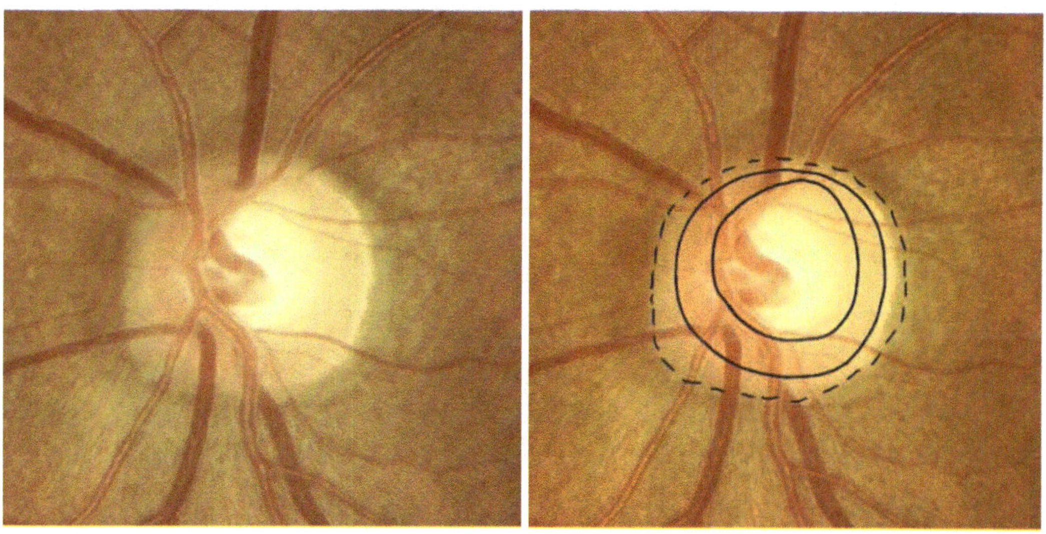

Fig. 5.15 (**c**) This is a regular sized and shaped nerve without any significant tilt. There is a focal superior rim defect in a typical location at 1 o'clock. There is an associated RNFL defect but no focal PPA. The defect was detected by experienced observers but infrequently by less experienced ones

high levels of vertical tilting with exaggerated areas of PPA and partial deficits of the peripapillary sclera. Tilted discs are also addressed in Chap. 7.

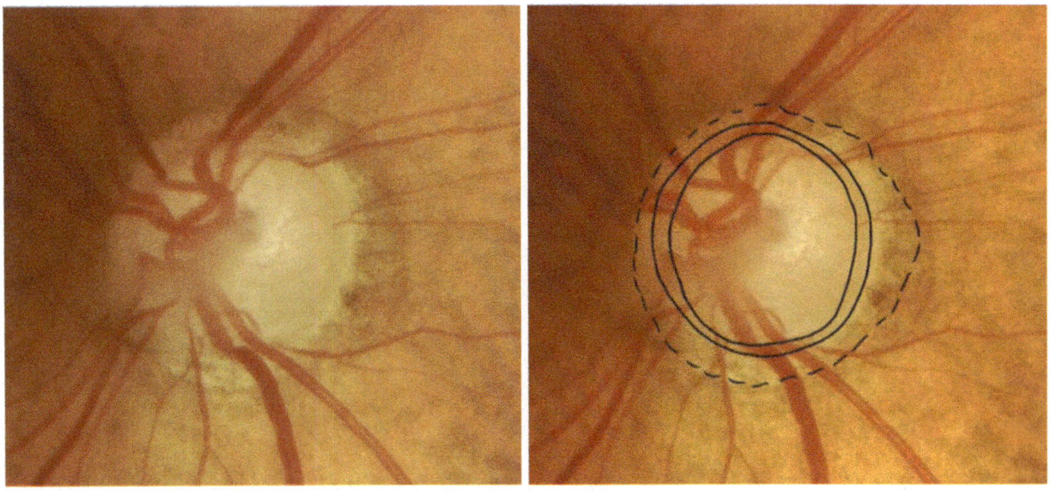

Fig. 5.15 (**d**) This is a normally shaped disc with no significant tilting. It has extensive rim loss in all areas, and extensive visual field loss. There is marked nasal rim loss as well. The presence of a vitreous opacity over the central and nasal part of the image may have distracted. Although less experienced observers agreed that the nerve likely had glaucomatous changes, they frequently underestimated the severity. Experienced observers correctly identified this as advanced glaucoma

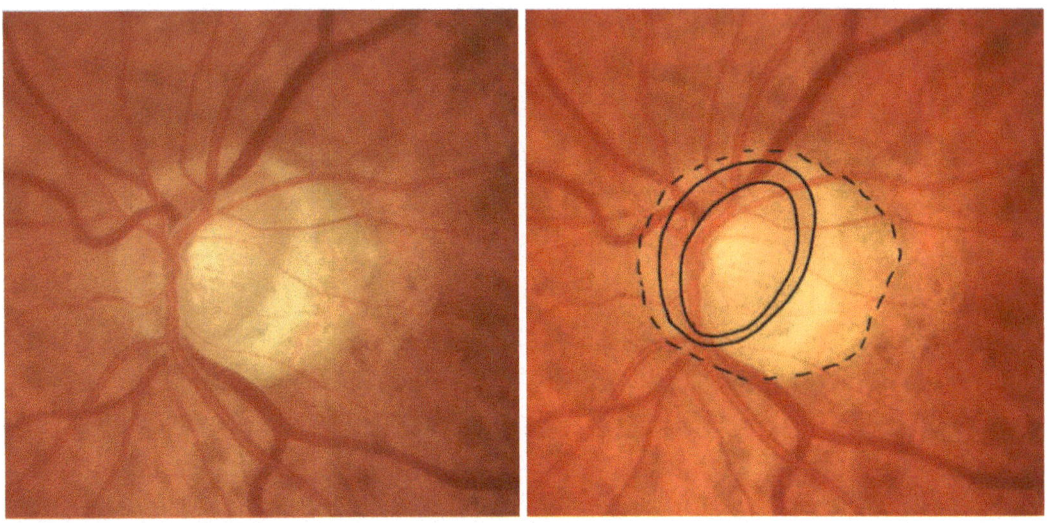

Fig. 5.15 (**e**) This is a smaller nerve, tilted and rotated, and is ovoid vertically. In addition, there is marked PPA (consistent with the tilting) but without accentuation at the area of maximal rim loss (inferiorly). This disc has a shallow cup and the vascular pattern inferiorly does not help to describe the rim margin

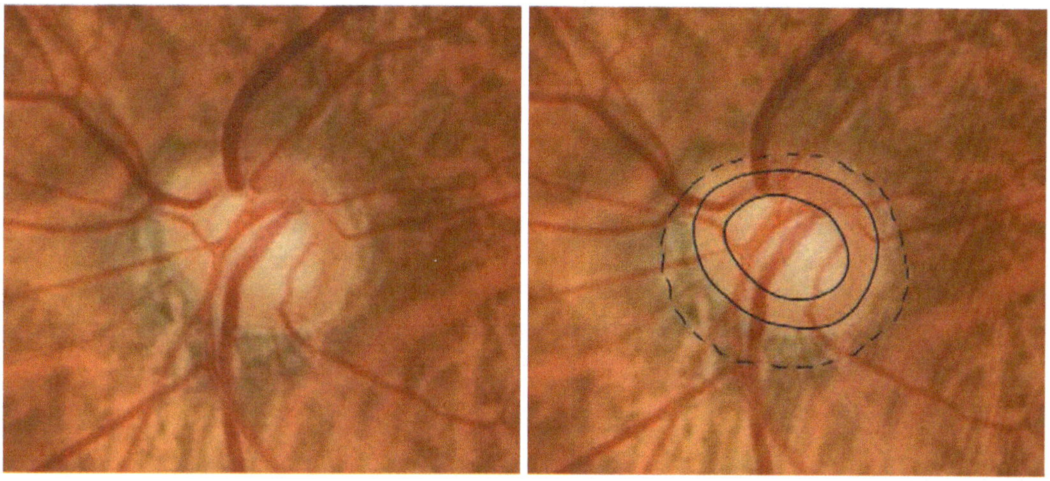

Fig. 5.16 (**a**) This disc features marked vertical and slightly nasal tilting. The rim of the nerve is readily assessable and is normal. This is a little unusual as most discs with this structure have marked inferior PPA. Solid lines mark the NRR and dashed lines show the area of subtle peripapillary changes

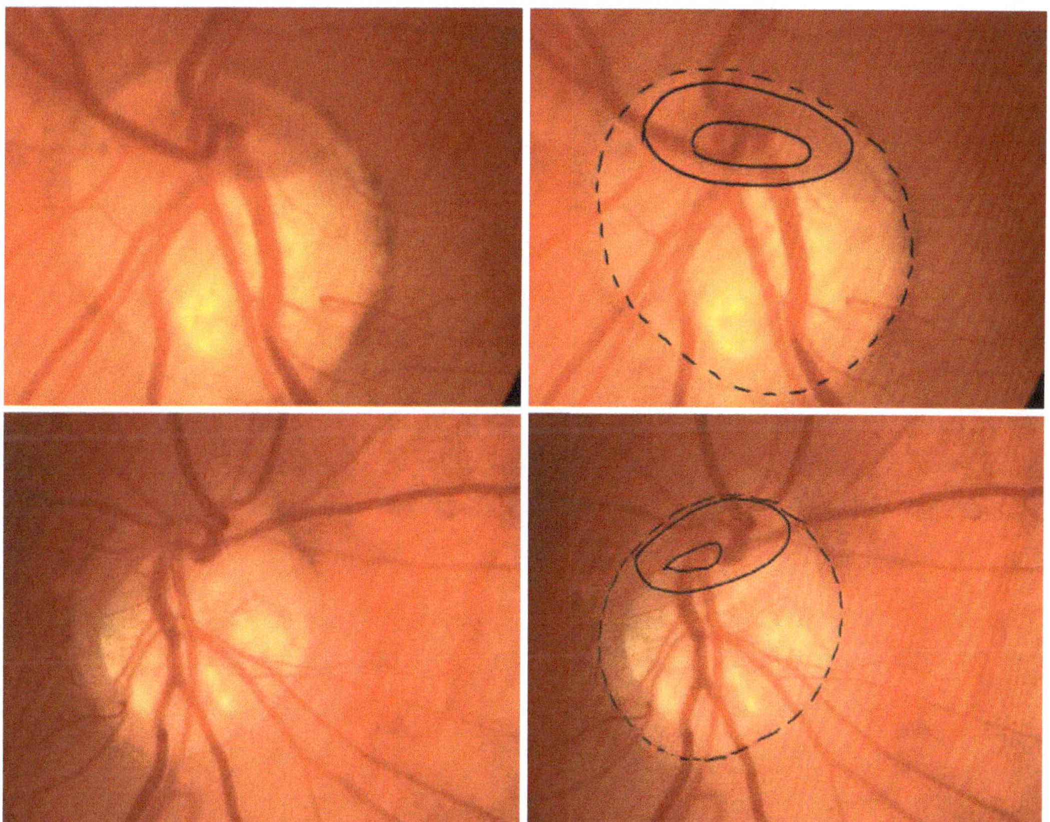

Fig. 5.16 (**b**) Very high levels of vertical tilting lead to disc structures which are difficult to interpret. There may be exaggerated areas of PPA with partial deficits of the peripapillary sclera. Defining the limits of the disc and clearly identifying areas that can be followed for rim loss needs experience

5.7.2 Structurally Abnormal Discs

5.7.2.1 Congenital Disc Pit

Figure 5.17a shows a large disc with congenital optic disc pit. Disc pits are also addressed in detail in Chap. 7.

5.7.2.2 Glaucomatous Discs with Coincidental Retinal Disorders

Retinal vein occlusions are associated with glaucoma [92], and when they occur it can be difficult to identify progression in the glauco-

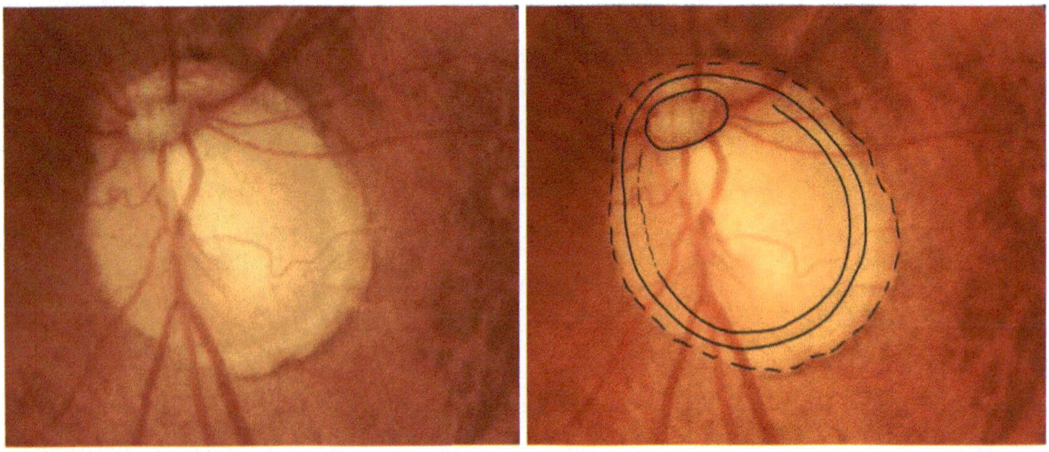

Fig. 5.17 (**a**) This is a macrodisc with a congenital disc pit in the superotemporal pole. There is an associated inferior field defect as there is loss of RNFL associated with the pit. But the patient also has steroid-induced glaucoma and has had some RNFL loss and reduction in rim inferiorly

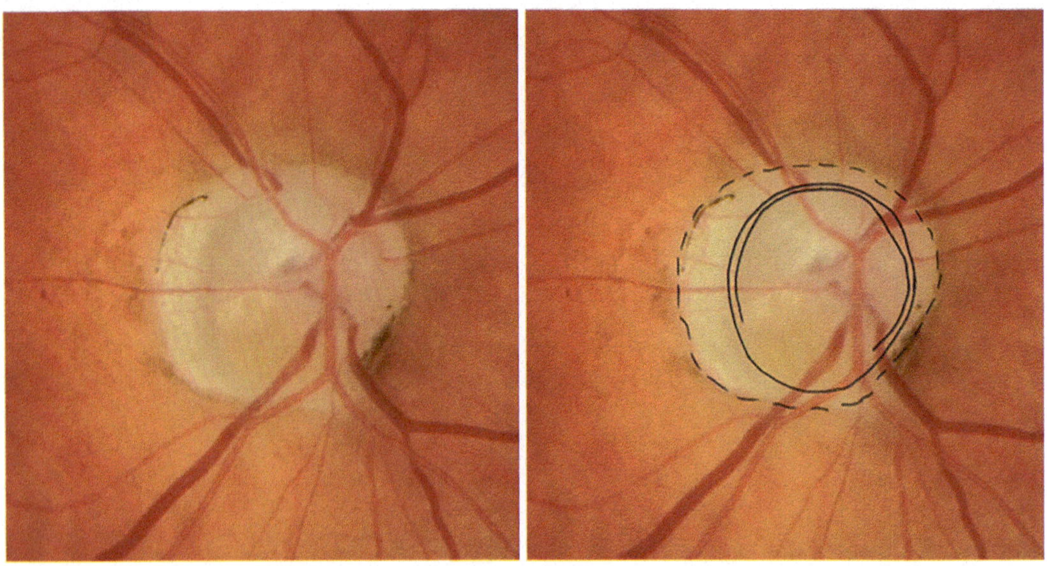

Fig. 5.17 (**b**) Drusen can produce visual field defects, presumably related to focal areas of axonal compression [90]. In ONH drusen the level of VF defect is linked to the amount of crowding of the pre-laminar optic nerve [91]. Drusen can co-exist with glaucoma, as in these discs, where the drusen is not material to the visual loss. Note that the inferior branch retinal artery travels over the drusen and hence does not alert the examiner that the rim is missing inferiorly. A shallow lamina position makes the extreme rim loss superiorly less obvious

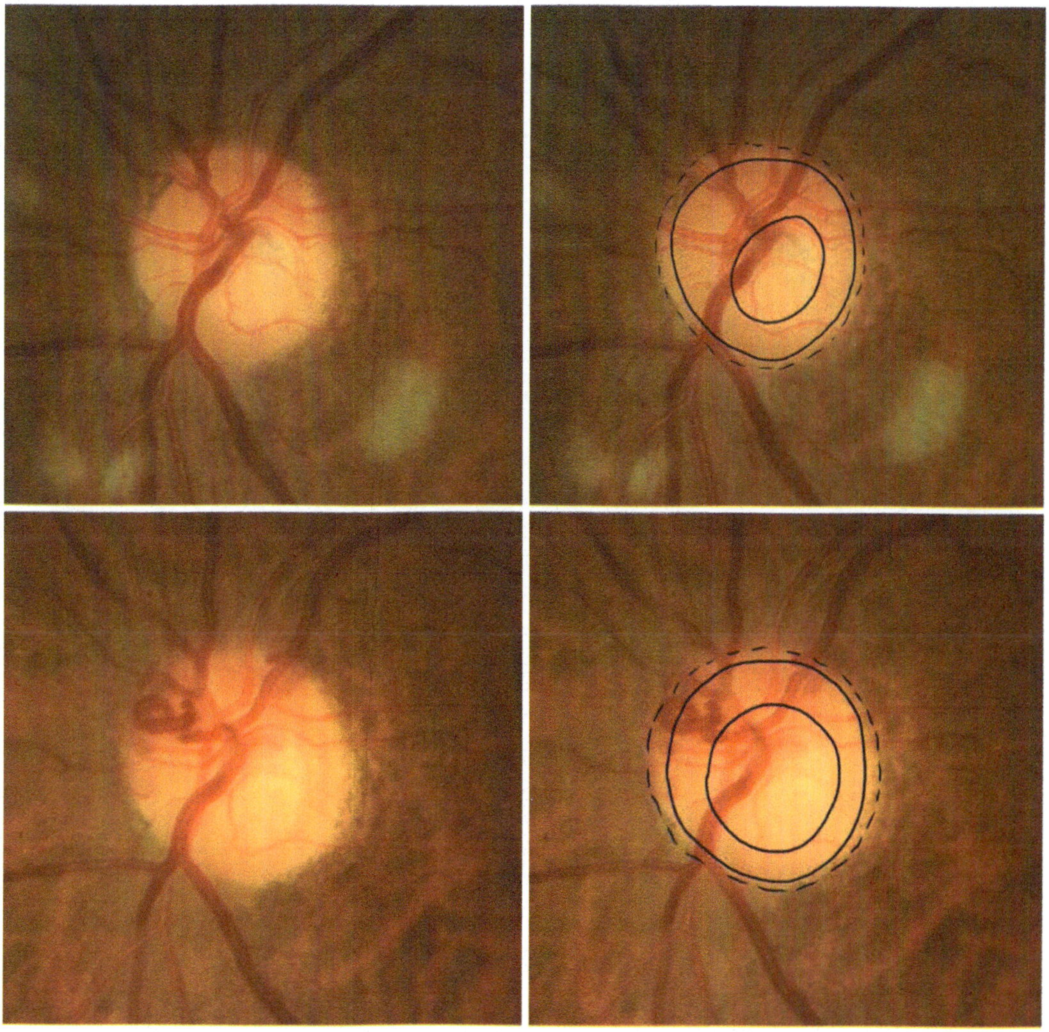

Fig. 5.17 (c) Patient with early glaucoma following a superior BRVO, with subsequent worsening of the glaucoma and the development of a collateral vessel at the superior pole

matous changes in the ONH. Figure 5.17b shows optic discs of a patient with early glaucoma who also developed superior branch retinal vein occlusion (BRVO) and subsequent collateral vessels (Fig. 5.17c).

5.7.3 Myopic Discs

Myopia varies from relatively normally structured discs to very abnormal discs with tilting, unusual shape and often entwined in peripapillary scleral changes (usually a posterior staphyloma) as shown in Fig. 5.18a, 5.18b, 5.18c.

5.7.4 Unusual PPA

With experience we are drawn to eccentric PPA as it is often associated with rim loss in the adjacent section of the disc [65–67]. Occasionally PPA can disguise the margin of the disc and encourage the clinician to see the outer margin of

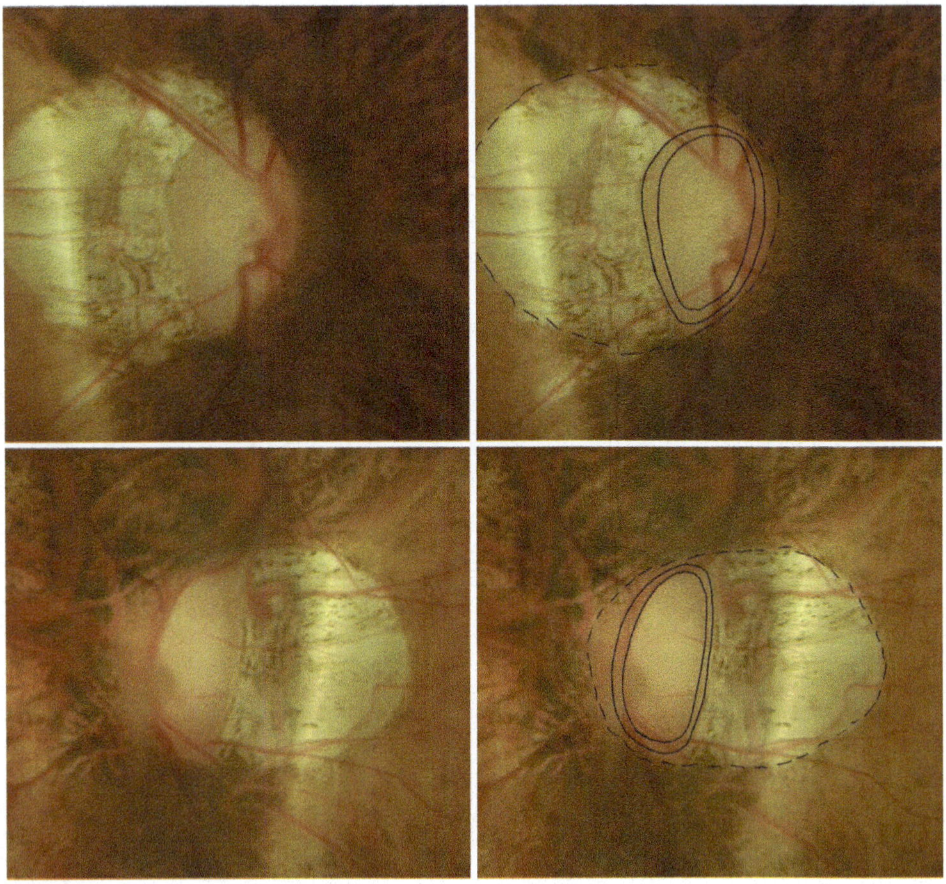

Fig. 5.18 (**a**) In these two discs the axial length is over 30 mm. There is marked temporal tilting and an ovoid scleral canal structure. Extensive PPA blends with macular changes of myopic posterior staphyloma

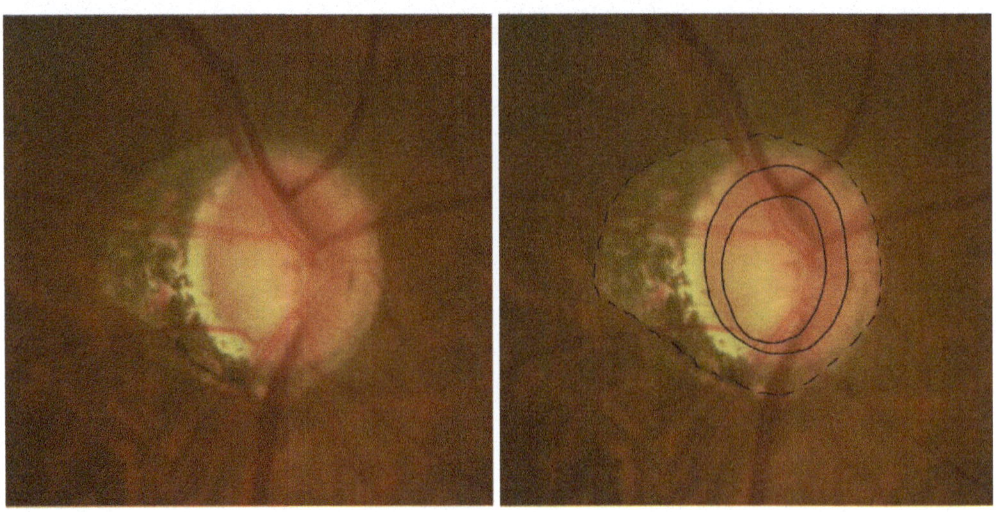

Fig. 5.18 (**b**) Some myopic eyes have smaller than normal scleral canals. The accurate recognition of the extent of 'cupping' and hence the extent of NRR loss is made more unreliable in the smaller disc, and was a cause of error in the GONE Project [18]. In this example there is significant inferior rim loss which was under-appreciated when this image was presented to trainees. Small discs are less likely to have posterior bowing of the lamina, which can help differentiate the rim, and the CDR underestimates the severity of the rim loss

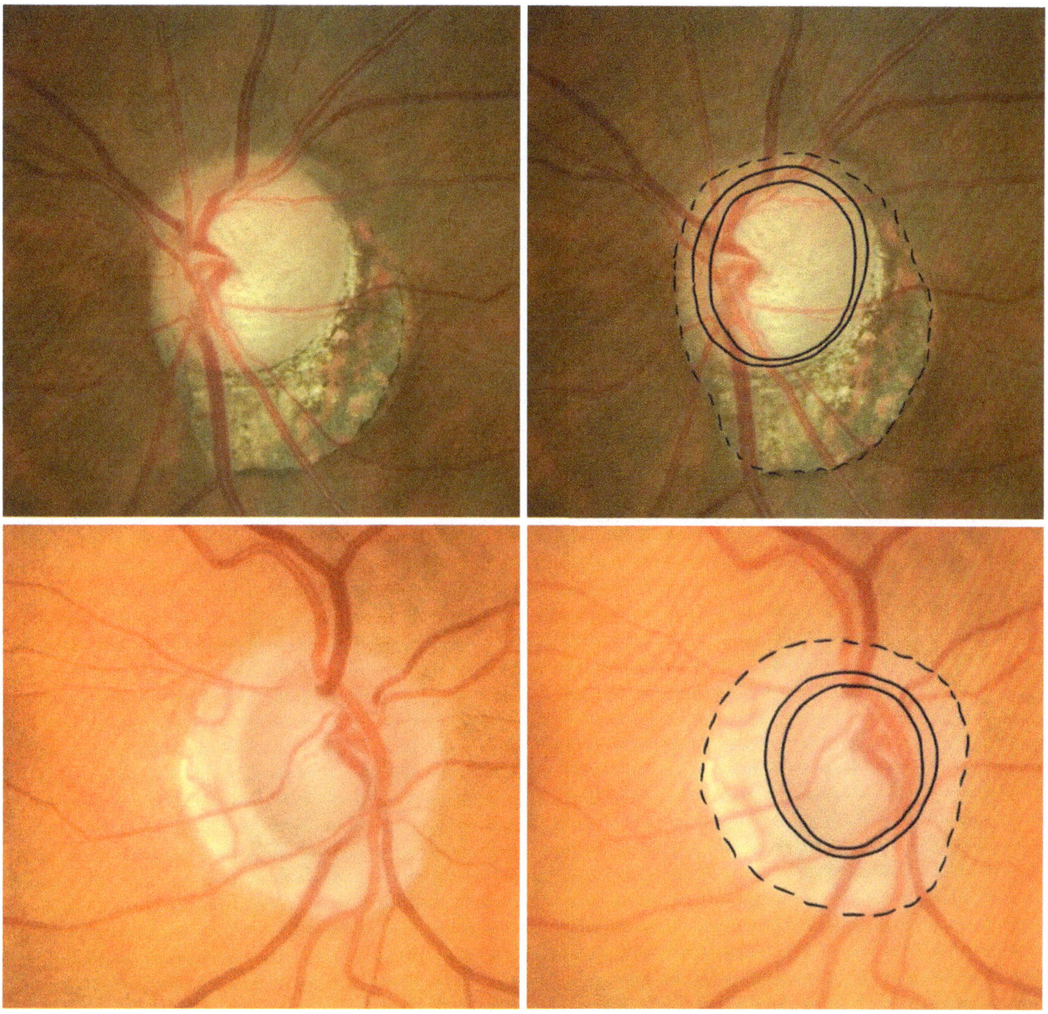

Fig. 5.18 (**c**) Myopia with shallow cups. In significant axial myopia it is unusual to have significant posterior bowing of the lamina cribrosa which leads to a shallower cup with a sloping rim. This reduces the ease of delineation of the inner margin of the NRR, a feature that was significantly associated with a lack of appreciation of the extent of the glaucomatous rim loss. In both of these examples there is a shallow cup, smooth sloping internal margin of the NRR and significant PPA

the rim (the scleral canal). In these examples the margins of the scleral canal can easily be mistaken (Fig. 5.19a, 5.19b, 5.19c).

5.7.5 Pallor without Cupping

Rapid elevation of the IOP causes damage but it may have a different appearance if it is not superimposed on pre-existing classic glaucomatous change. In many cases the development of cupping is as a result of prolonged posterior stress on the lamina, resulting in posterior bowing, deepening of the cup and thinning of the rim when there is axonal and glial loss [43, 73, 78]. Sudden pressure rise (or an abnormally rigid lamina) will produce pallor without the 'classic' cupping associated with glaucoma [55, 74] (Fig. 5.20).

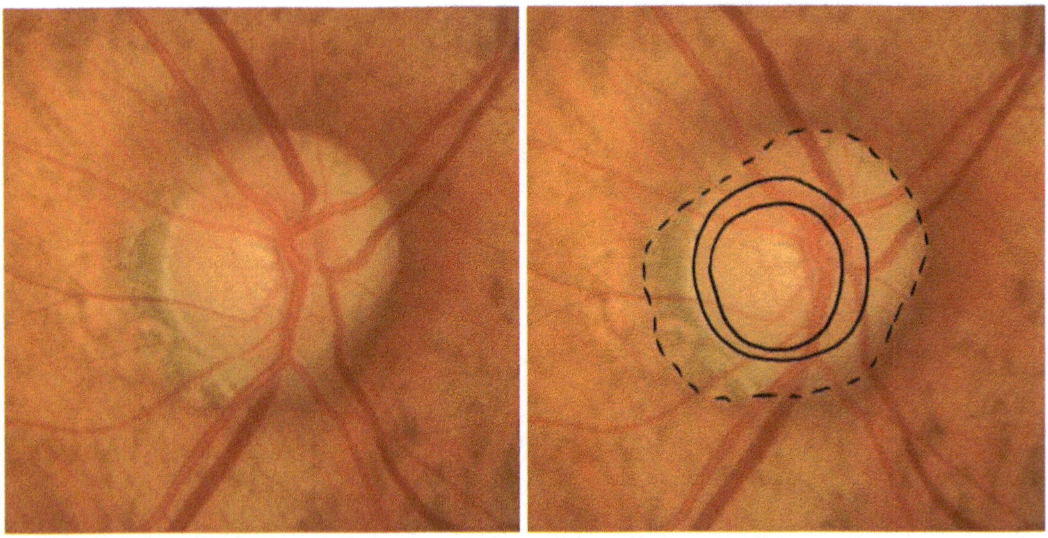

Fig. 5.19 (**a**) This is a small to medium disc with minor PPA inferotemporally and more marked PPA superonasally. The pattern of PPA is unusual and tends to make the scleral canal look larger than it is, and therefore the CDR smaller than it is

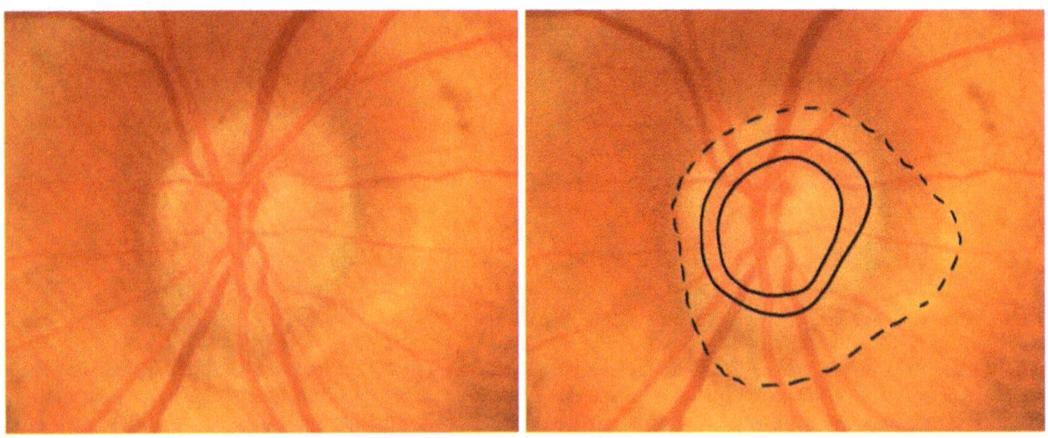

Fig. 5.19 (**b**) In this disc, the PPA tends to disguise the shape of the disc, which is not regular, being ovoid vertically with a wider superior half. Failure to appreciate the underlying shape of the scleral canal is likely to lead to incorrect assessment of the rim

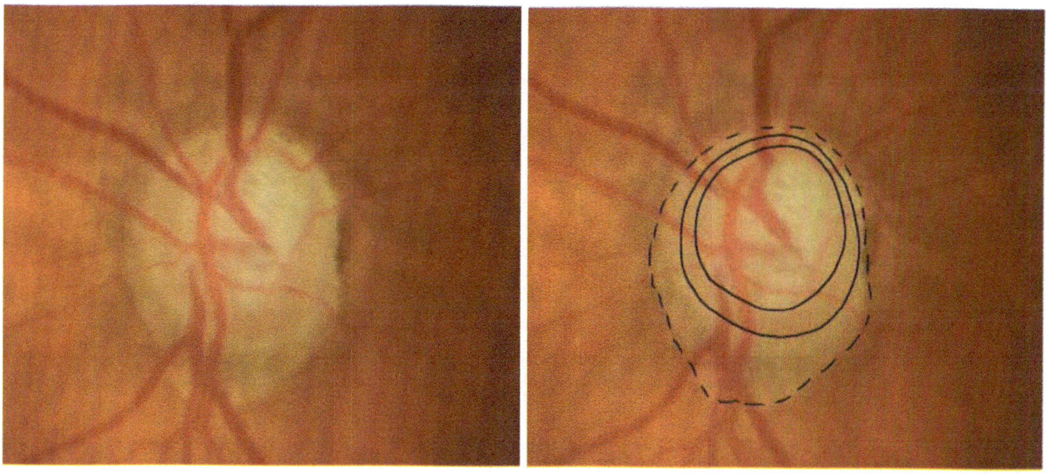

Fig. 5.19 (c) Classically, PPA is more significant in the area of greatest rim loss [67]. On occasion this pattern is not followed and it invites the clinician to under-appreciate the rim loss. In this example the PPA in inferior, extending a little nasally. But the maximal area of rim loss is superior where there is little PPA

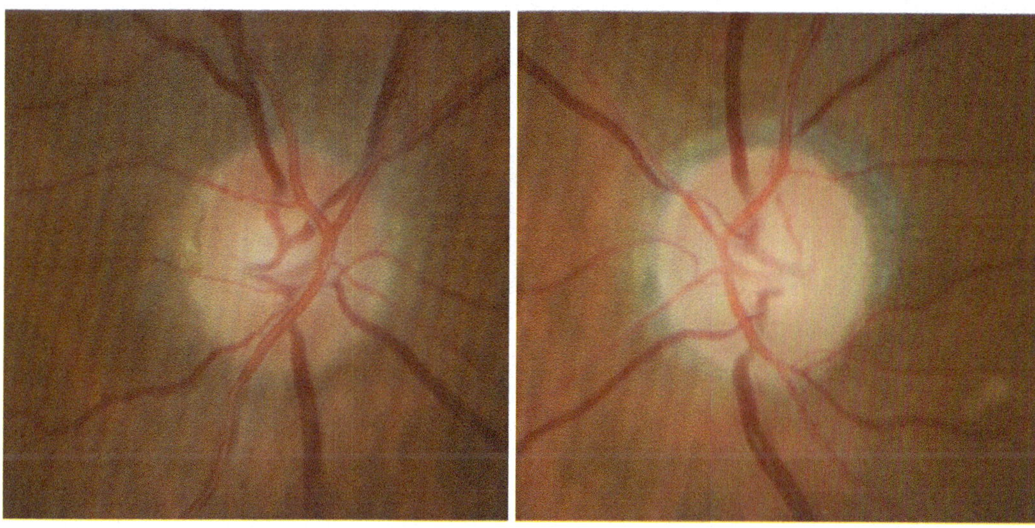

Fig. 5.20 In this example the left eye has suffered from Acute Angle Closure which has caused marked disc damage. But it has not deformed the lamina and excavated the central part of the nerve, hence there is no discernible increase in the CDR. Note there is pallor and an increase in the PPA compared to the fellow eye

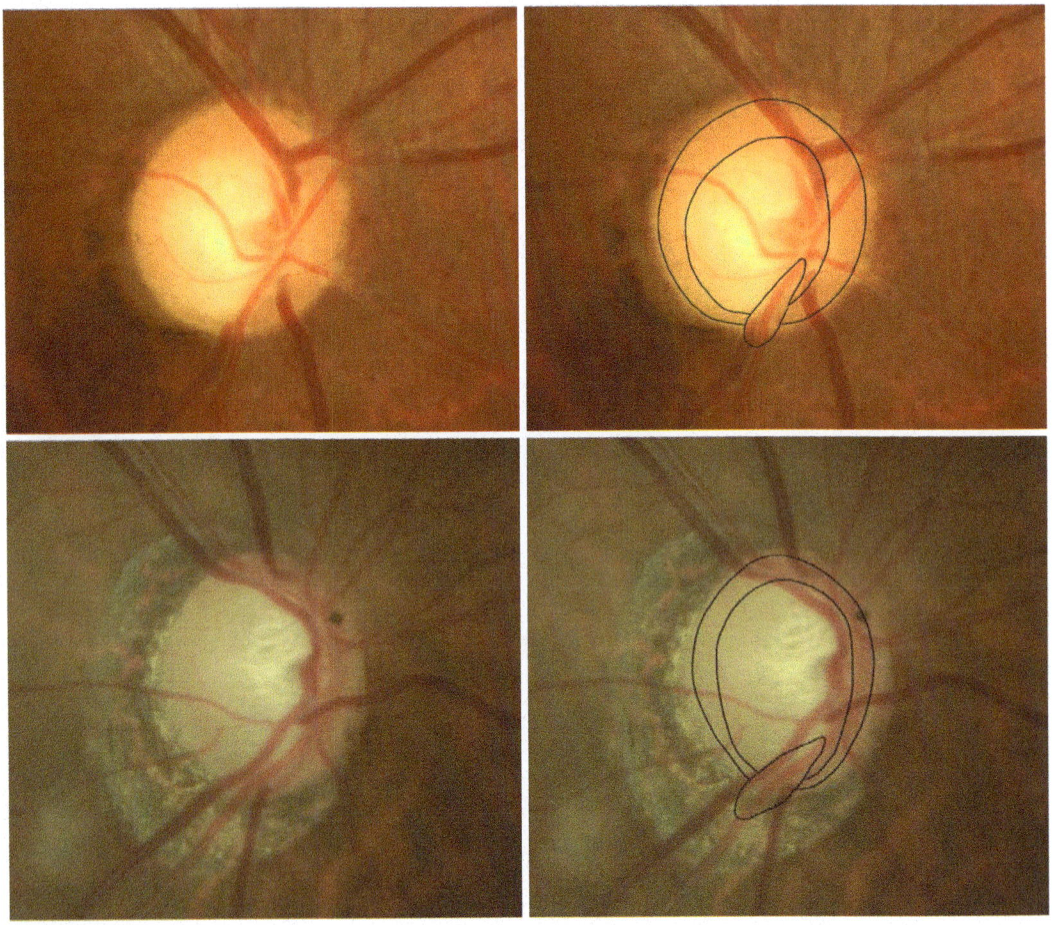

Fig. 5.21 (**a**) Examples of vessel contour not reflecting the NRR contour

5.7.6 Detecting Contour Can Be Difficult if the Vessel(s) Do Not Follow It

The inner margin of the NRR (or the 'inside') is usually detected by the colour change and the contour. The contour is possible to see when there is true stereopsis, but this will not be possible all the time (Fig. 5.21a. Indirect information about the rim can be gleaned from the vessel direction and bend (Fig. 5.21b). The vessels crossing the NRR will usually follow the shape of the rim. It is prudent to be aware that on occasion the vessels do not follow the surface, and thus can lead the examiner to believe the rim is wider than it is. This phenomenon was called 'overpass cupping' by Hitchings and Spaeth in 1976 [93] (Fig. 5.21c).

5.8 Conclusion: How Do We Get Better At Disc Examination?

Examination of the ONH is a complex skill. To err is common, and with formal testing we have identified some of the causes of inaccurate assessment. Avoiding error—getting better at ONH examination—is important for the early diagnosis of glaucoma and the detection of disease progression, and therefore key to the prevention of visual loss. It is a key expertise of the eyecare professional and an expected competency.

The GONE Project found that trainees who incorrectly assessed individual disc features were more likely to err in overall assessment of glaucoma likelihood. This suggests that teaching a

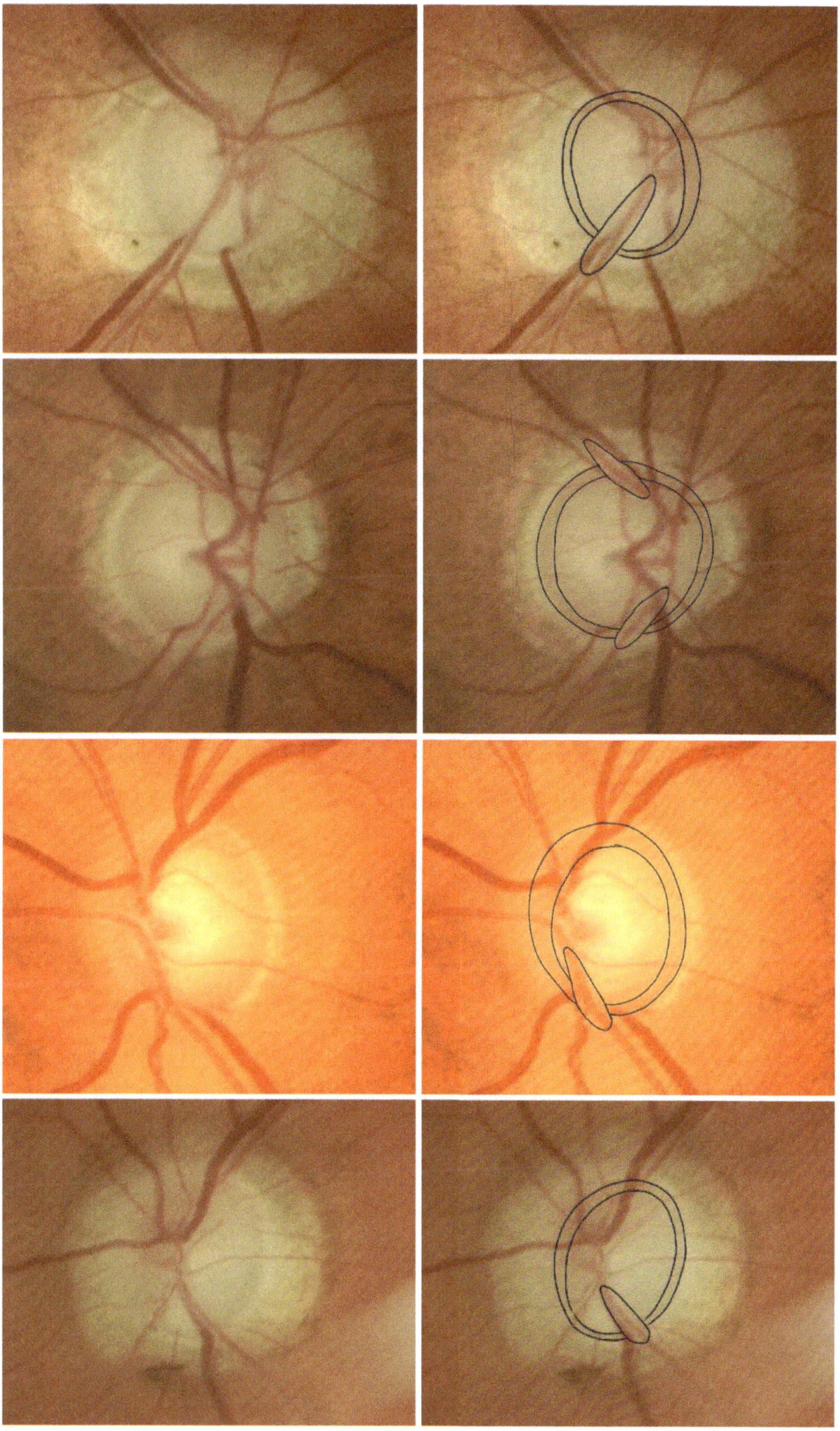

Fig. 5.21 (**a**) (continued)

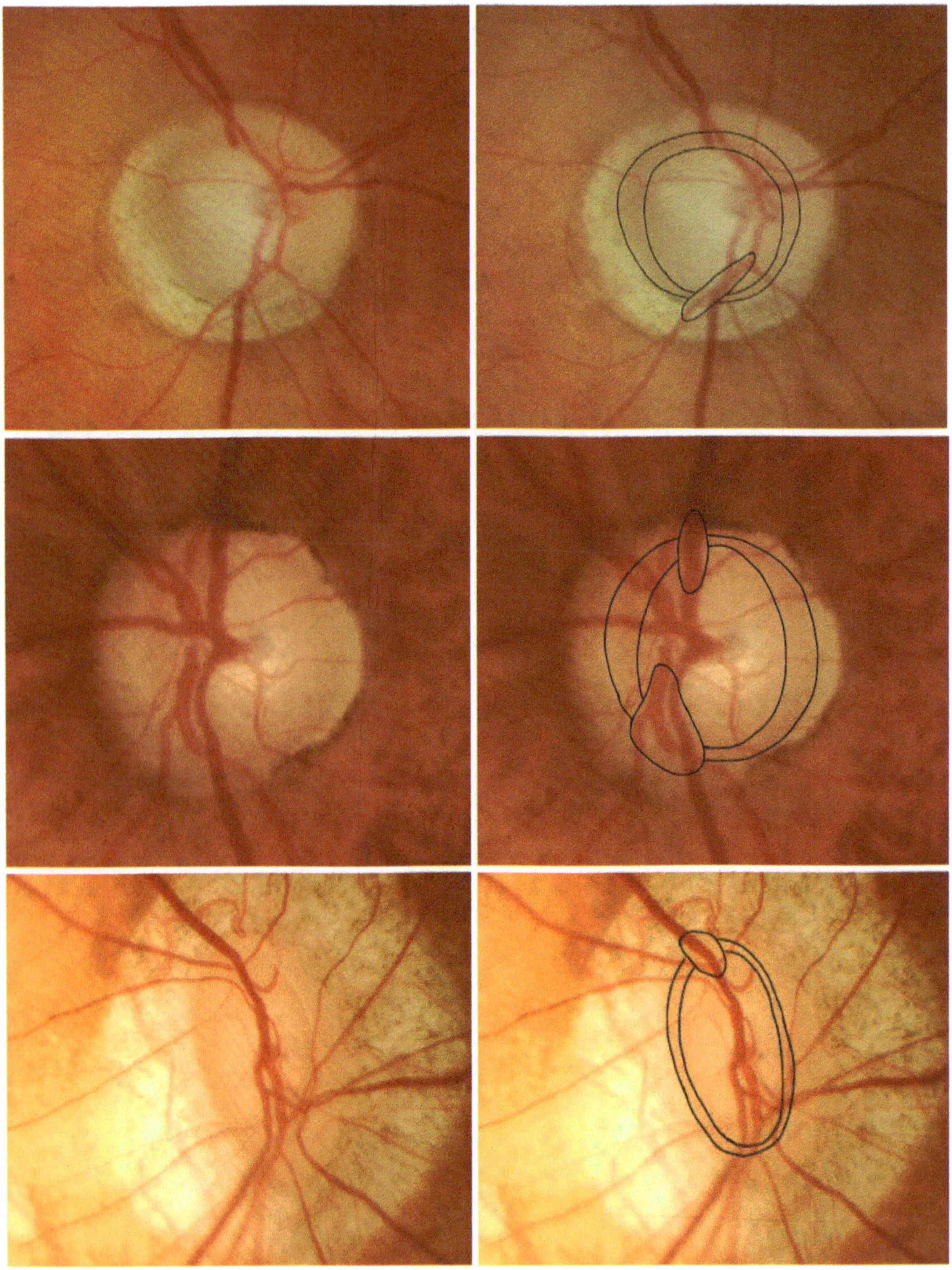

Fig. 5.21 (**a**) (continued)

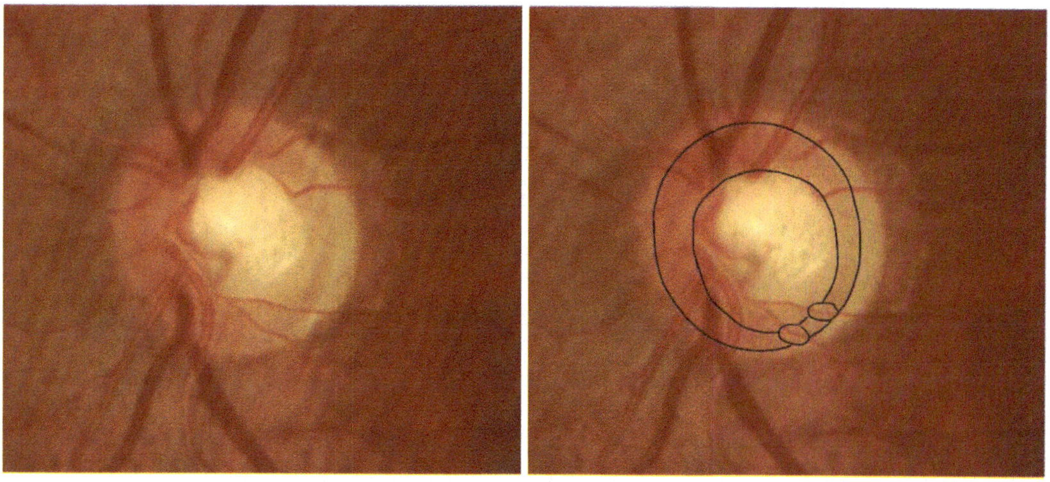

Fig. 5.21 (**b**) This disc is an example of the opposite phenomenon. Here the colour of the rim suggests the inferotemporal rim is wider than it is. The contour of the vessels indicates where the inner part of the rim is, now revealing significant inferior rim thinning

systematic approach to the disc exam (such as the WGA method) may be helpful. Teaching and learning this systematic approach are more easily performed outside the eye clinic using disc photos and directed feedback. However, all clinical skills must be practised to achieve expertise, and in the busy eye clinic it is important for trainees to slow down to examine a disc methodically, and to seek the opinion of expert colleagues when confronted with uncertainty.

In general, it is better to be able to learn from the errors of others than by making them all yourself. The systematic approach we recommend is based upon detecting and codifying these errors. The examples in this chapter are real eyes and the missed diagnosis or lack of recognition of extent of damage, as well as the over-treatment of others, has caused real and avoidable harm. Understanding and practising recognition of the structure of the ONH, combined with testing and training will reduce your chance of making errors. When we combine knowledge and diligence, we do our best in our fight against avoidable blindness.

The GONE Project is available for free online at *www.gone-project.com*.

References

1. Quigley HA. Glaucoma. Lancet. 2011;377:1367–77.
2. Weinreb RN, Leung CK, Crowston JG, et al. Primary open-angle glaucoma. Nat Rev Dis Primers. 2016;2:16067.
3. Flaxman SR, Bourne RRA, Resnikoff S, et al. Global causes of blindness and distance vision impairment 1990–2020: a systematic review and meta-analysis. Lancet. 2017;5(12):E1221–34.
4. Leske MC. Open-angle glaucoma—an epidemiologic overview. Ophthalmic Epidemiol. 2007;14(4):166–72.
5. Walland MJ. On the lookout: how to save the sight of Australians who have glaucoma. Med J Aust. 2008;188:269–70.
6. Sommer A, Pollack I, Maumenee AE. Optic disc parameters and onset of glaucomatous field loss. I. Methods and progressive changes in disc morphology. Arch Ophthalmol. 1979;97:1444–8.
7. Pederson JE, Anderson DR. The mode of progressive disc cupping in ocular hypertension and glaucoma. Arch Ophthalmol. 1980;98:490–5.
8. Quigley HA, Addicks EM, Green WR. Optic nerve damage in human glaucoma. III. Quantitative correlation of nerve fiber loss and visual field defect in glaucoma, ischemic neuropathy, papilledema, and toxic neuropathy. Arch Ophthalmol. 1982;100:135–46.
9. Sommer A, Katz J, Quigley HA, et al. Clinically detectable nerve fiber atrophy precedes the onset of glaucomatous field loss. Arch Ophthalmol. 1991;109:77–83.

10. Quigley HA, Katz J, Derick RJ, et al. An evaluation of optic disc and nerve fiber layer examinations in monitoring progression of early glaucoma damage. Ophthalmology. 1992;99:19–28.
11. Airaksinen PJ, Tuulonen A, Alanko HI. Rate and pattern of neuroretinal rim area decrease in ocular hypertension and glaucoma. Arch Ophthalmol. 1992;110:206–10.
12. Gordon MO, Beiser JA, Brandt JD, et al. The ocular hypertension treatment study: baseline factors that predict the onset of primary open-angle glaucoma. Arch Ophthalmol. 2002;120(6):714–20.
13. Tielsch JM, Katz J, Sommer A, et al. Family history and risk of primary open angle glaucoma. The Baltimore eye survey. Arch Ophthalmol. 1994;112:69–73.
14. Johnson CA, Sample PA, Zangwill LM, et al. Structure and function evaluation (SAFE): II. Comparison of optic disk and visual field characteristics. Am J Ophthalmol. 2003;135:148–54.
15. Michelessi M, Lucenteforte E, Oddone F, et al. Optic nerve head and fibre layer imaging for diagnosing glaucoma. Cochrane Database Syst. 2015;11:CD008803.
16. Kong YX, Coote MA, O'Neill EC, et al. Glaucomatous optic neuropathy evaluation project: a standardized internet system for assessing skills in optic disc examination. Clin Exp Ophthalmol. 2011;39:308–17.
17. O'Neill EC, Kong YX, Connell PP, et al. Gaze behavior among experts and trainees during optic disc examination: does how we look affect what we see? Invest Ophthalmol Vis Sci. 2011;52:3976–83.
18. O'Neill EC, Gurria LU, Pandav SS, et al. Glaucomatous optic neuropathy evaluation project: factors associated with underestimation of glaucoma likelihood. JAMA Ophthalmol. 2014;132:560–6.
19. Kong YXG, Crowston JG, Coote M, et al. Understanding glaucoma optic nerve assessment through systemic observation: the GONE project. SAOJ. 2016;11(4):20–5.
20. Gaasterland DE, Blackwell B, Dally LG, et al. The advanced glaucoma intervention study (AGIS): 10. Variability mong academic glaucoma subspecialists in assessing optic disc notching. Tr Am Ophth Soc. 2001;99:177–85.
21. Abrams LS, Scott IU, Spaeth GL, et al. Agreement among optometrists, ophthalmologists, and residents in evaluating the optic disc for glaucoma. Ophthalmology. 1994;101(10):1662–7.
22. Hadwin SE, Redmond T, Garway-Heath DF, et al. Assessment of optic disc photographs for glaucoma by UK optometrists: the Moorfields optic disc assessment study (MODAS). Ophthalmic Physiol Opt. 2013;33:618–24.
23. Reus NJ, Lemij HG, EODAT group. Characteristics of misclassified discs in the European optic disc assessment trial (EODAT) [abstract from ARVO annual meeting]. Invest Ophthalmol Vis Sci. 2008;49:3627.
24. Varma R, Steinmann WC, Scott IU. Expert agreement in evaluating the optic disc for glaucoma. Ophthalmology. 1992;99:215.
25. Lichter PR. Variability of expert observers in evaluating the optic disc. Trans Am Ophthalmol Soc. 1976;74:532–72.
26. Harper R, Reeves B, Smith G. Observer variability in optic disc assessment: implications for glaucoma shared care. Ophthalmic Physiol Opt. 2000;20(4):265–73.
27. Nicolela MT, Drance SM, Broadway DC, et al. Agreement among clinicians in the recognition of patterns of optic disk damage in glaucoma. Am J Ophthalmol. 2001;132(6):836–44.
28. Reus NJ, de Graaf M, Lemij HG. Accuracy of GDx VCC, HRT I, and clinical assessment of stereoscopic optic nerve head photographs for diagnosing glaucoma. Br J Ophthalmol. 2007;91(3):313–8.
29. Reus NJ, Lemij HG, Garway-Heath DF, et al. Clinical assessment of stereoscopic optic disc photographs for glaucoma: the European optic disc assessment trial. Ophthalmology. 2010;117(4):717–23.
30. DeLeon-Ortega JE, Arthur SN, McGwin G, et al. Discrimination between glaucomatous and nonglaucomatous eyes using quantitative imaging devices and subjective optic nerve head assessment. Invest Ophthalmol Vis Sci. 2006;47(8):3374–80.
31. Taylor HR. Eye care for the future: the Weisenfeld lecture. Invest Ophthalmol Vis Sci. 2003;44(4):1413–8.
32. Mitchell P, Smith W, Attebo K, et al. Prevalence of open-angle glaucoma in Australia. The blue mountains eye study. Ophthalmology. 1996;103(10):1661–9.
33. Sommer A, Tielsch JM, Katz J, et al. Relationship between intraocular pressure and primary open angle glaucoma among white and black Americans: the Baltimore eye survey. JAMA Ophthalmol. 1991;109(8):1090–5.
34. Cedrone C, Mancino R, Cerulli A, et al. Epidemiology of primary glaucoma: prevalence, incidence, and blinding effects. Prog Brain Res. 2008;173:3–14.
35. Wensor MD, McCarty CA, Stanislaosky YL, et al. The prevalence of glaucoma in the Melbourne visual impairment project. Ophthalmology. 1998;105:733–9.
36. Keeffe JE, Weih LM, McCarty CA, et al. Utilisation of eye care services by urban and rural Australians. Br J Ophthalmol. 2002;86:24–7.
37. Wong EY, Keeffe JE, Rait JL, et al. Detection of undiagnosed glaucoma by eye health professionals. Ophthalmology. 2004;111:1508–14.
38. Van der Shoot J, Reus NJ, Garway-Heath D, et al. Accuracy of matching optic discs with visual fields: the European structure and function assessment trial (ESAFAT). Ophthalmology. 2013;120(12):2470–5.
39. Chauhan BC, Hutchison DM, Artes PH, et al. Optic disc progression in glaucoma: comparison of confocal scanning laser tomography to optic disc photographs in a prospective study. Invest Ophthalmol Vis Sci. 2009;50(4):1682–91.
40. Wilsey LJ, Fortune B. Electroretinography in glaucoma diagnosis. Curr Opin Ophthalmol. 2016;27(2):118–24.
41. Jonas JB, Gusek GC, Naumann GO. Optic disc, cup and neuroretinal rim size, configuration and corre-

lations in normal eyes. Invest Ophthalmol Vis Sci. 1988;29:1151–8.
42. Jonas JB, Budde WM, Panda-Jonas S. Ophthalmoscopic evaluation of the optic nerve head. Surv Ophthalmol. 1999;43:293–320.
43. Jonas JB, Budde WM. Diagnosis and pathogenesis of glaucomatous optic neuropathy: morphological aspects. Prog Retin Eye Res. 2000;19(1):1–40.
44. Sanfilippo PG, Cardini A, Hewitt AW, et al. Optic disc morphology -- rethinking shape. Prog Retin Eye Res. 2009;28:227–48.
45. Burgoyne C. The morphological differences between glaucoma and other optic neuropathies. J Neuroophthalmol. 2015;35:S8–S21.
46. O'Neill EC, Danesh-Meyer HV, Kong GX, et al. Optic disc evaluation in optic neuropathies: the optic disc assessment project. Ophthalmology. 2011;118:964–70.
47. Hewitt AW, Poulsen JP, Alward AL, et al. Heritable features of the optic disc: a novel twin method for determining genetic significance. Invest Ophthalmol Vis Sci. 2007;48(6):2469–75.
48. Healey PR, Carbonaro F, Taylor B, et al. The heritability of optic disc parameters: a classic twin study. Invest Ophthalmol Vis Sci. 2008;49(1):77–80.
49. Garway-Heath DF, Wollstein G, Hitchings RA. Aging changes of the optic nerve head in relation to open angle glaucoma. Br J Ophthalmol. 1997;81:840–5.
50. Vianna JR, Danthurebandara VM, Sharpe GP, et al. Importance of normal aging in estimating the rate of glaucomatous neuroretinal rim and retinal nerve fiber layer loss. Ophthalmology. 2015;122(12):2392–8.
51. Crowston JG, Hopley CR, Healey PR, et al. The effect of optic disc diameter on vertical cup to disc ratio percentiles in a population based cohort: the blue mountains eye study. Br J Ophthalmol. 2004;88:766–70.
52. Baniasadi N, Paschalis EI, Haghzadeh M. Patterns of retinal nerve fiber layer loss in different subtypes of open angle glaucoma using spectral domain optical coherence tomography. J Glaucoma. 2016;25(10):865–72.
53. Spaeth GL. A new classification of glaucoma including focal glaucoma. Surv Ophthalmol. 1994;38:S9–S17.
54. Nicolela MT, Drance SM. Various glaucomatous optic nerve appearances: clinical correlations. Ophthalmology. 1996;103(4):640–9.
55. Sng CC, See JS, Ngo CS, et al. Changes in retinal nerve fibre layer, optic nerve head morphology, and visual field after acute primary angle closure. Eye. 2011;25(5):619–25.
56. Ericsson A, Pool R. Peak: how all of us can achieve extraordinary things. Random House; 2016.
57. Coote MA, Crowston JG. Optic nerve head clinical examination. In: Basic course in glaucoma. World Glaucoma Association; 2017. Retrieved from https://wga.one/wga/basic-course-in-glaucoma/
58. Kirwan JF, Gouws P, Linnell AE, et al. Pharmacological mydriasis and optic disc examination. Br J Ophthalmol. 2000;84:894–8.
59. Parkin B, Shuttleworth G, Costen M, et al. A comparison of stereoscopic and monoscopic evaluation of optic disc topography using a digital optic disc stereo camera. Br J Ophthalmol. 2001;85(11):1347–51.
60. Morgan JE, Sheen NJ, North RV, et al. Digital imaging of the optic nerve head: monoscopic and stereoscopic analysis. Br J Ophthalmol. 2005;89(7):879–84.
61. Chan HH, Ong DN, Kong YX, et al. Glaucomatous optic neuropathy evaluation (GONE) project: the effect of monoscopic versus stereoscopic viewing conditions on optic nerve evaluation. Am J Ophthalmol. 2014;157:936–44.
62. Garway-Heath DF, Ruben ST, Viswanathan A, et al. Vertical cup/disc ratio in relation to optic disc size: its value in the assessment of the glaucoma suspect. Br J Ophthalmol. 1998;82:1118–24.
63. Sheen NJ, Morgan JE, Poulsen JL, et al. Digital stereoscopic analysis of the optic disc: evaluation of a teaching program. Ophthalmology. 2004;111(10):1873–9.
64. Scheetz J, Koklanis K, McGuinness M, et al. A randomized trial to increase the assessment accuracy of glaucoma and optic disc characteristics by orthoptists. J Contin Educ Health. 2019;39(3):161–7.
65. Jonas JB, Fernandez MC, Naumann GO. Glaucomatous parapapillary atrophy. Occurrence and correlations. Arch Ophthalmol. 1992;110:214–22.
66. Jonas JB. Clinical implications of peripapillary atrophy in glaucoma. Curr Opin Ophthalmol. 2005;16(2):84–8.
67. Teng CC, CG DM, Prata TS, et al. β-zone parapapillary atrophy and the velocity of glaucoma progression. Ophthalmology. 2010;117(5):909–15.
68. Hoffman EM, Zangwill LM, Crowston JG, et al. Optic disc size and glaucoma. Surv Ophthalmol. 2007;52(1):32–49.
69. Jonas JB, Zach FM, Gusek GC, et al. Pseudoglaucomatous physiologic large cups. Am J Ophthalmol. 1989;107:137–44.
70. Girkin CA, McGwin G Jr, Long C, et al. Subjective and objective optic nerve assessment in African Americans and whites. Invest Ophthalmol Vis Sci. 2004;45(7):2272–8.
71. Wang Y, Xu L, Zhang L, et al. Optic disc size in a population based study in northern China: the Beijing eye study. Br J Ophthalmol. 2006;90:353–6.
72. Jonas JB, Kling F, Grundler AE. Optic disc shape, corneal astigmatism, and amblyopia. Ophthalmology. 1997;104(11):1934–7.
73. Yang H, Ren R, Lockwood H, et al. The connective tissue components of optic nerve head cupping in monkey experimental glaucoma part 1: global change. Invest Ophthalmol Vis Sci. 2015;56(13):7661–78.
74. Azuara-Blanco A, Harris A, Cantor LB, et al. Effects of short term increase of intraocular pressure on optic disc cupping. Br J Ophthalmol. 1998;82:880–3.
75. Harizman N, Oliveira C, Chiang A, et al. The ISNT rule and differentiation of normal from glaucomatous eyes. Arch Ophthalmol. 2006;124:1579–83.

76. Chan EW, Liao J, Wong R, et al. Diagnostic performance of the ISNT rule for glaucoma based on the Heidelberg retinal tomograph. Trans Vis Sci Tech. 2013;2(5):2.
77. Poon LY, Sola-Del Valle D, Turalba AV, et al. The ISNT rule: how often does it apply to disc photographs and retinal nerve fibre layer measurements in the normal population? Am J Ophthalmol. 2017;184:19–27.
78. Jung KI, Jung Y, Park KT, et al. Factors affecting plastic lamina cribrosa displacement in glaucoma patients. Invest Ophthalmol Vis Sci. 2014;55(12):7709–15.
79. Drance SM, Fairclough M, Butler DM. The importance of disc hemorrhage in the prognosis of chronic open angle glaucoma. Arch Ophthalmol. 1977;95(2):226–8.
80. Healey PR, Mitchell P, Smith W, et al. Optic disc hemorrhages in a population with and without signs of glaucoma. Ophthalmology. 1998;105(2):216–23.
81. Budenz DL, Anderson DR, Feuer WJ, et al. Detection and prognostic significance of optic disc hemorrhages from during the ocular hypertension treatment study. Ophthalmology. 2006;113(12):2137–43.
82. Leske MC, Heijl A, Hyman L, et al. Predictors of long-term progression in the early manifest glaucoma trial. Ophthalmology. 2007;114(11):1965–72.
83. De Moraes CG, Prata TS, Liebmann CA, et al. Spatially consistent, localized visual field loss before and after disc hemorrhage. Invest Ophthalmol Vis Sci. 2009;50(10):4727–33.
84. Budenz DL, Huecker JB, Gedde SJ, et al. Thirteen-year follow-up of optic disc hemorrhages in the ocular hypertension treatment study. Am J Ophthalmol. 2017;174:126–33.
85. Parikh RS. Normal age-related decay of retinal nerve fiber layer thickness. Ophthalmology. 2007;114(5):921–6.
86. Dias DT, Ushida M, Battistella R, et al. Neurophthalmological conditions mimicking glaucomatous optic neuropathy: analysis of the most common causes of misdiagnosis. BMC Ophthalmol. 2017;17:2.
87. Fraser CL, White AJ, Plant GT, et al. Optic nerve cupping and the neuro-ophthalmologist. J Neuroophthalmol. 2013;33(4):377–89.
88. Feldman RM, Cioffi GA, Liebmann JM, et al. Current knowledge and attitudes concerning cost-effectiveness in glaucoma pharmacotherapy: a glaucoma specialists focus group study. Clin Ophthalmol. 2020;14:729–39.
89. Chan CC, Crowston JG, Tan R, et al. Burden of ocular surface disease in patients with glaucoma from Australia. Asia Pac J Ophthalmol. 2013;2(2):79–87.
90. Palmer E, Gale J, Crowston JG, et al. Optic nerve head drusen: an update. Neuroophthalmology. 2018;42(6):367–84.
91. Noval S, Visa J, Conteras I. Visual field defects due to optic nerve head drusen in children. Graefes Arch Clin Exp Ophthalmol. 2013;251(10):2445–50.
92. Yin X, Li J, Zhang B, et al. Association of glaucoma with risk of retinal vein occlusion: a meta-analysis. Acta Ophthalmol. 2019;97(7):652–9.
93. Hitchings RA, Spaeth GL. The optic disc in glaucoma. Br J Ophthalmol. 1976;60:778–85.

6 What Imaging Errors Occur When Evaluating the Optic Nerve Head?

Gábor Holló

6.1 Is Conventional Fundus and Optic Nerve Head Assessment Still Necessary?

Since in the last decade diagnostics in ophthalmology became increasingly technical one may think that modern instruments are able to take over diagnostic decision making from ophthalmologists, thus clinical evaluation of the optic nerve head (ONH) and the retina is unnecessary. This, however, is a misconception. Ophthalmologists need to know which disease or diseases are present, and when they decide about imaging they need to select the appropriate instrument and scan type accordingly. They also need to consider the typical imaging artifacts caused by the current fundus abnormalities and other ocular conditions. For example, imaging via a vitreous body that contains vitreous floaters in front of the retinal area of interest, or measuring peripapillary retinal nerve fiber layer thickness (RNFLT) of an eye in which the measuring ellipse overlaps with severe peripapillary atrophy (PPA) provides no useful information. In ONH and peripapillary area imaging quantitative information (exact parameter values) is needed. Therefore, images free of artifacts and optimal image quality are required.

G. Holló (✉)
Glaucoma and Perimetry Service, Semmelweis University, Budapest, Hungary
e-mail: hollo.gabor@med.semmelweis-univ.hu

A detailed clinical assessment of the ONH and the ocular fundus is always necessary prior to imaging, even when a previously examined patient returns for a new imaging visit [1]. As it is discussed later in this chapter the current status of the disc and the peripapillary area may considerably differ from that seen earlier, which may result in imaging artifacts and incorrect treatment decisions.

Imaging of the ONH cannot substitute a proper clinical investigation. In addition, printed imaging reports, which summarize and classify the measured parameter values, are not suitable to identifying most of the imaging artifacts. Therefore, clinicians are expected to examine the ONH and the fundus before imaging; review the acquired images on the instrument's screen for artifacts; delete images with insufficient quality or artifacts; and only then print the selected report for the patient or the file [2].

6.2 Operator Related Errors in Optic Nerve Head and Peripapillary Imaging

When a new imaging instrument becomes available in the office all ophthalmologists who will work with it need to carefully read the manual or online manual, and undergo a training session by the manufacturer's representative. Then they need to gain sufficient experience in image

S. Pandav et al. (eds.), *The Optic Nerve Head in Health and Disease*,
https://doi.org/10.1007/978-981-33-6838-5_6

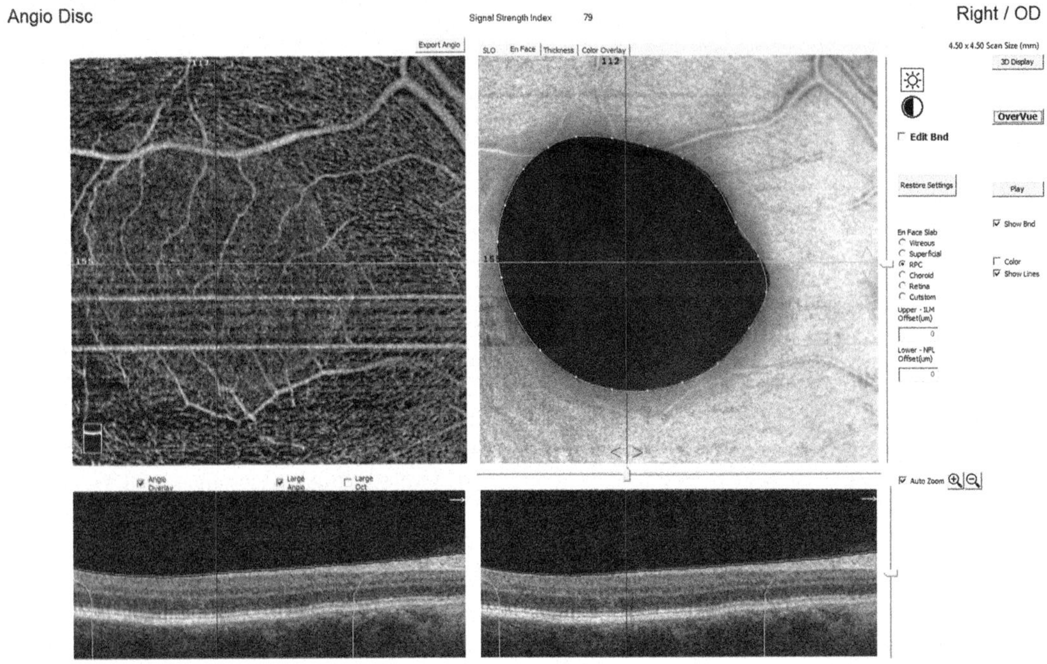

Fig. 6.1 Inappropriate scan selection. The selected scan is an optic nerve head scan (Angio Disc Scan), but the imaged retinal area is the macula. The resulting image and measurement values are useless, and the erroneous scan has to be deleted

acquisition and evaluation of the results of normal eyes. Lacking appropriate education and training may lead to basic errors in real life clinical practice. Figure 6.1 shows an image acquired using an ONH scan (Disc Angio Scan) for macular imaging. Surprisingly, the instrument's software "detects" a disc area, and the scan results in measurement values. These data, however, are incorrect and useless. The incorrect image needs to be deleted, and a new, correctly selected scan is required.

Motion artifacts (vertical or horizontal lines due to eye movements) are common in optical coherence tomography (OCT) disc imaging (Fig. 6.2). They cause false values in the area of the artifact. The operators are expected to recognize the motion artifact lines, delete the image, and substitute it with a high-quality new scan.

Correct definition of the ONH border is essential to all disc and peripapillary OCT measurements. The different instrument systems use different protocols for disc margin determination. In some systems the instrument offers the "best" (most precise) disc margin definition in one cross sectional plane. This can be modified by the operator. As a result, the disc margin is defined in one of the several section plains, and the center of the optic nerve head is automatically determined. Peripapillary RNFLT measurement is made along a measuring ellipse at a preset distance from the center of the disc. This method works well for most discs, but in large myopic disc the definition in one direction is considerably different from that in another direction. Figure 6.3 shows a myopic glaucoma eye with a large and oval disc. The operator correctly defined the disc margin in one plain, but this definition is incorrect for the perpendicular plain. In similar cases it is important to always use the same plane for disc definition in the follow-up examinations during long-term assessment (e.g. in glaucomatous RNFLT progression analysis). Figure 6.4 shows what happens if different disc definition planes are used for a large oval disc in the follow-up visits. RNFLT values show greater long-term variability (Fig. 6.4a), compared to the inner macular

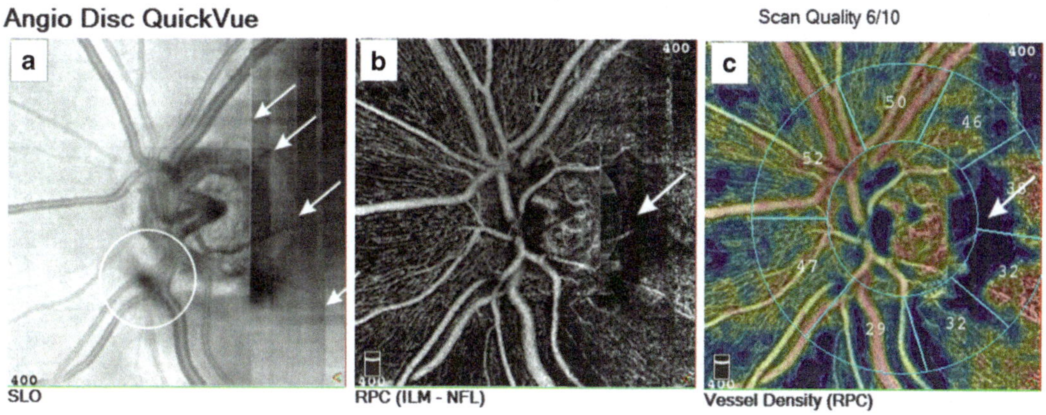

Fig. 6.2 Motion artifacts (arrows) and a small vitreous floater with shadow effect (encircled) (**a**) Scanning laser ophthalmoscopy (SLO) image; (**b**) OCT angiography image of the retinal nerve fiber layer (radial peripapillary capillaries, RPC), (**c**) color-coded perfusion image. On images (**b**) and (**c**) the arrows point at the area in which perfusion is not detected by the software due to the motion artifact on image (**a**) (arrows)

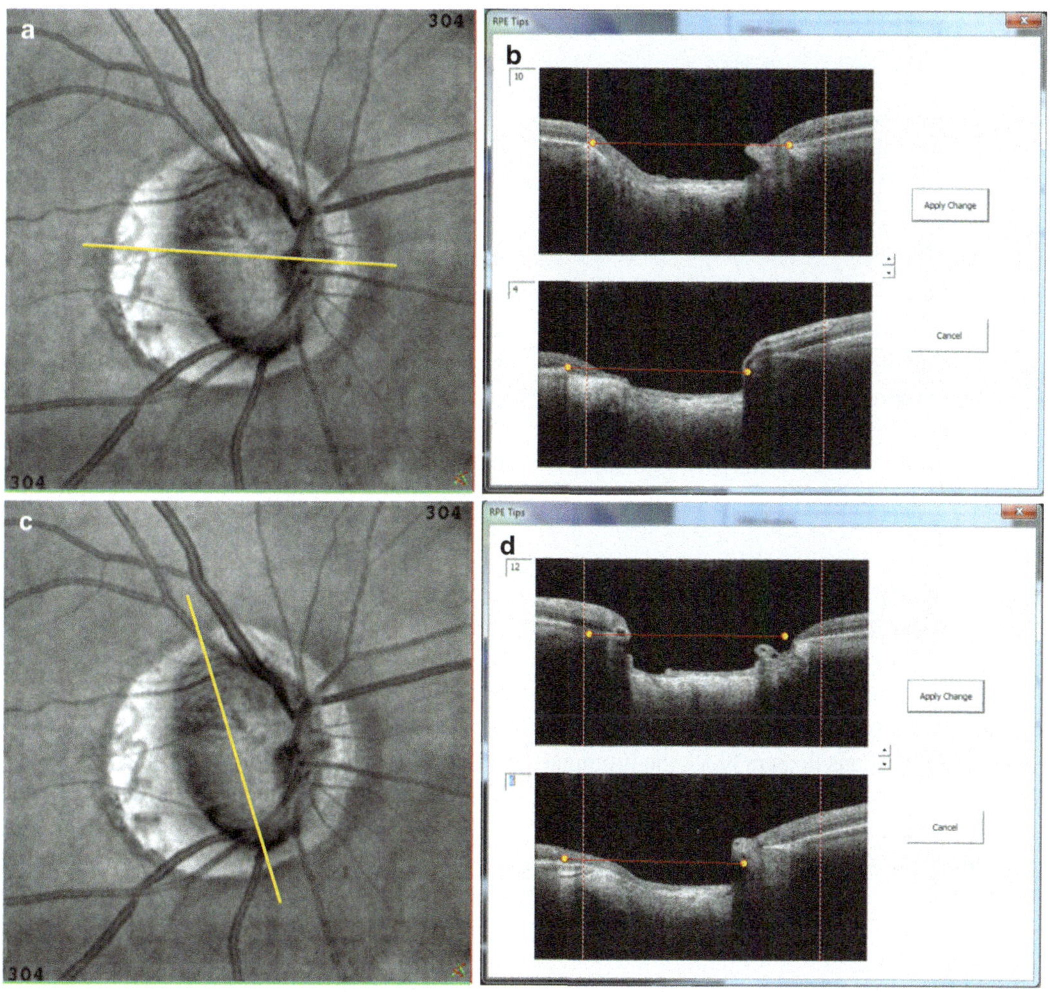

Fig. 6.3 Influence of plane selection on disc border definition in a large oval disc: (**a** and **b**) The margin is correctly defined in an almost horizontal plane; (**c** and **d**) this definition is incorrect in the close to vertical plane

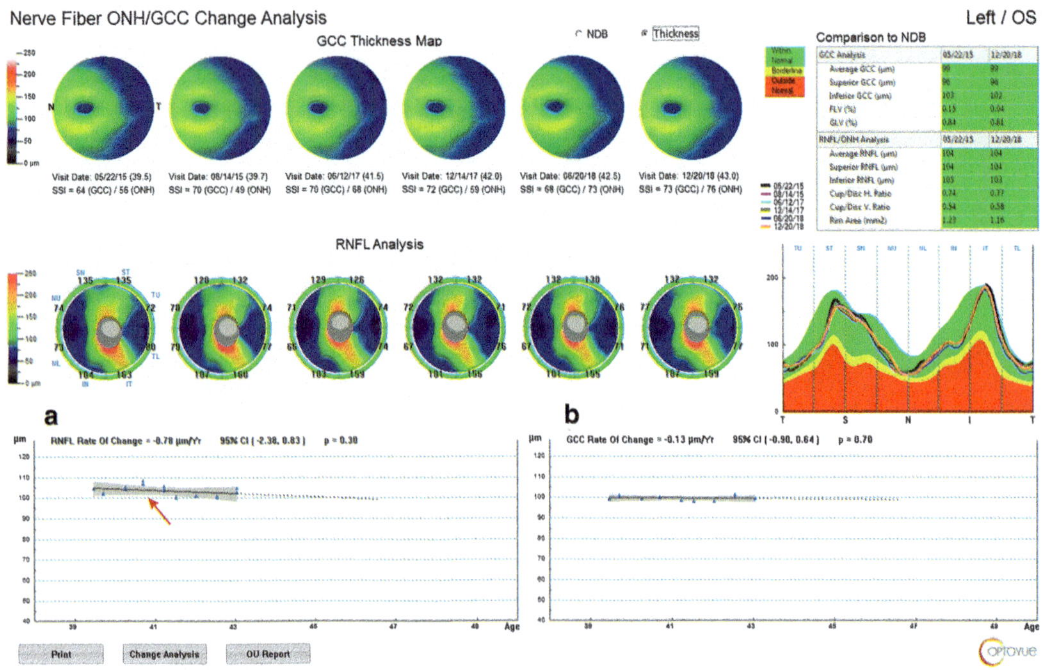

Fig. 6.4 Retinal nerve fiber layer thickness (RNFLT) and inner macular retina thickness (ganglion cell complex, GCC) progression report of an eye with a large and oval disc: (**a**) Due to the inconsistent use of disc margin definition plains in the different follow-up visits the stable (non-progressive) peripapillary RNFLT shows increased fluctuation (arrow) and (**b**) the corresponding inner macular retina thickness (GCC) values show less fluctuation than RNFLT

retina thickness (ganglion cell complex, GCC) values (Fig. 6.4b). In the presented case no glaucomatous progression is seen. But when progression occurs, increased measurement variability may delay the detection of significant progression by the instrument's software.

6.3 Imaging Errors Due to Ocular Abnormalities

Vitreous floaters are common in myopic and glaucomatous eyes and in the general elderly population. Vitreous floaters block the illuminating and reflected light during OCT examination [2]. Therefore, they cause segmentation errors and falsely low measured values (shadow effect). Complete elimination of vitreous floaters from an image area is not always possible. Asking the patient to blink may help to remove the floaters from the image area. Figure 6.5 shows an optic nerve head image acquired for OCT angiography analysis. The large vitreous floater in the superotemporal part of the vitreous body causes shadow effect over the superotemporal peripapillary sector and the superotemporal ONH, which results in a falsely low (practically zero) measured perfusion in these areas. This image cannot be used for global peripapillary or disc perfusion measurement, but can be used for perfusion measurement in those peripapillary sectors which are outside the area of the artifact. Some vitreous floaters have an arcuate shape which imitates a retinal nerve fiber bundle defect on the printed OCT report when the floater is close to the ONH [3].

Figure 6.6 shows a small vitreous floater that causes a localized shadow effect and a segmentation error when RNFLT is measured. This scan is not suitable to 360° peripapillary RNFLT measurement since the measured RNFLT is falsely low in the affected area.

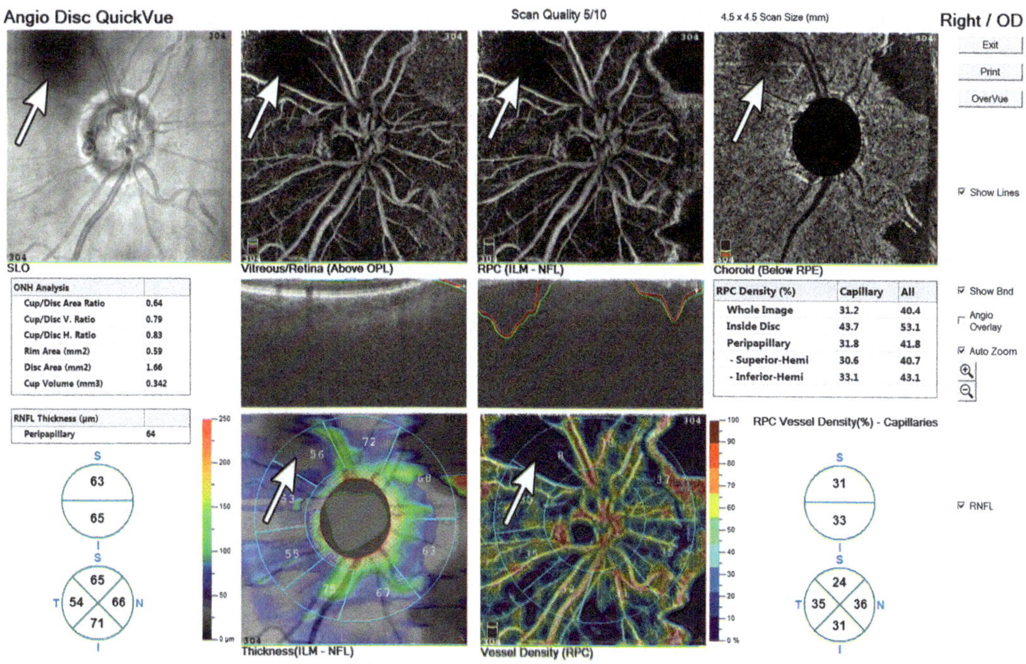

Fig. 6.5 Shadow artifact caused by a large vitreous floater on the scanning laser ophthalmoscopy (SLO), vessel density and retinal nerve fiber layer thickness images and maps (arrow) on an optical coherence tomography angiography scan

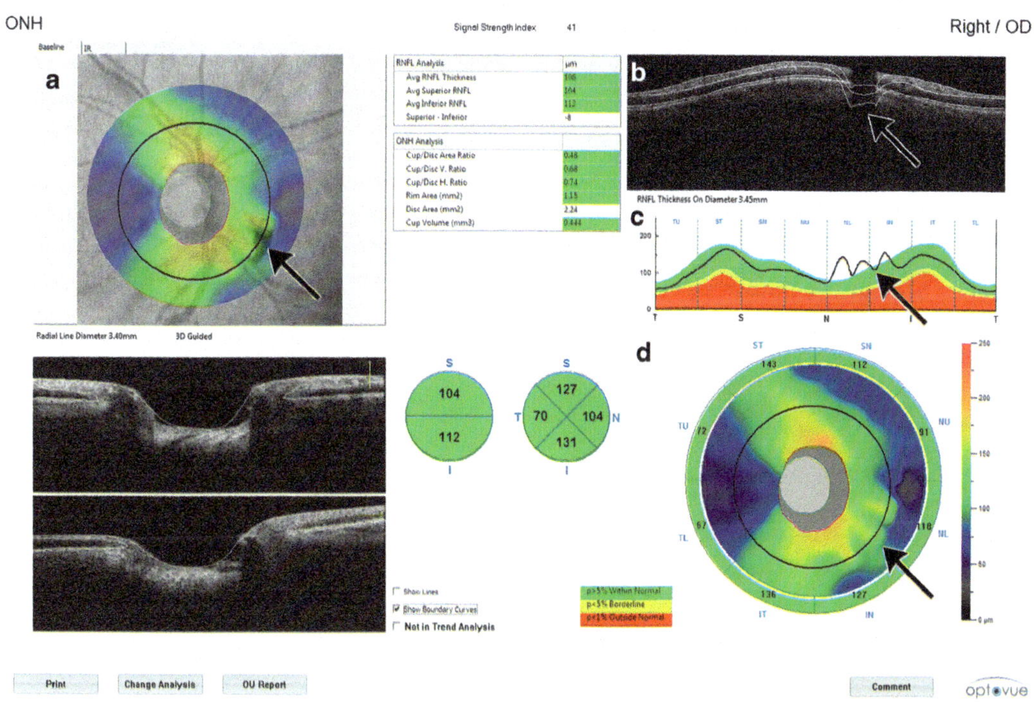

Fig. 6.6 Segmentation artifact and shadow effect caused by a small vitreous floater on a RNFLT scan. (**a**) The vitreous floater (arrow) is located in front of the inferonasal section of the RNFLT measuring ellipse; (**b** and **c**) Due to the floater's shadow effect the RNFLT signal is missing (arrow), and the segmentation is erroneous (arrow) in the inferonasal peripapillary area. (**d**) The color-coded RNFLT map also shows an RNFLT artifact in the corresponding position (arrow)

It is important to note that the measured thickness values are not always tissue specific on the OCT images. Any additional volume in the retina is automatically considered by the software as a part of the anatomically expected tissue layer [2]. If a detailed fundus examination is not performed prior to ONH imaging the nature of the alteration remains unrecognized, and the pathology's effect on the image falsely suggests normal thickness even when the true thickness is low. Such cases are most commonly seen in the peripapillary retina, where the pathologies cause falsely high RNFLT values [2]. Figure 6.7 illustrates how myelinated nerve fibers cause a circumscribed increase of the measured peripapillary RNFLT. The myelin sheets represent an additional volume. Therefore, the myelinated nerve fibers increase the spatially corresponding RNFLT value [4]. In addition, they cause a shadow artifact in the deep peripapillary retinal layers. Myelinated nerve fibers (and various other retinal pathologies) may also block the OCT angiography signals. This results in a falsely low or absent perfusion result in the corresponding image area [2, 4].

In contrast to myelinated nerve fibers several other pathologies are not stable conditions, and the artifacts caused by them also change with time. The most common sources of such artifacts are peripapillary retinal bleedings. Figure 6.8

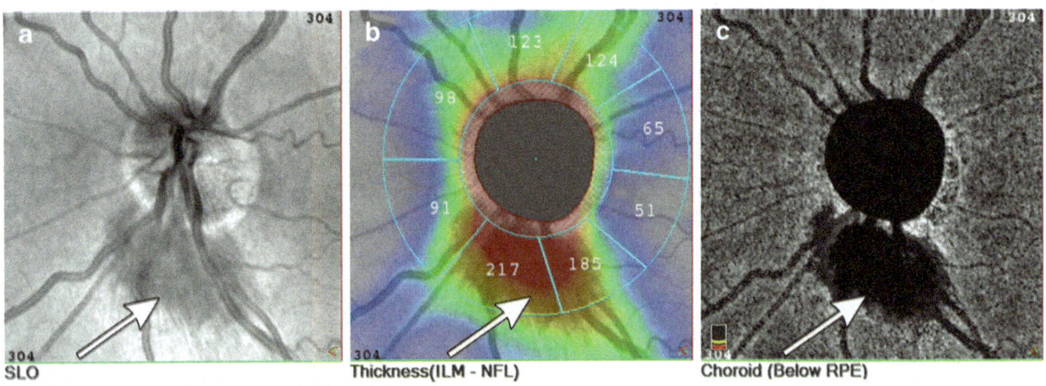

Fig. 6.7 Influence of myelinated nerve fibers on the measured RNFLT and the choroid: (**a**) Scanning laser ophthalmoscopy (SLO) image shows myelinated retinal nerve fibers (arrow) adjacent to the optic nerve head; (**b**) Myelinated fibers are considered as a part of the RNFLT by the optical coherence tomography software. This results in an increased RNFLT in the inferior peripapillary sectors (arrow); (**c**) In the choroid, the myelinated fibers cause a localized shadow effect (arrow)

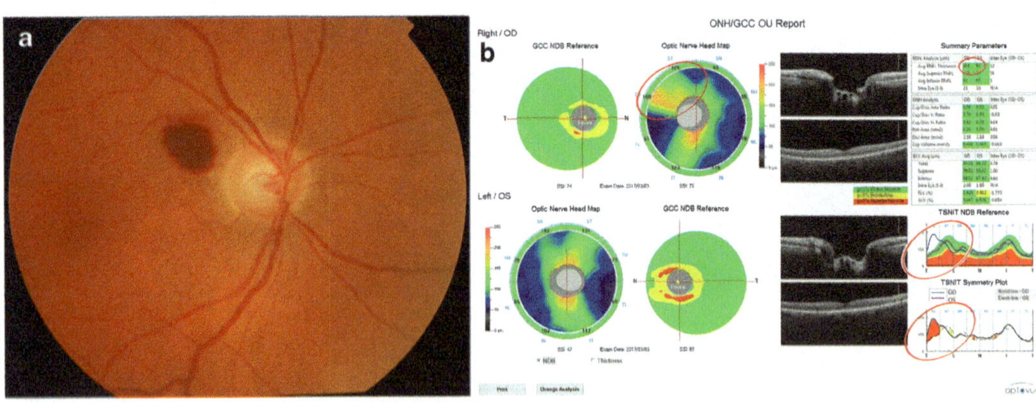

Fig. 6.8 Influence of a localized hemorrhage under the internal limiting membrane on the retinal nerve fiber layer thickness (RNFLT) measurement: (**a**) The hemorrhage is located in the superotemporal peripapillary sector of the right eye; (**b**) The corresponding sector RNFLT is erroneously high on the RNFLT map, the RNFLT symmetry plot and in the summary parameters table (encircled)

shows a localized superficial peripapillary hemorrhage, which was an incidental finding. The artifact causes supernormal RNFLT value in the temporal upper peripapillary sector. In a glaucoma eye a similar artifact can mask glaucomatous retinal nerve fiber layer thinning, make diagnosing glaucoma more difficult, or prevent detecting glaucomatous RNFLT progression.

Reflective posterior lens capsule opacities developing after cataract surgery may cause strange and irregular signals, which make the images clinically unusable. These effects, however, may disappear after laser capsulotomy, which makes the eye once again suitable to imaging. When long-term progression analysis is made in a glaucoma eye the technically incorrect images must not be included in the analysis. If they are included in the analysis, the extreme variability of the values widens the confidence interval (Fig. 6.9), which makes it impossible to detect or exclude true changes, e.g. glaucomatous progression.

6.4 Errors Due to Misinterpretation of ONH Images

There are typical cases in which OCT imaging is technically correct, but the results are difficult to interpret, in particular when detailed clinical disc assessment is not performed. Healthy large optic nerve heads (macrodiscs) are commonly classified as "outside normal limits" or "borderline" by the OCT software [2]. Ophthalmologists need to know that the software-based classifications are not clinical decisions but simple comparisons of the actual measured parameter values with the corresponding age corrected normal parameter ranges. Thus, "outside normal limits" classification does not mean that the measured parameter is pathological. It means that the measured parameter is lower than 95% or 99% (as defined) of the reference values measured on healthy eyes. Since the optic disc is particularly variable in size and shape, [1] large and unusually shaped discs are commonly classified as "outside the normal limits." Treatment of such eyes only because they were labeled with a red ("outside normal limits") or a yellow ("borderline") flag by the software is incorrect. In these cases, clinical disc size assessment and use of other OCT parameters (e.g. RNFLT, macular inner retina thickness, or OCT angiography vessel density) are needed.

Edema of the disc leads to extreme RNFLT values on OCT examination. Since in most OCT systems the extremely high RNFLT values are not flagged, the color code remains green ("within normal limits"). However, these thickness values are in fact abnormal (Fig. 6.10). To recognize these cases, it is not enough to consider the color code on the printed report, but the actual thickness values have also to be evaluated. In order to do so clinicians need to be familiar with the healthy RNFLT values.

For each OCT parameter there is a minimal measurable value. Values below this limit cannot be measured (floor effect). The reason of this phenomenon is that below the floor the measurement noise exceeds the true parameter value, which therefore becomes undetectable. For RNFLT measurements the floor level is around 60 μm. In advanced glaucoma the true RNFLT values are also around 60 μm. Therefore, in the follow-up of advanced glaucoma the stability of RNFLT is not informative, and does not guarantee that the patient's glaucoma is well-controlled (Fig. 6.11).

There are pathologies which are difficult to interpret based on OCT imaging results. In these conditions the preset definitions of the various retinal layers and the real position of the layers do not match each other. Figure 6.12 shows a retinoschisis adjacent to the ONH. The superficial retinal layers are displaced towards the vitreous body. This causes segmentation errors and an abnormally high RNFLT value. In the measurement depth, where the retinal nerve fibers are expected by the software, only fluid is found. Since in the fluid there is no red blood cell movement, the OCT angiography image and the color-coded OCT angiography map falsely show lack of peripapillary capillary perfusion.

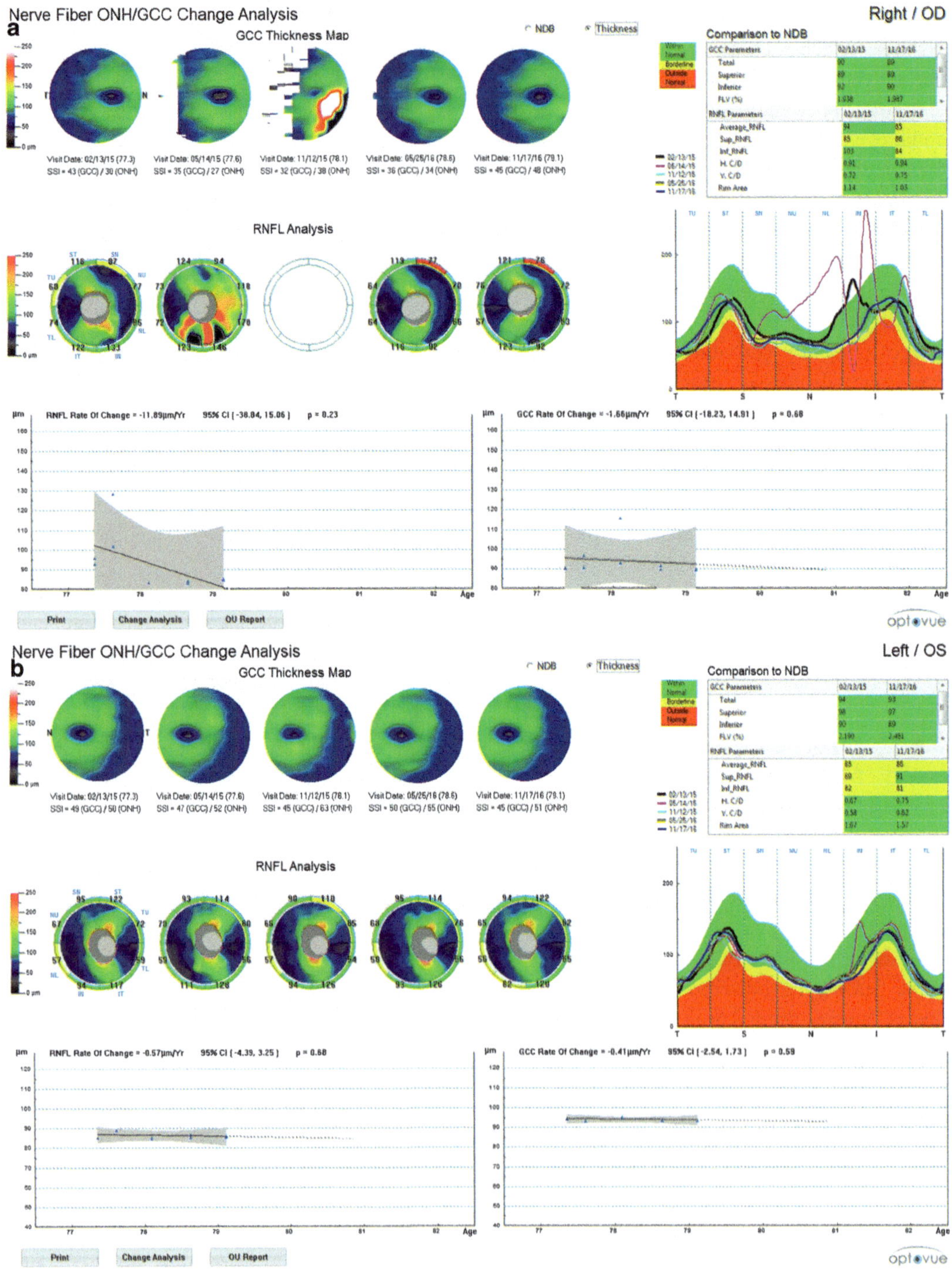

Fig. 6.9 Influence of highly reflective artifacts on peripapillary RNFLT progression analysis with OCT. (**a**) For the right eye, the first scan and the last two scans are technically correct, but the second and third scans are seriously influenced by reflective artifacts due to posterior lens capsule opacification, which developed after cataract surgery. The opacification was solved with laser capsulotomy, which resulted in the disappearance of the artifact. The erroneous scans were not excluded from the analysis. Therefore, the results are chaotic and not valid, and the confidence interval of the measurements (gray zone) is extremely wide. No conclusion can be drawn on the RNFLT stability. (**b**) In contrast, for the left eye of the same patient all RNFLT measurements are free from artifacts, the confidence interval of the thickness values is narrow, and the long-term stability of the RNFLT is proven

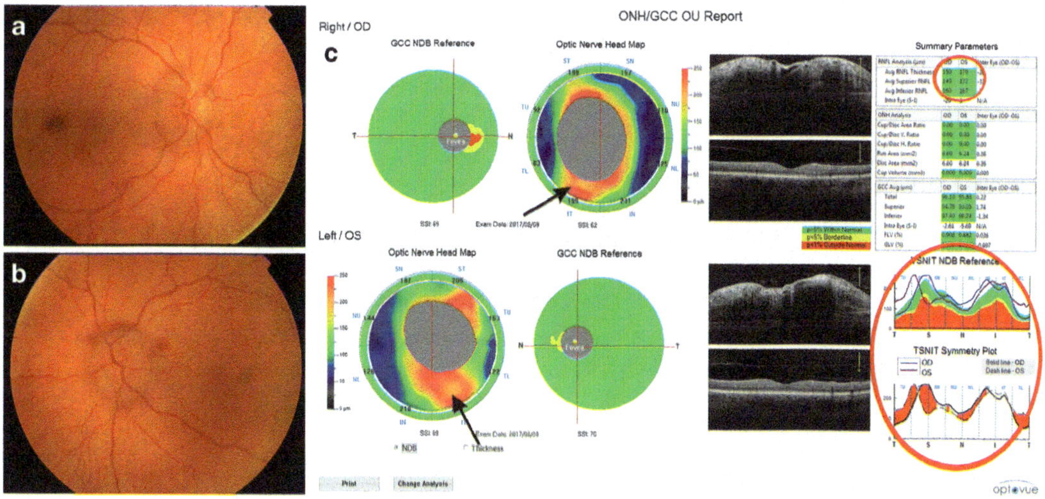

Fig. 6.10 Influence of disc swelling (bilateral chronic papilledema) due to an intracranial tumor on the optic disc and peripapillary thickness values with optical coherence tomography. (**a** and **b**) Fundus photograph of the swollen discs; (**c**) The abnormally high peripapillary RNFLT is indicated with arrows on the optic nerve head maps, and encircled on the RNFLT plots. The average RNFLT values in the summary parameters box (encircled) are clearly pathologically high values, but the color code is green ("within normal limits") because the software flags only the low RNFLT values

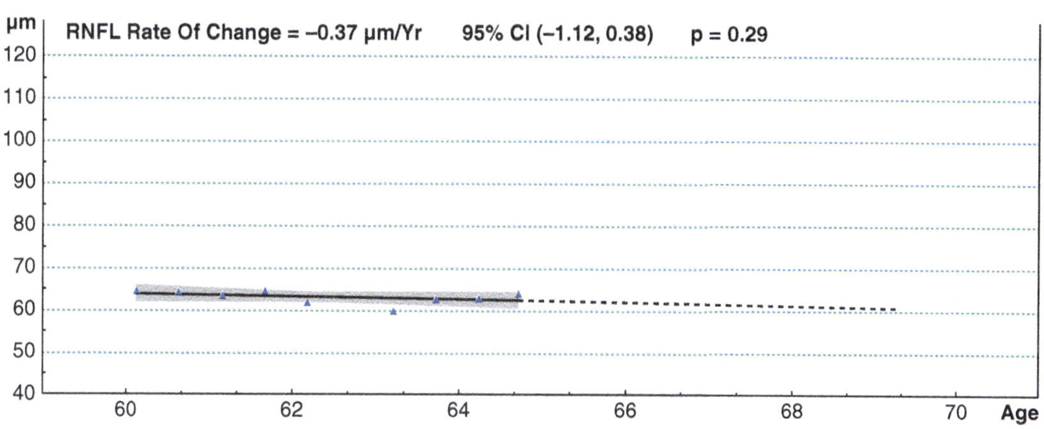

Fig. 6.11 RNFLT progression analysis in advanced glaucoma. The RNFLT values are stable, and there is no progression on the plot. Still, we cannot be sure about the true RNFLT stability since the RNFLT values have reached the measurement floor level, thus the software cannot detect any further RNFLT decrease

6.5 How to Prevent Errors in Disc and Peripapillary Imaging?

In order to prevent errors and artifacts in optic nerve head imaging use of a simple protocol is recommended (Table 6.1). Ophthalmologists have to be familiar with the imaging instruments available in the office [5]. They need to complete the clinical eye and fundus examination before they decide about the necessity of disc imaging and select the scan type. Imaging without a well-defined purpose, routine imaging before the eye is clinically examined, and acquiring the same scan type for all patients and eyes are not efficient, and result in artifacts and misinterpretations in a considerable number of the cases.

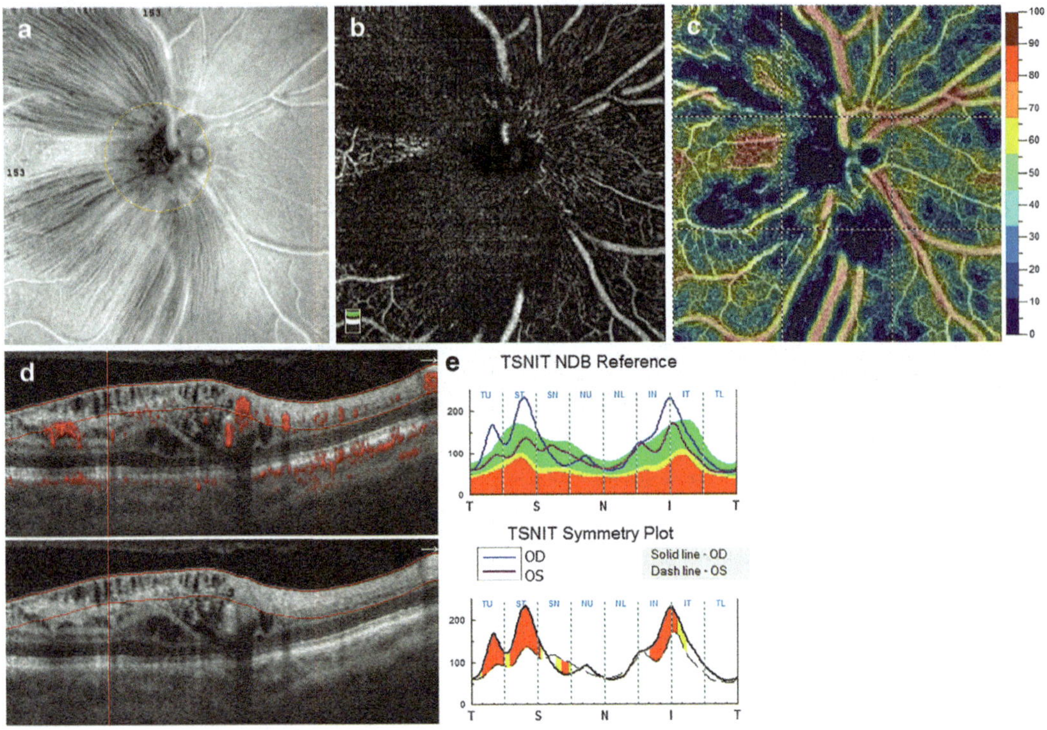

Fig. 6.12 Optical coherence tomography artifacts caused by a retinoschisis adjacent to the optic nerve head. (**a**) The superficial retinal layers are displaced towards the vitreous, which results in falsely high RNFLT values (**e**) and segmentation errors (**d**). In the plain where the retinal nerve fibers are expected by the software only fluid is found, which does not provide the expected red blood cell movement signals. Therefore, on the perfusion image (**b**) and the color-coded perfusion map (**c**) falsely low perfusion is shown for the retinal nerve fiber layer

Table 6.1 Proposed protocol to prevent using images with artifacts and making incorrect decision on disc images

Action	What to do?	Why to do it?
1.	Get familiar with the OCT instrument and its scan types available in the office, and read the instruction manual. In order to familiarize yourself with the technique acquire various scan types on healthy individuals with clear optical media	One cannot apply an instrument for clinical purposes on patients without understanding its function and limits, and being familiar with the scan options
2.	Complete the detailed eye examination including the disc and fundus evaluation before imaging even if the patient was examined earlier	In order to define information expected from OCT imaging one has to be able to set specific questions and select the scan types. The status of the eye might have altered since the last visit, which may influence the current image content and the measured values.
3.	When the images have been acquired, review them for artifacts and quality using the OCT instrument's screen and the software provided options. If necessary, delete the insufficient scans and substitute them with high-quality images	Artifacts and poor image quality lead to incorrect interpretation of the results, which may result in incorrect clinical decisions
4.	Evaluate the disc, the peripapillary image parameter values and the clinical eye examination results together in a comprehensive manner	No software provided parameter value or classification is meaningful, if the clinical picture is unknown or incorrectly understood
5.	If necessary, go for complementary scans to clarify any unanswered questions	Clinical questions may arise when the images provide new information. Additional scan types may clarify the situation and help to answer the clinical questions.

When the scans are completed a trained person (ideally the ophthalmologist who performed the clinical investigation) needs to review the result for artifacts and image quality, and substitute the insufficient images with high-quality scans. If acquiring a high-quality image for a fundus or disc area is impossible, one must accept that imaging in the particular case is not successful. One should not use misleading scans for clinical decision making. Unfortunately, many ophthalmologists use only printed OCT reports, and do not participate in the image analysis on the OCT instrument's screen. This practice does not allow detecting several artifact types presented in this chapter, since the printed report is only a simplified document, in which only selected information pieces are given.

References

1. Holló G. The optic nerve in glaucoma. In: Choplin NT, Traverso CE, editors. The atlas of glaucoma. 3rd ed. London: Informa Healthcare; 2013. p. 61–72.
2. Holló G. How to overcome imaging artifacts and prevent misinterpretation of imaging results? In: Bhartiya S, Ichhpujani P, editors. Clinical cases in glaucoma. An evidence-based approach. Delhi and New York: Jaypee Brothers; 2017. p. 145–52.
3. Holló G. Optical coherence tomography angiography and glaucoma. In: Chow DR, de Olivieria RPC, editors. OCT angiography. New York: Thieme Medical Publishers Inc.; 2017. p. 112–26.
4. Holló G. Influence of myelinated retinal nerve fibers on retinal vessel density measurement with AngioVue OCT angiography. Int Ophthalmol. 2016;36:915–9.
5. Holló G. What's new in optical coherence tomography angiography for glaucoma. In: Ichhpujani P, editor. Singapore: Springer Nature Singapore Pte Ltd; 2019. p. 91–106.

How to Interpret Difficult Optic Discs?

7

Parul Ichhpujani, Faisal TT, and Surinder Pandav

7.1 Introduction

Accurate assessment of both the optic disc or optic nerve head (ONH) and the visual field is crucial for the diagnosis of glaucoma. Optic disc assessment is more important out of the two because the visual field is usually only tested when the optic disc appears suspicious for glaucoma. Some studies have shown that the ability of ophthalmologists to discriminate between healthy and glaucomatous eyes is limited [1–3]. This chapter addresses some basic aspects that pose difficulty in interpretation and some aberrant discs that pose a diagnostic dilemma.

A recent European study explored the ability of many general ophthalmologists to judge optic disc photographs for the detection of glaucoma. The overall diagnostic accuracy of ophthalmologists was 80.5% but there was large variability in diagnostic accuracy among and agreement within clinicians [4]. This variability is likely to be more marked in discs with anatomical variations.

The Glaucomatous Optic Neuropathy Evaluation (GONE) Project (www.gone-project.com) was developed to benchmark optic disc examination among eye care professionals and the researchers found that even among ophthalmologists, the diagnostic accuracy was variable [5]. Ophthalmology trainees and comprehensive ophthalmologists were twice as likely to underestimate glaucoma as overestimate it. In optic discs that glaucoma subspecialists graded as probable or definite glaucoma, ophthalmology trainees and comprehensive ophthalmologists underestimated glaucoma likelihood in a mean of 22.1 and 23.8%, respectively. For the optic discs graded as possible or unlikely glaucoma by glaucoma subspecialists, ophthalmology trainees and comprehensive ophthalmologists overestimated glaucoma likelihood in a mean of 13.0 and 8.9%, respectively. Errors in the assessment of Vertical Cup: Disc Ratio (VCDR), Retinal nerve fiber layer (RNFL), neuroretinal rim (NRR) loss, and disc hemorrhage were the most influential factors that led to incorrect estimation of glaucoma likelihood [5].

Neural rim seemingly has the maximum variability as shown by Ramrattan et al. who have reported a three-fold variation in their study participants of the Rotterdam Eye Study [6], and Jonas et al. who have reported almost a six-fold variability in their study of 457 normal Caucasian eyes [7].

Horizontally ovoid optic discs were at a higher risk of having glaucoma likelihood underestimated by ophthalmology trainees, due to the influence of disc shape on other VCDR or cup

P. Ichhpujani
Glaucoma Service, Department of Ophthalmology, Government Medical College and Hospital, Chandigarh, India

F. TT · S. Pandav (✉)
Advanced Eye Centre, Post Graduate Institute of Medical Education and Research, Chandigarh, India

S. Pandav et al. (eds.), *The Optic Nerve Head in Health and Disease*,
https://doi.org/10.1007/978-981-33-6838-5_7

shape in these discs [5]. These errors can be minimized by using more thorough disc evaluation nomograms such as Disc Damage Likelihood Scale (DDLS).

Disc characteristics, such as the shape and size of the optic disc and the presence or absence of peripapillary atrophy (PPA), can influence the diagnostic accuracy. Eyes with moderate to severe PPA make it difficult to identify the outer margin of optic disc. One must identify the scleral rim and not the zone of sclera visible due to PPA. Scleral rim appears as a white ring, about the size of a small artery, and is most visible on the nasal and temporal margins. The identification of this feature becomes difficult with aging, as the NRR becomes sloped and its color changes from orange-pink to yellow-gray due to media changes [8].

It is apparent that ONH appearance can vary significantly in glaucomatous as well as non-glaucomatous eyes. This creates difficulties in correct classification of the discs from glaucoma point of view, more so where the underlying structure is unexpected or not clearly identified.

This brings us to the question how we can overcome these difficulties to minimize errors in diagnosis. There are a number of ways described to examine discs for glaucoma. Classical approach described by Armaly is to systemically look for signs of glaucoma such as the cup-to-disc ratio (CDR), NRR thinning, notching or the rim, nasalization of vessels, bayoneting, etc. [9]. As we know, CDR is the ratio of cup diameter to disc diameter, and depends on the size of the optic disc and cup. The CDR also shows interindividual variability being higher in large discs and lower in smaller discs. Additionally, the application of the evaluation rules of CDR is not appropriate for subjects with an optic nerve or disc anomaly (tilted, hypoplastic, dysplastic nerves).

The way to discern the CDR is to define the inner margins of the scleral canal and neural rim. Point of deviation of small blood vessels on the surface of the ONH (contour method) and not the area of pallor in the center of the optic disc (color contrast method) helps delineate the rim margin [7, 10].

R Sussana proposed study of **5R**s to diagnose glaucoma—**R**ing (identification of scleral ring), **R**im (neuroretinal rim), **R**etinal nerve fiber layer, **R**egion of PPA, **R**etinal/disc hemorrhages [11]. This approach was originally published as a PowerPoint monograph entitled FORGE (Focusing Ophthalmology on Reframing Glaucoma Evaluation). This approach had a flaw that it did not consider disc size.

DDLS developed by George Spaeth aims to minimize the issues with the CDR estimation, by taking into account the rim configuration, adjusted for the disc size. It is a ten stage system that grades the optic disc according to amount of damage based on the narrowest width of the rim and on the vertical disc diameter [12, 13]. The DDLS formalizes the process of examining the NRR as the examiner is forced to examine the NRR throughout its circumference. The method has a learning curve and is best practised with the DDLS nomogram at hand while evaluating ONH.

More recently, the "outside-in" approach has been proposed to better differentiate glaucomatous discs from the normal (Chap. 5). Optic disc evaluation for glaucoma is a clinical skill which has been taught for many decades in different ways. This skill seems to be difficult to acquire as rates of underdiagnosis are still high as about half of glaucoma patients in the community remain undiagnosed [14].

Many years of learning is required to become proficient in the art of examining optic discs. In this chapter, we propose a different approach where we emphasize on focusing on what is important. Here we emphasize on qualitative assessment of the neural tissue for its adequacy, any regions of tissue loss, and signs suggestive of ill health. Glaucomatous optic neuropathy can be identified by distinctive patterns of disc damage that forms the cornerstone of clinical diagnosis of glaucoma. This chapter builds on our innate ability to identify patterns. Human beings are naturally good in recognizing patterns around us—we recognize people from their faces almost instantaneously. With practice this trait can be utilized to recognize glaucomatous optic discs as well.

7.2 Where Is the Money?

A number of variables are considered while examining discs for glaucoma. Even normal discs can vary a lot as discussed earlier (see Chap. 1). Therefore, identifying a glaucomatous change within "variable normality" is a challenge. This gets further compounded in discs with obvious anatomical defects or uncertain underlying structure. In this context it helps if we focus on structures that are most important for visual function. Structure–function relationship in glaucoma is well documented but not that well understood [15]. Structural change in the ONH and RNFL can largely predict the occurrence and location of visual field defects [16]. However, some patients can have disc changes suggestive of glaucoma without detectable field defect and vice versa. The most important structure to look for, that we can examine clinically, is the neural tissue which is represented by NRR and RNFL. The classical optic disc signs of glaucoma are basically clues that help us decide whether there is loss of neural tissue or not. These signs are meant to lead us towards the correct diagnosis—thinning of NRR or notching suggests loss of neural tissue. Enlargement of the cup or bayoneting of vessels is indicative of thinning of neural rim and deepening of the cup. But sometimes, if these signs are not interpreted in proper context, it can lead to incorrect conclusions. PPA is often associated with glaucoma but all eyes with PPA do not have glaucoma. Obvious PPA thus can also bias us towards glaucoma diagnosis [5]. Therefore, it is important to examine the NRR especially in the region adjacent to PPA. Similarly, disc size will influence the assessment of neural tissue present in the disc. Same amount of neural tissue will fill discs of different shapes and sizes differently. Since neural tissue is distributed along the periphery of the disc, in a large disc there will be a large area in the center devoid of nerve fibers (cup) and NRR will appear thin. Such discs can be mistaken for glaucomatous discs. On the contrary, same amount of neural tissue will fill a small disc completely without leaving any space without nerve fibers (cup). Loss of neural tissue in this small disc is difficult to ascertain as we are accustomed to see some cup in the discs. A stereotype image of the disc is that with a cup in the center. So a small disc with a cup is likely to be passed off as normal. Thus, consideration must be given to the amount of neural tissue present in the disc. Therefore, first thing to do is to identify the neural tissue and assess how much tissue is there. Keeping disc size in mind, irrespective of the shape of the disc or presence of tilt or other anomalies a, reasonable estimate can be made to say whether neural tissue is adequate or less or scanty or absent. Agreed that it is a subjective way of assessment but once we have consciously "dissected" the neural tissue it is possible to say whether the tissue is enough or less (Figs. 7.1, 7.2, 7.3, 7.4, 7.5, 7.6).

Second important thing to consider while evaluating the neural tissue in the disc is to look for its distribution. Neural tissue is not distributed evenly over the optic disc even in a normal disc. Rim tissue is most abundant in the inferior half of the disc. ISNT rule (the thickest part of a healthy neural rim is located in the inferior quadrant, followed by the superior, nasal, and temporal quadrants) is applicable to normal discs and is considered as a good guide to assess neural tissue distribution in the disc [7, 17]. Neural tissue loss in glaucoma is not uniform. Superior and/ or inferior poles of the disc are often the first to manifest changes (Figs. 7.7 and 7.8). When that happens normal distribution of neural tissue is altered. Clinically, it would be seen as thinning of the NRR or rim notch. Diffuse loss of neural tissue may lead to concentric enlargement of the cup making it hard to detect changes. Therefore, it is very important to look for any areas of thinning, notching, or irregularities in the NRR tissue. The typical sequence of NRR loss in glaucoma is the inferotemporal and supero-temporal, followed by the temporal, inferonasal, superonasal and, finally, the nasal sectors [18]. NRR notching usually does not occur in the temporal or nasal quadrant. Temporal NRR notching without other tell-tale signs of glaucomatous damage is likely to be associated with an optic disc insertion anomaly. Some studies have shown that ISNT rule has poor specificity for detecting

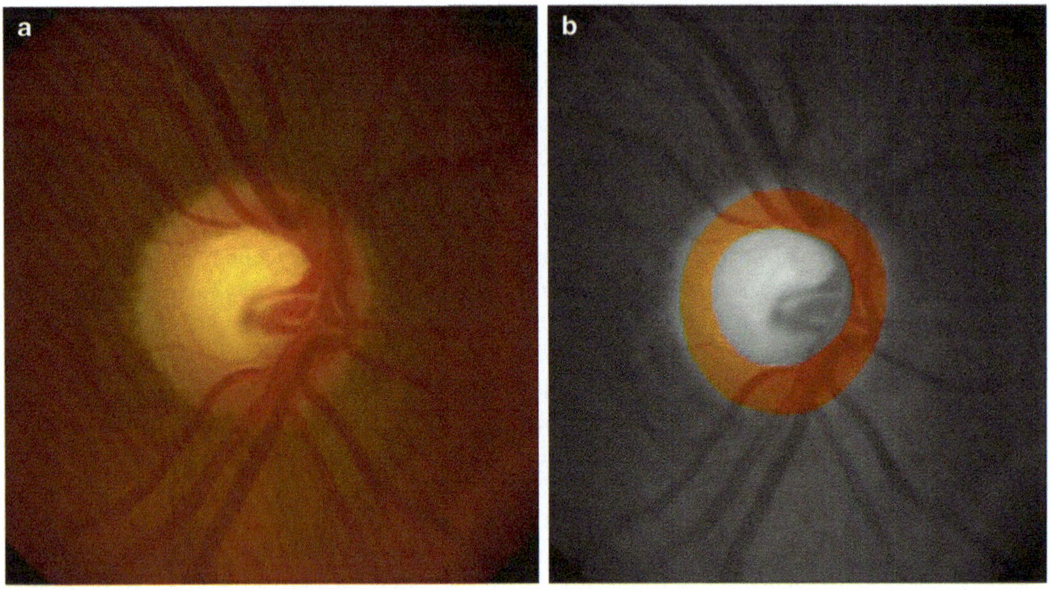

Fig. 7.1 Disc with adequate neural tissue. (**a**) Normal size disc with moderately deep cup. NRR is well defined with regular and smooth contour. (**b**) This figure emphasizes "mental dissection" of the neural tissue to isolate it from other structures. That way we can focus better on the structure that is most important and pick up abnormalities if any

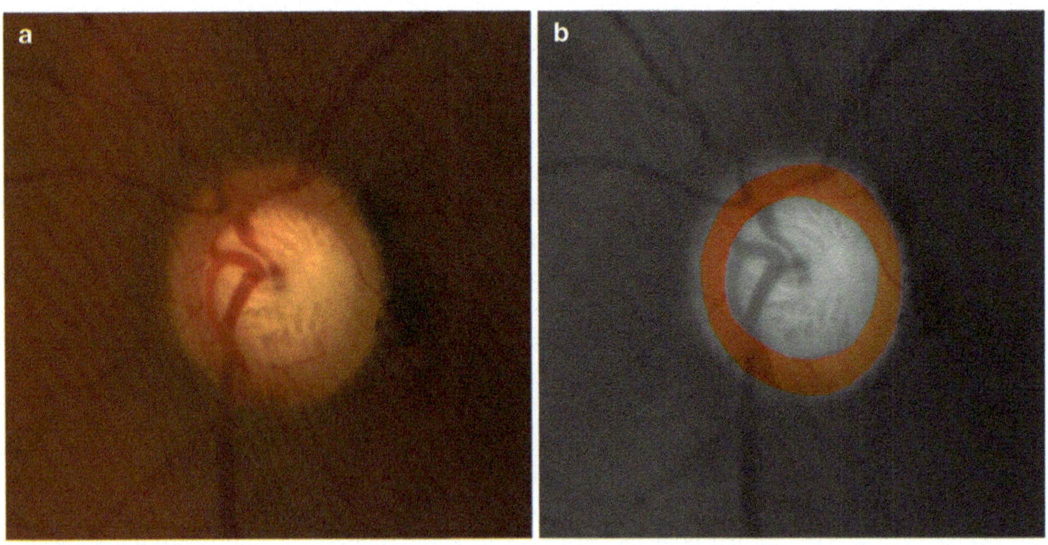

Fig. 7.2 (**a**) Slightly large disc (upper side of normal) with deep cup. Laminar dots are visible. There is good amount of NRR with well-defined smooth contour. (**b**) There is subtle irregularity at the inner margin of the superior NRR. This disc is somewhat different from the "normal disc" as seen in Fig. 7.1, but glaucoma is unlikely as there is enough neural tissue without any clear evidence of rim loss or damage (glaucoma unlikely)

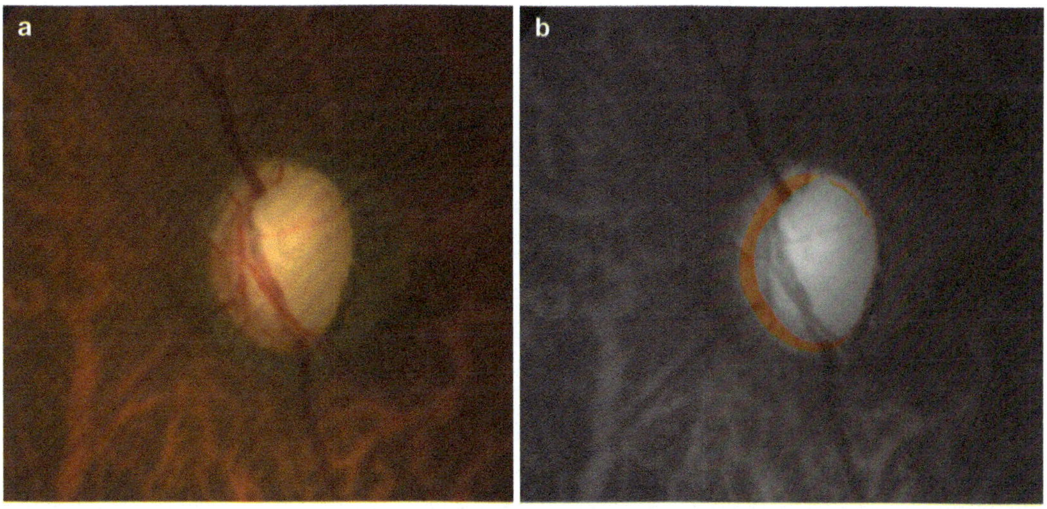

Fig. 7.3 (**a** and **b**) There is very small amount of NRR visible in this disc indicative of marked loss of neural tissue. This along with other signs like large deep cup, nasal shifting of vessels, presence of PPA are indicative of advanced glaucomatous damage

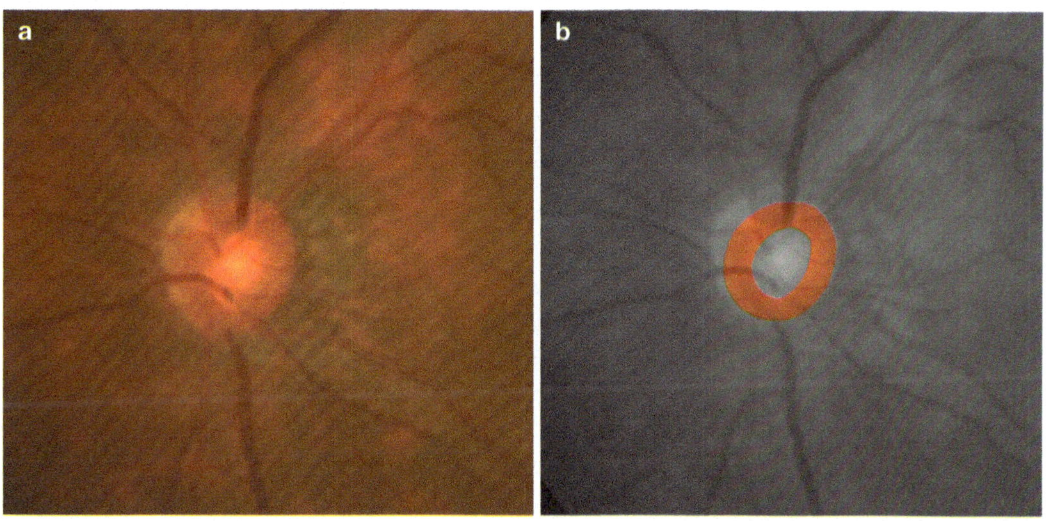

Fig. 7.4 (**a**) Small disc with cup. NRR is well defined and regular with shallow cup which can be easily missed. (**b**) On dissecting the NRR, overall amount of neural tissue appears less. This disc does not look obviously glaucomatous but possibility remains (glaucoma possible)

glaucomatous damage due to the confounding effects of optic disc size, variability of tilt, and vascular trunk location [19, 20]. Therefore, in anatomically different discs such as tilted discs, very large discs, discs with pits, colobomatous or hypoplastic discs, ISNT rule is not helpful. In these situations a careful delineation of the NRR tissue to look for any unexpected areas of thinning is important and can give clues to the diagnosis.

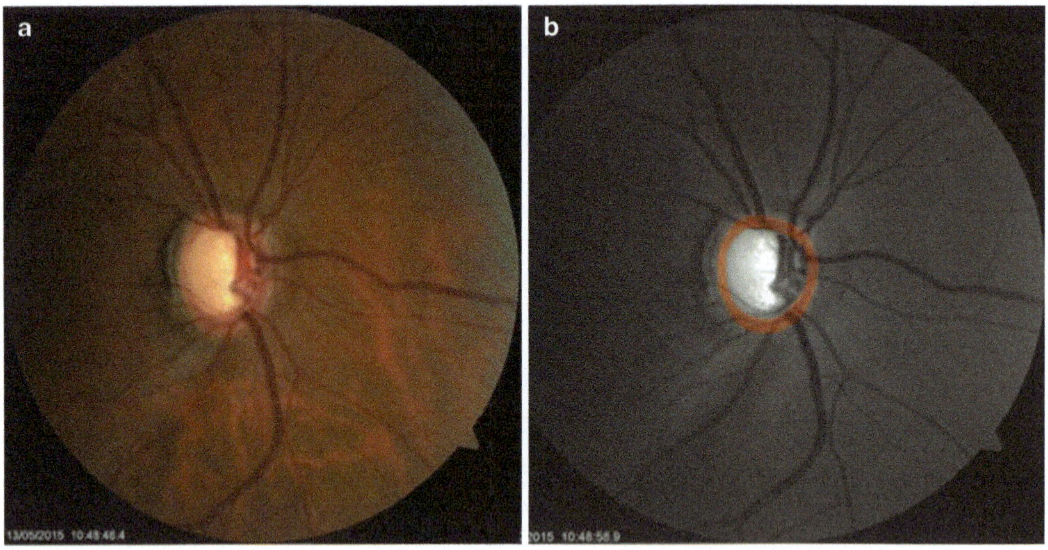

Fig. 7.5 (**a**) Large disc with large cup and mild concentric thinning of rim tissue. Also there is baring of circumlinear vessel along the inferior rim margin. (**b**) On dissecting the NRR, concentric NRR loss is seen along with RNFL defect inferiorly (glaucoma likely)

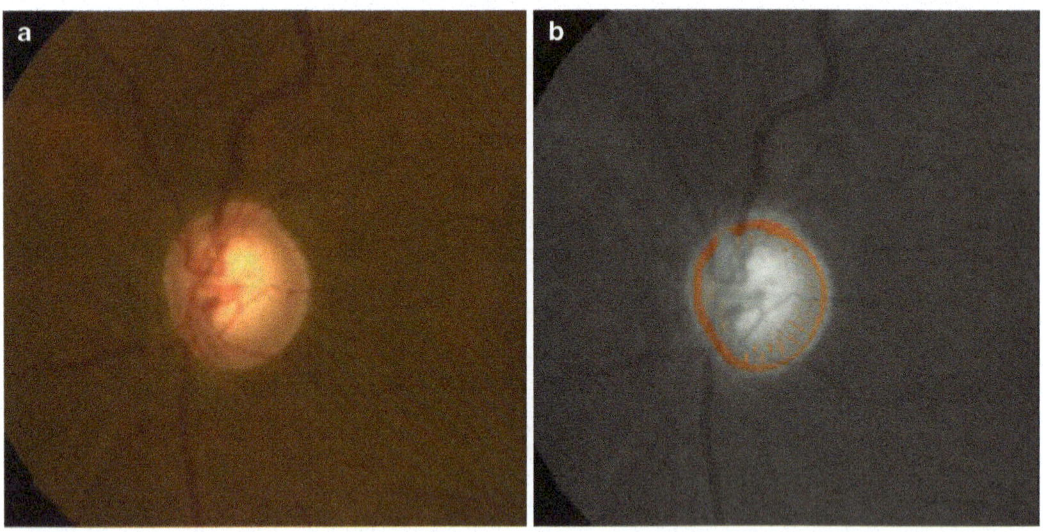

Fig. 7.6 (**a**) Average size disc with large cup and marked thinning of the NRR. There is marked discrepancy between "cup by colour" and "cup by contour." In such discs glaucoma damage is underestimated or even missed. (**b**) Rim margin is hard to define due to marked saucerization in all quadrants. RNFL is not visible—diffuse loss

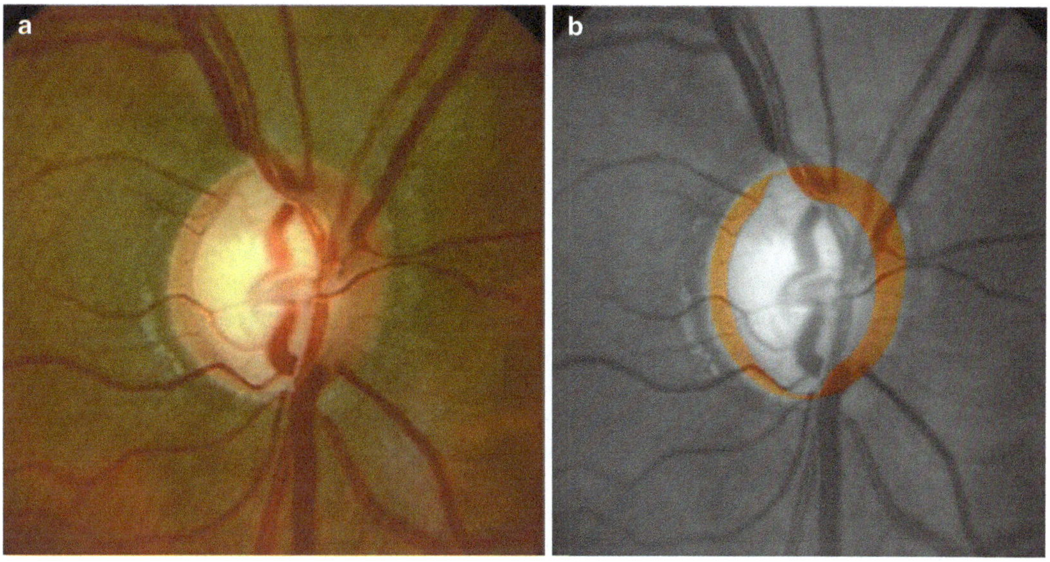

Fig. 7.7 (**a**) Disc size is towards upper side of normal with good amount of rim tissue on nasal and temporal sides. Neural tissue is missing at superior and inferior poles of the disc. (**b**) There is overall reduction in the amount of neural tissue with superior and inferior notch. This pattern of NRR loss along with large VCDR, deep cup, and defects in the RNFL is certainly suggestive of glaucoma

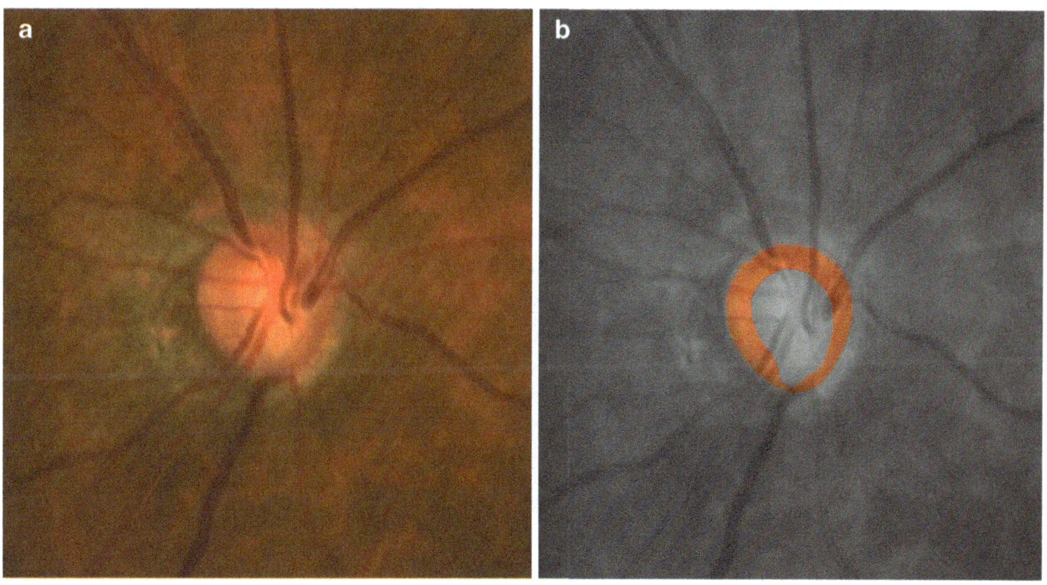

Fig. 7.8 (**a**) Small disc with cup and focal rim loss. It is easy to miss disc cupping and rim notch in a small disc if you are not careful. Casual observer may pass this disc as normal. (**b**) If you "mentally dissect" this disc, loss of neural tissue inferiorly is quite evident, suggestive of glaucoma

7.3 Where to Dig for the Treasure?

We need to ask three questions about the disc.

1. Is there enough neural tissue?
2. Is the neural tissue distributed normally?
3. Is it healthy?

To answer these questions the key skill required is delineation of boundaries of the neural tissue. This is a clinical skill and can be mastered with practice. The outer limit of the NRR is defined by the inner edge of the scleral canal; therefore, identifying the anatomy of the scleral canal is important (Fig. 7.9). Special care is needed in defining scleral canal in patients with marked PPA or with myopic degeneration. The demarcation between the rim and the cup, i.e., inner edge of the NRR may not be clearcut due to sloping nature of the rim in certain parts in many discs. Course of smaller blood vessels over the disc is used as a guide to define the NRR edge, as mentioned earlier. Vessels bend as they pass over the edge of the rim, the point of bending is taken as inner limit of the NRR. Stereoscopic view is helpful in detecting the point where nerve fibers dip down towards lamina cribrosa creating a cliff of neural tissue. Central disc pallor also indicates extent of the disc cupping; however, it is not very reliable in itself. When it corresponds with the stereoscopic clues and vessel bending, all add up to a reliable inner limit of the NRR. Inner margin of the NRR is easier to define in discs with moderate to deep cups but difficult if the cup is very shallow.

Discs with unusual anatomy are difficult to interpret as various clues we use may be placed differently and sometimes it is hard to identify various landmarks. Focusing primarily on neural tissue is helpful as its variations then can be explained on the basis of altered anatomy and distinguish them from pathological state.

Here are a few examples of such discs:

7.3.1 Tilted Discs

Usually, an optic disc is considered torted when the vertical axis of the optic disc is rotated >15° from the vertical meridian and is considered tilted when there is (three-dimensional) angulation of the (anteroposterior) optic cup axis (best commented on a stereo photograph after the clinical examination).

In the tilted optic disc syndrome, the superior pole of the optic disc may appear elevated with

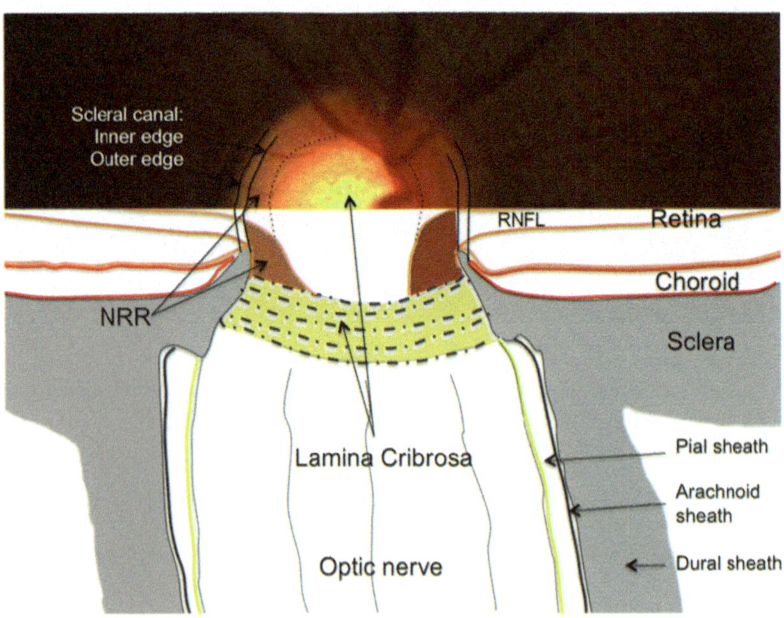

Fig. 7.9 Schematic anatomy of the optic nerve head. Accurate definition of inner edge of the scleral canal and inner margin on the NRR is important. Scleral canal margins are somewhat indistinct on the nasal side. Disc margin may further be obscured in small discs, discs with variable anatomy, presence of drusens and PPA

posterior displacement of the inferonasal disc, or the disc can be horizontally tilted, resulting in an oval-appearing optic disc with an obliquely oriented long axis [21].

It may be accompanied by an inferior or inferonasal scleral crescent, situs inversus (a nasal detour of the temporal retinal vessels as they emerge from the disc before turning back temporally), and posterior ectasia of the inferior nasal fundus. Figures 7.10, 7.11, and 7.12 show vertical and horizontal tilt.

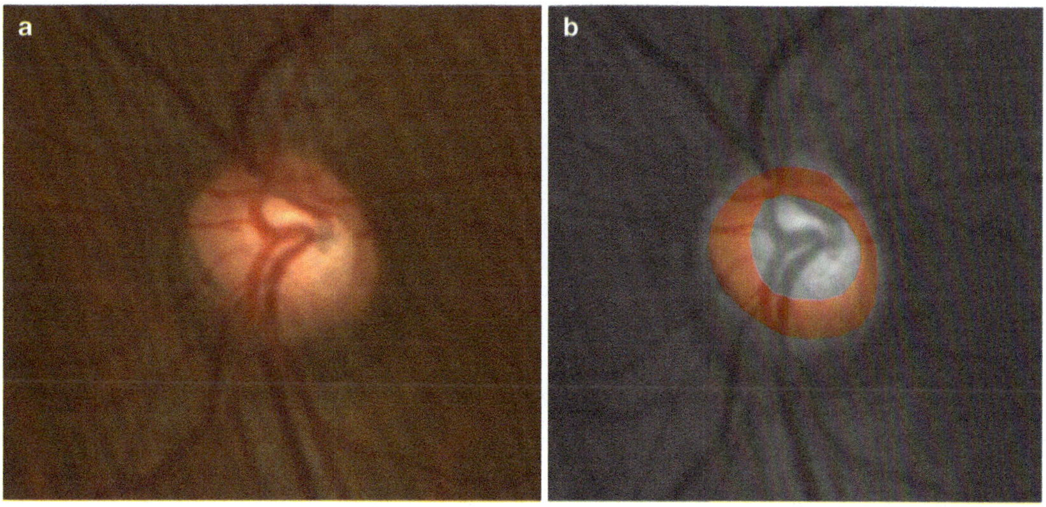

Fig. 7.10 (**a**) The disc is tilted obliquely. Good amount of neural tissue is there. The temporal rim is seen more prominently due to the tilt. (**b**) On mental dissection of NRR, inferior rim looks more like "normal" temporal side. There is no evidence of focal tissue loss. However, the disc is a bit on smaller side and has shallow cup (glaucoma unlikely)

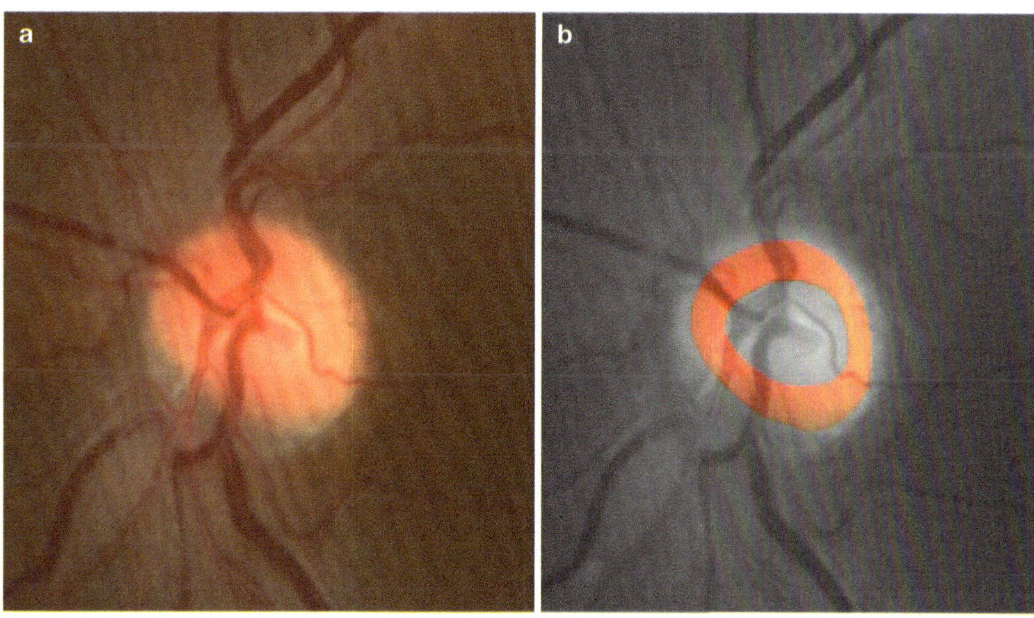

Fig. 7.11 (**a**) The disc has mild vertical tilt with altered pattern of vessels. (**b**) There is enough neural tissue with shallow, not so well-defined cup. Unlikely to have glaucoma

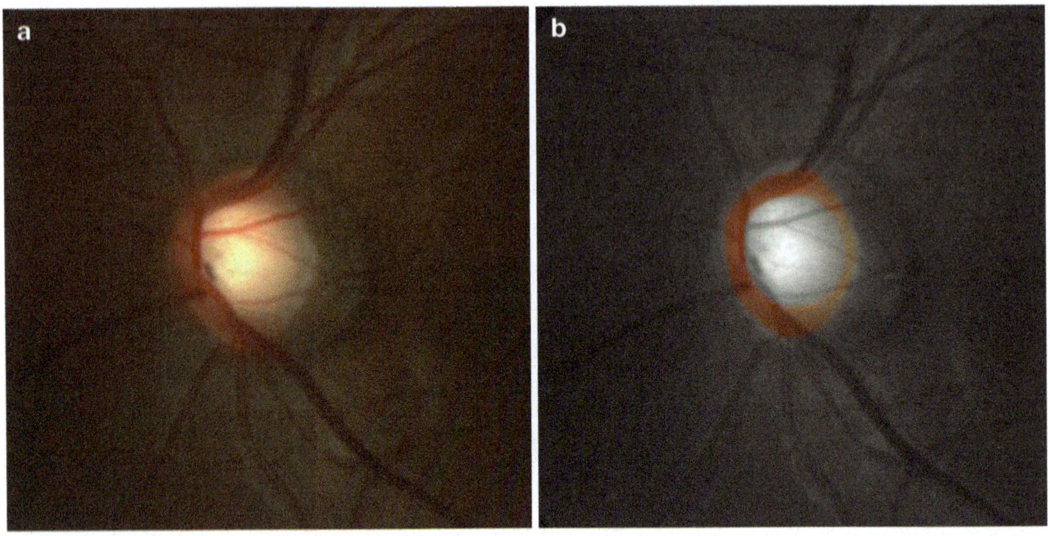

Fig. 7.12 (**a**) This disc shows marked horizontal tilt. The main vascular trunk is hidden under the nasal rim. NRR is well defined nasally, superiorly, and inferiorly. It looks a bit thin but contour is smooth and regular. NRR on temporal is difficult to define which is usually the case in tilted discs. Rim details are obscured due to more reflective background on temporal side. B. On focusing at the NRR, good amount of neural tissue without any evidence of focal loss is noted. Peripapillary RNFL does not show any defects. Glaucoma is unlikely

7.3.2 Situs Inversus of the Disc (Discus Inversus)

Situs inversus of the optic disc is a rare, usually bilateral, developmental abnormality associated with high myopia or myopic astigmatism due to anomalous curvature of the posterior segment, tilted optic disc or optic disc coloboma. It may also be seen in otherwise normal, healthy eyes as an incidental finding. It is characterized by dysversion of the optic disc with emergence of the retinal vessels in an anomalous direction (Fig. 7.13) [22].

7.3.3 Medullated Nerve Fibers

The typical appearance of myelinated or medullated nerve fibers is of a distinct peripapillary white striated patch with feathered borders approximately one disc diameter or larger in size (Fig. 7.14). Interestingly, these medullated fibers may also disappear with time in patients with several neurologic, inflammatory, and retinal diseases [23]. It is hypothesized that the disappearance of these fibers signals pathological degeneration of the retinal nerve axons. The neurological disease associations include pituitary adenoma, optic neuritis, and primary open angle glaucoma [24]. These fibers maybe associated with relative afferent pupillary defect, visual field deficits, optic disc drusen, and optic nerve hypoplasia. OCT will not be reliable in measuring RNFL thickness or disc parameters.

7.3.4 Morning Glory Anomaly

Morning glory anomaly is a congenital malformation of the optic nerve, wherein increased number of straight retinal vessels arises from the disc margin with or without associated peripapillary pigmentation (Fig. 7.15) [25].

7.3.5 Optic Disc Coloboma

Optic disc colobomas present as a white excavation involving the inferior part of the optic disc (Fig. 7.16) and extending to the choroid and retina. Typically, optic nerve colobomas lack the

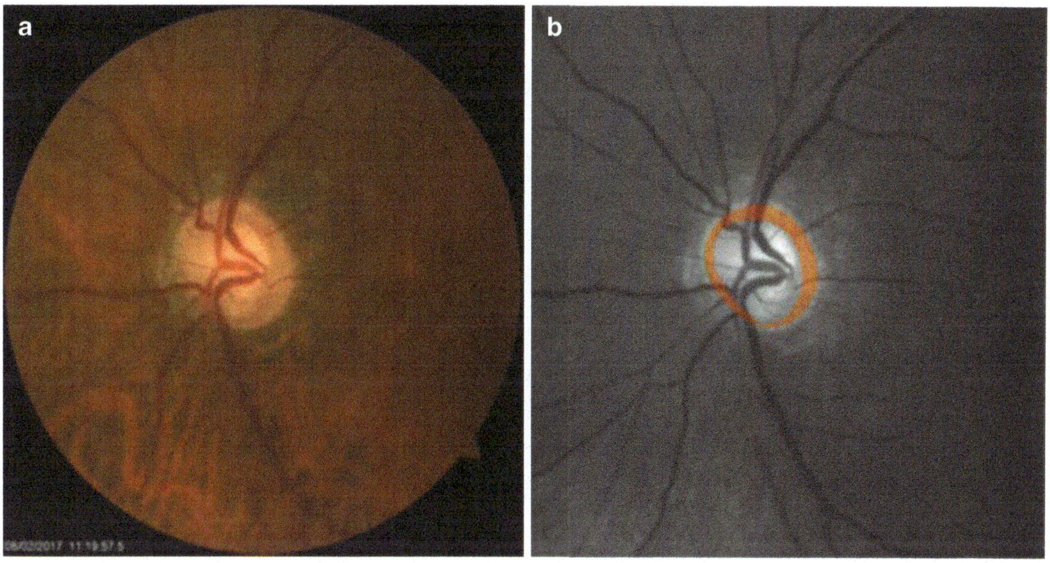

Fig. 7.13 (**a**) This left disc is showing discus inversus. Temporal rim has appearance of nasal rim whereas nasal rim looks like temporal rim with corresponding change in vascular trunks. (**b**) Neural tissue is on lesser side with inferior thinning. Inferior RNFL too appears thin—likely glaucoma

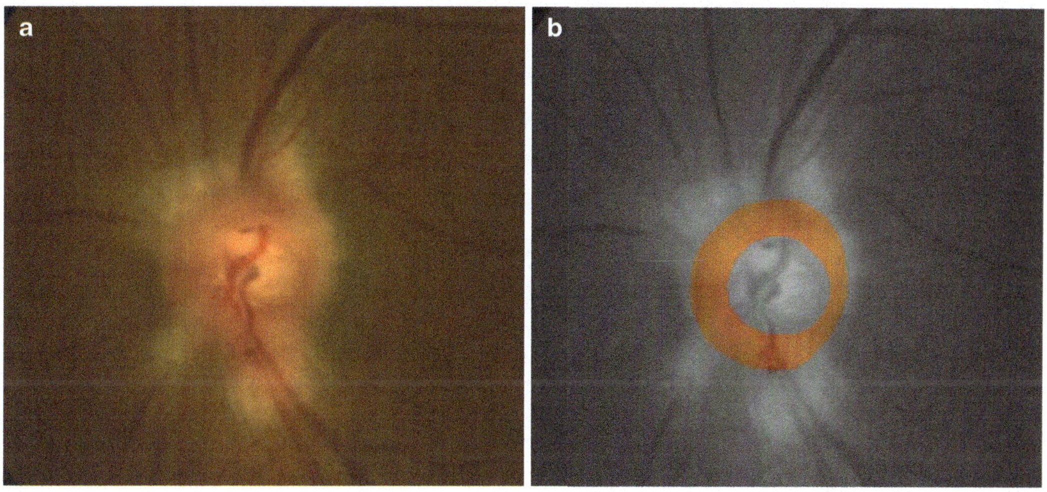

Fig. 7.14 Medullated nerve fibers. (**a**) Medullated retinal nerve fibers can obscure the landmarks of the disc making it hard to delineate NRR tissue. (**b**) A reasonable estimate about neural tissue and its health can be made by careful examination

central glial tuft and peripapillary pigmentation seen in morning glory disc anomalies [26]. It is important to differentiate from a morning glory disc anomaly because optic nerve colobomas can be associated with systemic syndromes such as CHARGE (coloboma of the eye, heart defects, choanal atresia, growth retardation, genitourinary abnormalities, and ear abnormalities). In addition to different faulty embryological causes, colobomas are usually genetically inherited, whereas the morning glory anomaly is never familial.

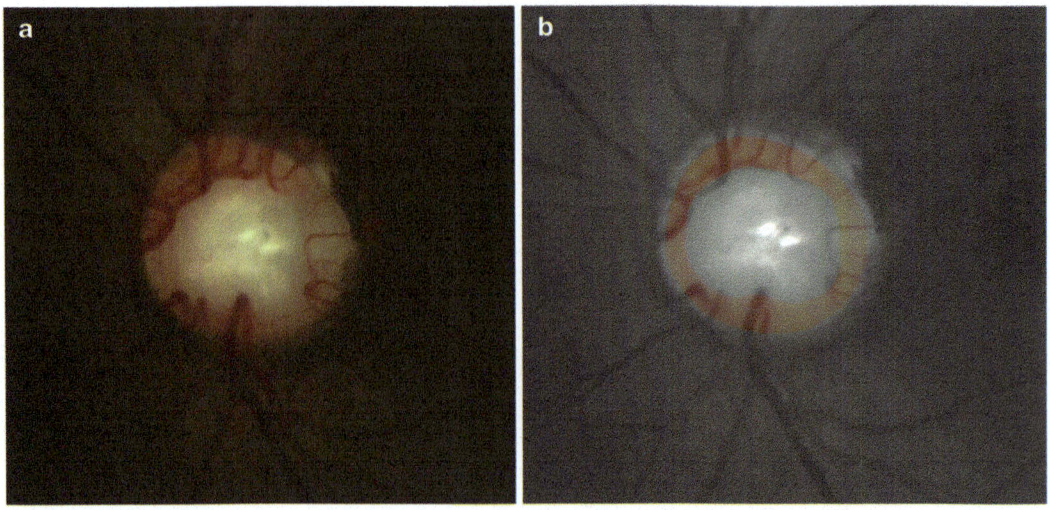

Fig. 7.15 Morning glory anomaly. (**a**) Large disc with abnormal vasculature. Cup is large and deep without any central retinal vasculature. (**b**) NRR is present all around in good amount without any focal loss or rim irregularity

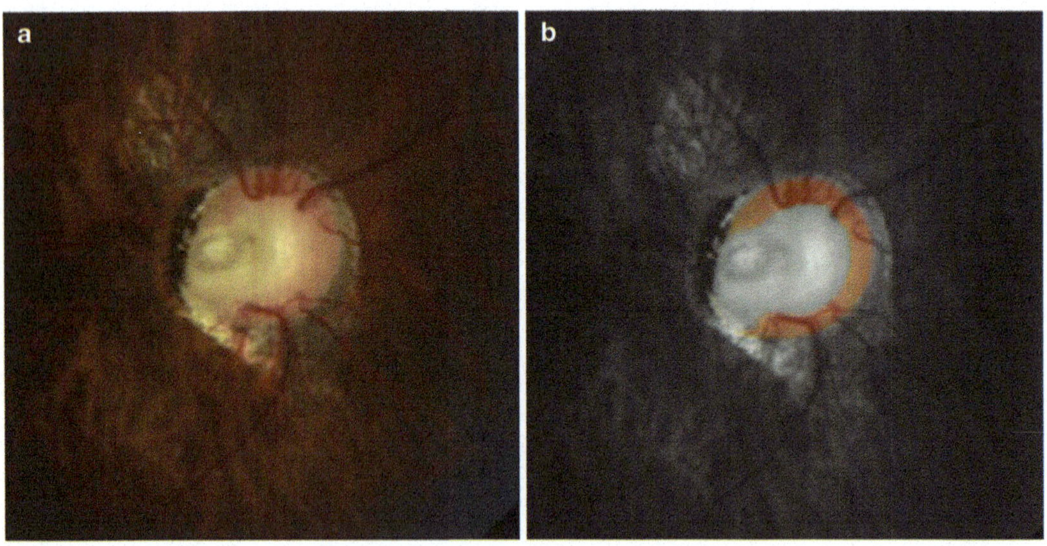

Fig. 7.16 Colobomatous disc. (**a**) This is big disc with coloboma involving the temporal rim and abnormal vasculature. (**b**) There is good amount of neural tissue with smooth regular contour except on temporal side where NRR is missing. There may be a visual field defect corresponding to rim loss in these eyes. Such field defects usually do not progress

7.3.6 Hypoplastic Optic Discs

Hypoplastic optic discs often present with a double ring, and a ring of hypopigmentation or hyperpigmentation surrounds the disc defining the area of the putative scleral canal (Figs. 7.17 and 7.18). The outer ring represents the normal junction between the sclera and the lamina cribrosa, while the inner ring represents the abnormal extension of retina and pigment epithelium over the outer portion of the lamina cribrosa [27]. Tortuous retinal arterioles, venules, or both may accompany the disc. The RNFL is variably thinned, and the disc itself may appear grayish in color.

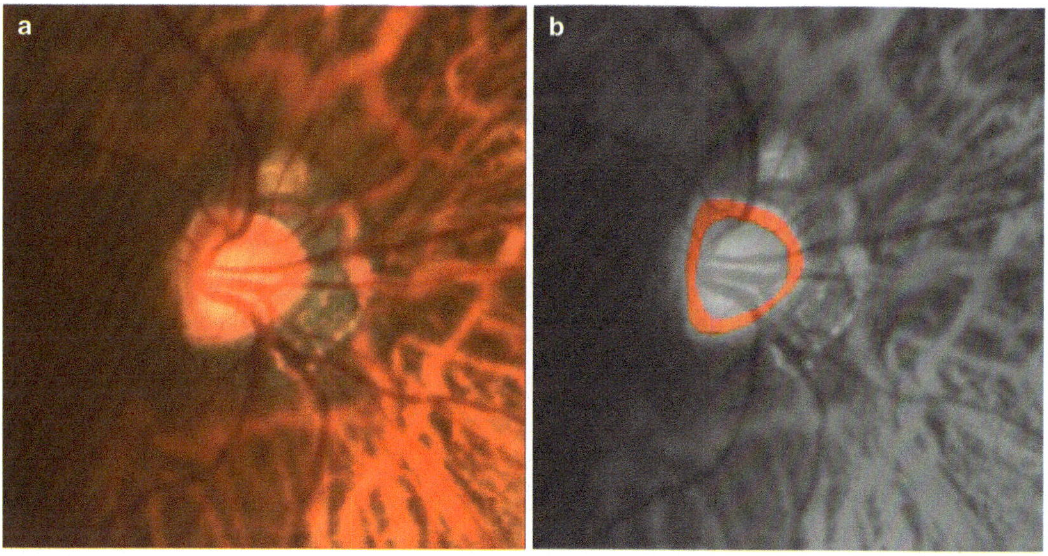

Fig. 7.17 Hypoplastic disc. (**a**) This is small disc with unusual shape (triangular). There is horizontal tilt and vessels appear to be dragged to one side. (**b**) The NRR follows the contour of the scleral canal, is regular, and has no focal areas of rim loss

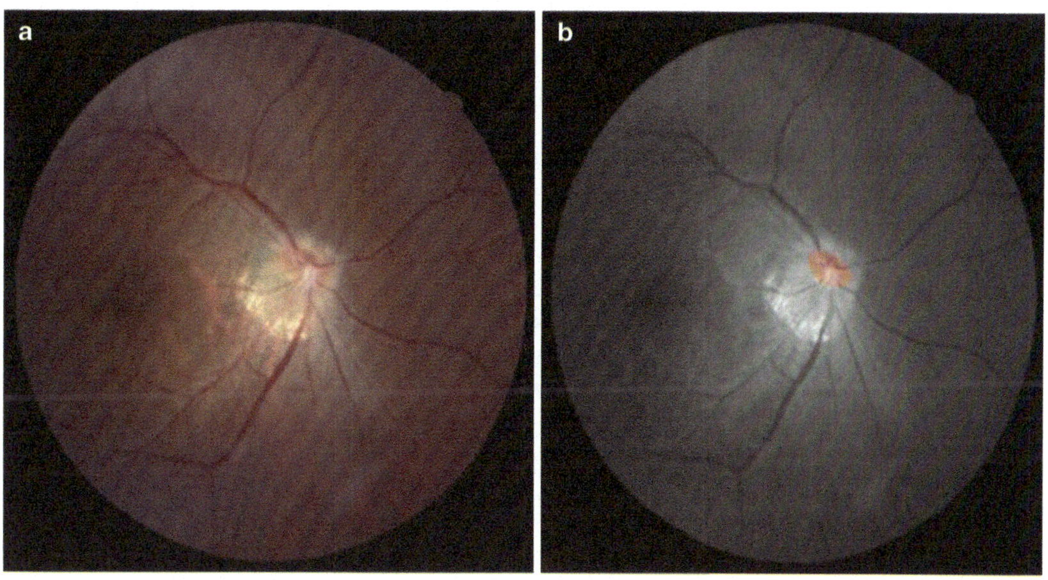

Fig. 7.18 (**a**) Hypoplastic disc with oblique tilt with grossly inadequate neural tissue. Disc is small with no cup and normal pink color. (**b**) On mentally dissecting the neural tissue, the second ring around the disc is clearly visible

One must remember that the observed size of an optic disc is dependent on magnification of the lens and the refractive error of the eye. Myopic refractive error can make even a hypoplastic disc appears normal in size, while the hyperopia may make even an average disc appear small.

7.3.7 Optic Disc Pit (ODP)

Optic disc pit is an optic disc cavitary anomaly, which is usually congenital but can be acquired in high myopes and patients with glaucoma.

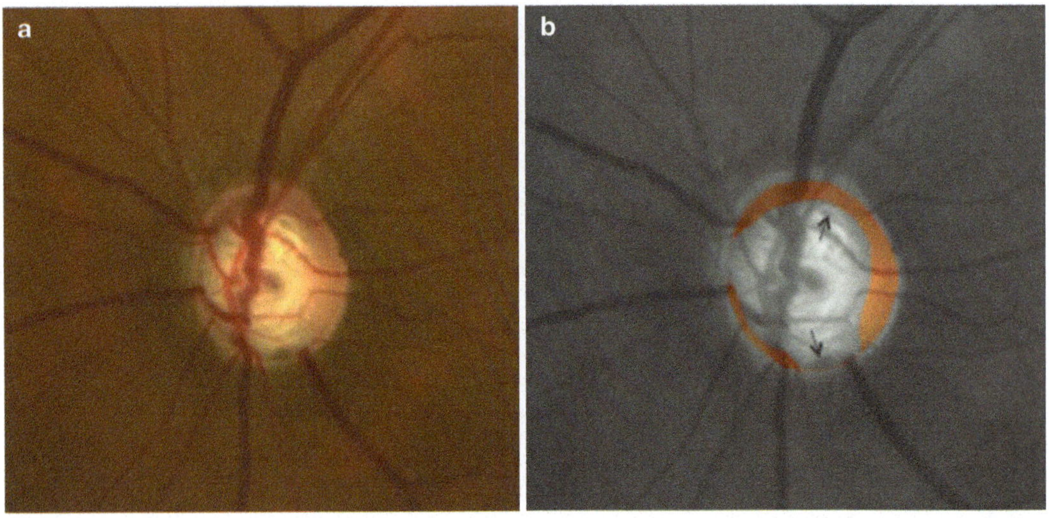

Fig. 7.19 Acquired optic disc pit. (**a**) Normal sized disc with large, deep cup. (**b**) Marked loss of neural tissue and disc pits (black arrows)

An acquired optic disc pit (AODP) develops in a localized area of the optic disc which is susceptible to the damaging effects of probably persistently elevated IOP. The affected is pale and little or no rim tissue remains adjacent to the disc edge (Fig. 7.19).

Studies have shown AODPs to be common in patients with normal-tension glaucoma (NTG), which contradicts the previous theory. It was then believed that biomechanical properties of the ocular tissues may play a pressure-independent role in the pathogenesis of AODP. Corneal hysteresis in primary open angle glaucoma (POAG) patients with AODP has been found to be significantly lower than in patients that did not have such structural changes of the optic disc [28]. AODP has been recently reported with angle closure [29].

AODPs are closely associated with the underlying pathologic process, and are more often located at the inferior optic disc unlike the congenital optic disc pits (CODP) which are usually seen in temporal part (but can occur in any part of the disc) (Fig. 7.20) and are a result of defective closure of the embryonic fissure of the eye and/or an impaired differentiation of the peripapillary sclera from the primary mesenchyme. Usually there is only one pit per disc; however, two to three pits have been described in the same optic nerve. They are usually unilateral, though 10–15% are bilateral [30]. AODPs are nearly always associated with visual field loss close to fixation, beta peripapillary atrophy, and/or optic disc hemorrhage.

Additionally, CODPs, just like morning glory discs, are seen alone or in combination with optic disc coloboma in same or contralateral eye. It is important to differentiate between an AODP and a CODP. Patients with CODP can be observed but patients with AODPs must be treated aggressively due to the progressive nature of vision loss secondary to maculopathy [31]. The fluid from the AODP can initially form a schisis-like cavity and later get complicated by an outer layer detachment and subretinal fluid, resulting in maculopathy and retinal pigment changes.

In addition to close clinical observation, OCT imaging is of utmost importance in appreciating the depth of pit and the potential conduit to the subsensory retinal space.

7.3.8 Optic Disc Drusen

Optic disc drusens are autofluorescent, calcified deposits that are seen in small and crowded optic discs giving them a lumpy, bumpy appearance. Drusen are most often concentrated in the nasal half of the disc with associated vascular anomalies such as tortuous and dilated veins, cilioretinal arteries, and optociliary shunt vessels.

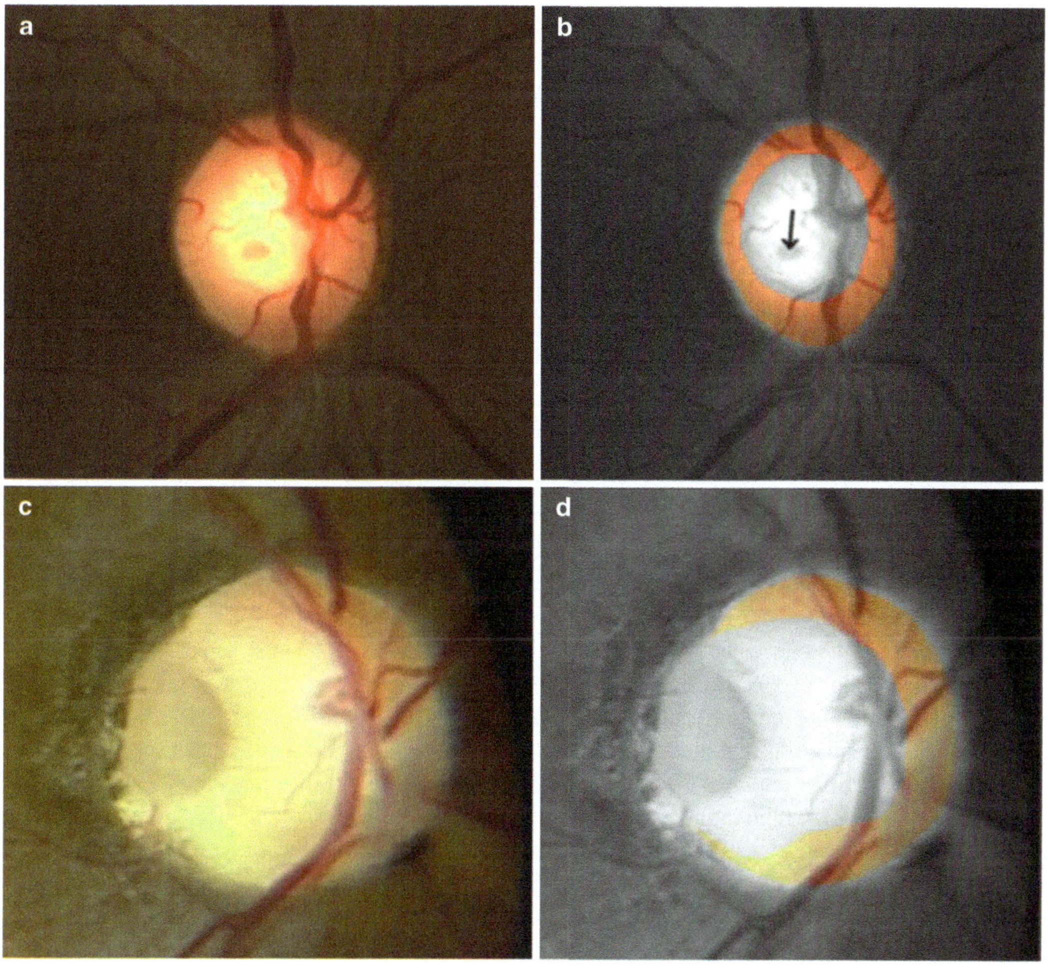

Fig. 7.20 (**a** and **b**) Isolated small central congenital optic disc pit in a young female. (**c** and **d**) Large temporal congenital optic disc pit in a young male with family history of glaucoma

There are two types of drusen: visible and buried. Visible optic disc drusen appear as refractile, whitish yellow, rounded crystalline deposits embedded within the optic disc.

Buried optic disc drusen are harder to visualize and the optic disc may have a variable appearance ranging from normal to pseudopapilledematous. Buried drusen are seen in younger individuals and cause obscuration of the optic disc margins.

These drusens exert a crowding effect that can lead to structural as well as functional ophthalmological changes (Fig. 7.21). In presence of RNFL thinning and visual field defects, glaucoma must be considered as an important differential. Additionally, patients with optic disc drusen have a family history of glaucoma more frequently compared to healthy controls [32].

Grippo et al. have shown that visual field defects are highly prevalent in eyes with optic disc drusens and concomitant ocular hypertension [33].

7.4 Is the Money Tainted?

There may be good amount of neural tissue in the disc with more or less normal distribution, still there could be signs on the ONH to indicate that tissue is not healthy. Therefore, third important

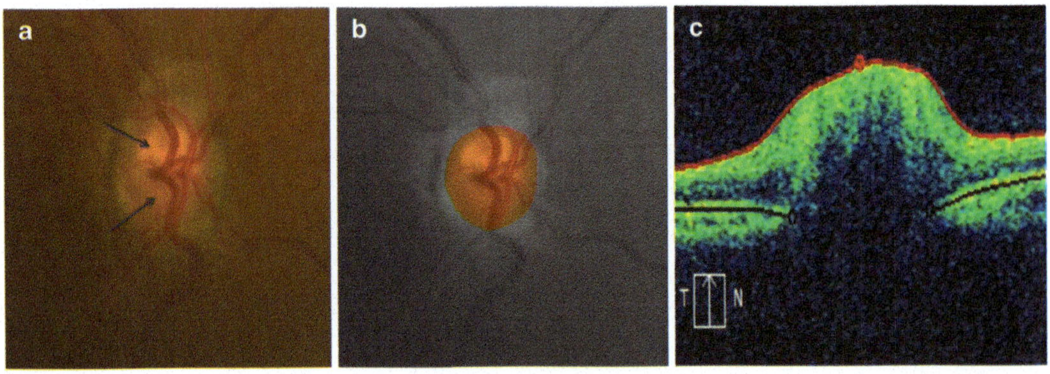

Fig. 7.21 Disc drusen. (**a**) Limits of the NRR are hard to define in this due to obliteration of the cup and irregular elevations of the disc surface due to underlying drusen (arrows). (**b**) There is marked PPA. Overall pinkish hue of the disc suggests presence of neural tissue. (**c**) OCT confirming the clinical diagnosis

question to be asked about the optic disc is: Is the neural tissue healthy? Here we look for any sign of sickness in the neural tissue. Diffuse pallor, segmental pallor, disc hemorrhages indicate the disc is not healthy. Pallor of the rim is distinct from absence of the rim. Mild temporal pallor is normal and can be exaggerated in myopic eyes or when the disc is tilted. Diffuse pallor of the NRR is seen after acute episode(s) of high intraocular pressure. More often it is indicative of a neurological cause such as compression or inflammation of optic pathways. Marked pallor (whitish appearance), segmental or diffuse is usually due to vascular insult to the disc like after anterior ischemic optic neuropathy. Also look for any abnormal vessels on the disc and PPA. PPA as such is not a disease of the neural tissue but its association with glaucoma is well known. PPA can be viewed as "something is not right" in the vicinity of the ONH. It can cause errors in delineation of disc margin leading to misdiagnosis (Fig. 7.22). PPA is especially significant when it is present in the area next to disc segment showing rim abnormalities.

Disc hemorrhages (DH) are frequently seen in glaucomatous discs especially in normal-tension glaucoma [34] and are indicative of microvascular abnormality in the ONH. These hemorrhages are characteristic linear, splinter or flame-shaped, located perpendicularly on the disc margin or within one disc diameter of ONH and in the RNFL, but never approaching the cup (Figs. 7.23, 7.24, 7.25). DH is more common in patients with large variations in IOP and typically resolves within 6–10 weeks of onset. These are usually missed in routine examination because of their resolving time. DH associated with early glaucoma is usually located on the superotemporal and inferotemporal regions of the optic disc, and is associated with localized RNFL defects and NRR notching [35]. The association with progression is similar for different types of glaucoma, for example, the hazard ratio for future progression was very similar in the Ocular Hypertension Treatment Study and the Collaborative Normal-Tension Glaucoma Study [34, 35]. The presence of a DH suggests that the disease is active.

One must remember that non-glaucomatous DH can occur in patients with posterior vitreous detachment, diabetic retinopathy, hypertensive retinopathy, branch retinal vein occlusion, and in patients with anaemia [36].

7.5 Connecting the Threads

Fourth and last questions to be asked about the neural tissue are about the RNFL. Is the RNFL normal? Retinal nerve fibers can be seen as whitish thread like striations radiating away from the disc margin. This happens as the long axons of the retinal ganglion cells form bundles and converge on to the optic disc. Thinning of RNFL causes loss of these striations in the affected area giving a rather "bland" and darker look as loss of RNFL exposes the underlying less reflective back-

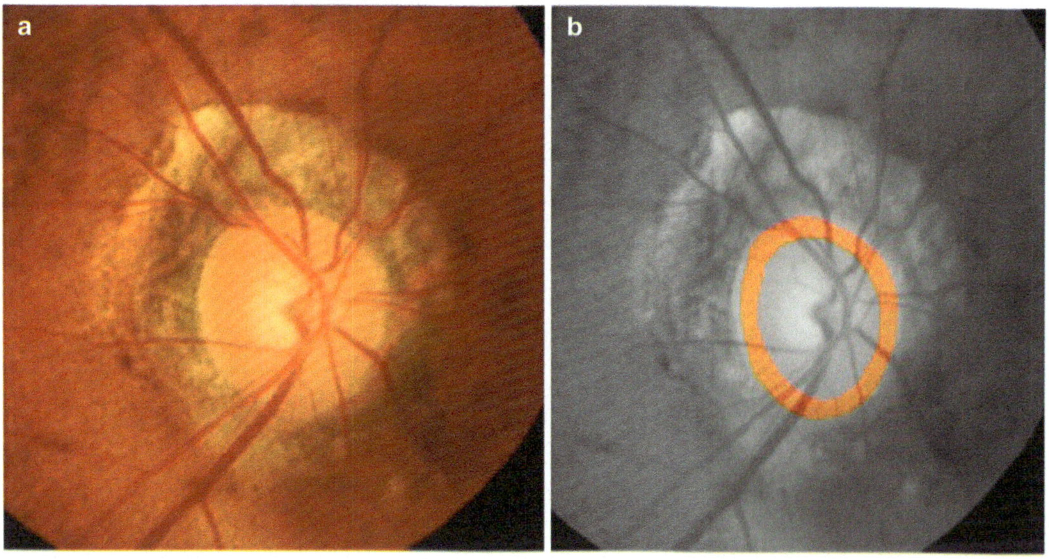

Fig. 7.22 (**a**) Marked PPA all around the disc. Disc margin is easily identifiable. Sometime in the presence of PPA it may be hard to define the scleral ring. (**b**) There is good amount of NRR with regular smooth contour. Inner limit of the NRR is difficult to define due to shallow cup

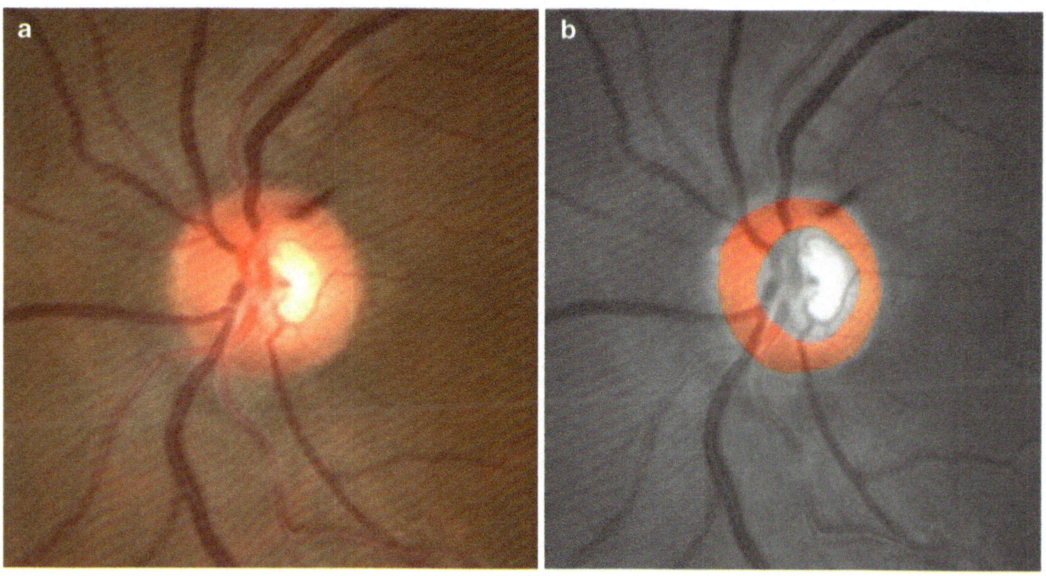

Fig. 7.23 (**a**) Averaged sized disc with adequate neural tissue. Difficult to define the inner limit of the NRR on nasal side due to vessels, but NRR looks regular. There is a splinter shaped disc hemorrhage in the superotemporal quadrant crossing the disc margin. (**b**) There is no RNFL defect adjacent to disc hemorrhage. There are arterio-venous changes suggestive of hypertensive retinopathy

ground (Fig. 7.26). There are two patterns of RNFL loss, focal (Slit or wedge defects) or diffuse defects. A slit defect is larger than an arteriole width in size and travels all the way back to the ONH, while wedge or sector shaped defects are relatively dark areas radiating from the disc margin usually on the temporal side arching over or under the macular area (Fig. 7.27). Wedge defects well correspond with visual field defects. Presence of RNFL

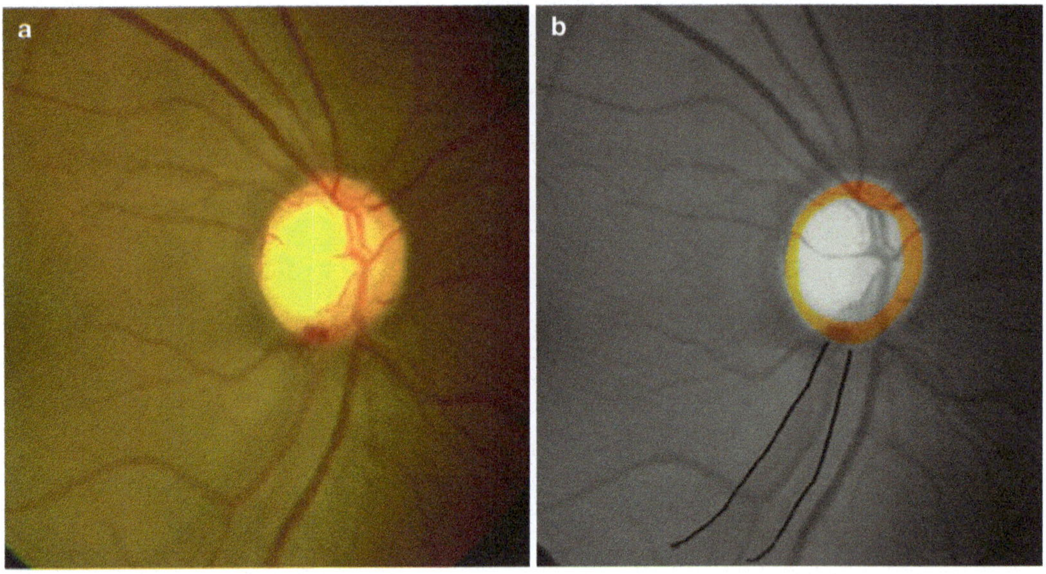

Fig. 7.24 (**a** and **b**) Thinning of NRR, large cup and disc hemorrhage with adjacent RNFL defect is suggestive of glaucoma

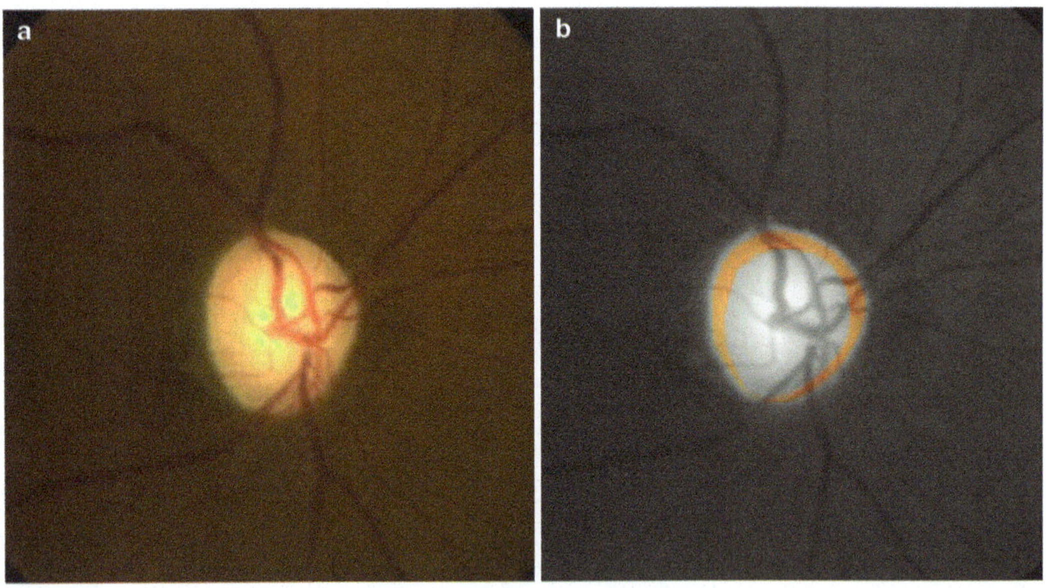

Fig. 7.25 (**a**) Average size disc with large cup. (**b**) NRR is thin, especially inferiorly with disc pallor involving rim tissue. This eye had an episode of acute angle closure. Severity of glaucoma damage is likely to be underestimated in this disc

defects usually corresponds with changes in the NRR. Diffuse loss is difficult to identify as compared to wedge defects. Asymmetry of the RNFL brightness between two zones may indicate diffuse RNFL loss. If one is facing difficulty to detect diffuse RNFL in one eye, but when both eyes are compared together then it is easily recognized as glaucoma atrophy is usually asymmetric.

NRR changes along with corresponding RNFL defects are a strong pointer towards glaucoma and subsequent progression [37].

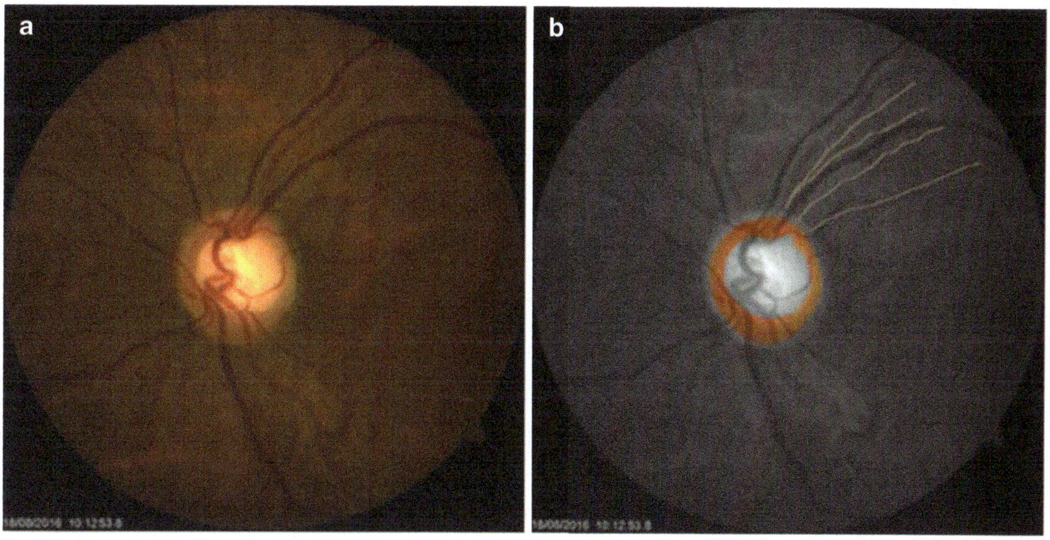

Fig. 7.26 (**a**) Average size disc with well-defined NRR which is thinner superiorly with a small notch. (**b**) RNFL shows subtle defects superotemporally, suggestive of glaucoma

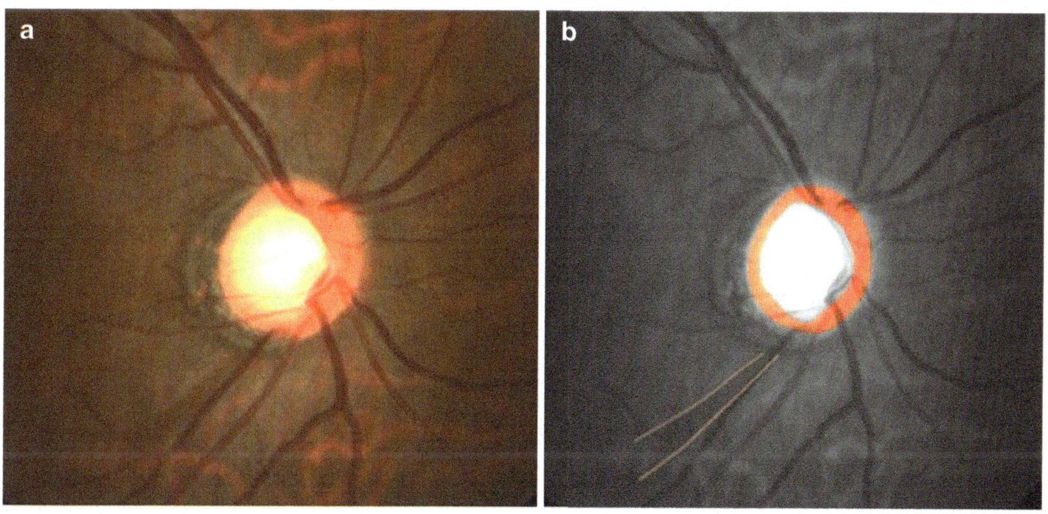

Fig. 7.27 (**a**) This is horizontally tilted disc showing good amount of NRR, but NRR is thin at both the poles. (**b**) Presence of RNFL defect infero-temporally clinches the diagnosis

7.6 Putting It Together

These four tests can be applied to any disc, normal or anatomically different. Depending on the answers a rough probability of it being glaucomatous or not can be assigned to the given disc. If disc has enough neural tissue with normal distribution, normal RNFL, and healthy NRR (yes to all questions), the disc would be considered normal. If the same disc is very large or too small or have some anatomical variation without any focal rim irregularity, it may be labeled as unlikely glaucoma. On the other hand if there is obvious thinning of NRR or loss of rim at the superior or inferior poles with corresponding nerve fiber layer defect (no to all questions), such discs will be classified as glaucomatous. Discs with enough amount of neural tissue but showing some irregularity or localized thinning of NRR or disc hemorrhage or having nerve fiber layer defect would be classified as possible or likely glaucoma. A clear answer as to whether patient has glaucoma or not is not always possible especially when dealing with discs that have unusual anatomy. Such patients are often labeled as "glaucoma suspects." Glaucoma suspect is someone who has one or more clinical features and/or risk factors associated with possibility of developing glaucoma in the future [38]. Clinically, they represent a gray zone where treatment needs to be individualized based on overall risk of glaucoma. Hodapp et al. regarded glaucoma suspect as presence of any of the following characteristics including elevated IOP, ONH, or RNFL appearance suggestive of glaucomatous damage, unexplained visual field defect consistent with glaucoma, abnormal angles, or strong family history of severe glaucoma and other risk factors [39]. In this chapter we are emphasizing only on optic disc-related features to figure out the chance of having glaucoma. This does not reflect the overall probability of having glaucoma or developing glaucoma in future. Evaluation of subtle changes in ONH and RNFL is of importance in labeling suspicious discs. An increase in CDR and asymmetry of 0.2 between the two eyes is most frequently associated with glaucoma suspects. CDR asymmetry is seen in 1% of the normal population [40]. Other suspicious findings include large cup, progressive enlargement of the cup, increasing pallor, and loss of ISNT rule [41]. Presence of disc hemorrhages in a patient with OHT increases the risk of conversion to POAG by six times [36]. Assigning a rough glaucoma probability in these cases is helpful in charting out further plan for the patient. On clinical examination every disc should be classified as normal, suspect, or glaucomatous. Based on the strength of the suspicion, suspected discs can further be split into three categories—glaucoma unlikely, glaucoma possible, glaucoma likely. Details of glaucoma probability based on disc appearance are given in Table 7.1.

This probability is in relation to optic disc appearance only. Overall risk of developing glaucoma is complex and depends on interplay of many other factors such as age, IOP, family history, corneal thickness/biomechanics, refractive status of the eye, etc. However, disc-related glaucoma probability assumes significance as very often optic disc is the first place where glaucoma is suspected, and triggers subsequent actions for glaucoma diagnosis and management.

7.7 How to Deal with Disc Suspects?

The information gathered has to be applied in some way for patients benefit. Glaucoma probability scale helps us to formulate recommendations for our patients. Clinically, we label various discs as normal, glaucoma or glaucoma suspects (disc suspects). There is no set protocol on how to proceed with disc suspects. How should they be investigated or monitored? Careful analysis of these discs allows us to subclassify them into unlikely glaucoma, possible glaucoma or likely glaucoma. This way 'unlikely glaucoma' can be grouped with normal discs whereas 'likely glaucoma' category can be pushed towards the glaucoma (glaucoma certain) group for investigations and treatment point of view. This leaves behind 'possible glaucoma' as true suspects. Possible glaucoma group would definitely need followup

Table 7.1 Disc-related glaucoma probability scale

Label	Characteristics
Normal	Adequate NRR, normal distribution, healthy neural tissue, normal RNFL. Answer is 'Yes' to all questions.
Unlikely	Large discs where NRR appears thin but clearly identifiable and regular. Abnormal anatomy of ONH where no defect in NRR or RNFL. Answer is 'Yes' to most questions.
Possible	NRR on thinner side, irregularities in NRR contour, disc hemorrhage without any other evidence. Small disc with a cup.
Likely	Typical NRR notch with corresponding RNFL defect. Disc hemorrhage with NRR changes, disc hemorrhage with RNFL defect, neural tissue assessed as inadequate with other signs.
Certain	Marked thinning of NRR, focal NRR loss with adjacent RNFL defect. With or without disc hemorrhage or PPA. 'No' is the answer to most questions.

Table 7.2 How to proceed based on the Disc-related glaucoma probability scale

Label	Action
Normal Unlikely	No action is required. Regular eye checkup suggested at yearly or longer intervals, depending on age and other risk factors.
Possible	Go into more details of patient history to assess risk of developing glaucoma. Emphasize on next checkup within a year. Can do baseline imaging and fields.
Likely	Investigate for glaucoma with intention to treat. Establish good baselines for VF, imaging, CCT/corneal biomechanics. Assess risk factors for developing glaucoma and its progressing. Follow up in next 6–12 months.
Certain	Baseline investigations, likely to be treated, regular follow ups depending on severity and response to therapy and risk of vision loss. Assess risk factors for progression.

but question remains should they be investigated? Decision to investigate or will be influenced by the presence or absence of other risk factors in a given case. Final recommendations are not made based on optic disc findings alone. We have to consider age, intraocular pressure, family history of glaucoma, and other risk factors. Assuming that other factors are favorable, following table (Table 7.2) can be used plan next steps based on disc findings.

7.8 Conclusion

Clinical evaluation of ONH for glaucoma is of fundamental importance as very often this is the first place to raise suspicion of glaucoma. Errors in evaluating ONH for glaucoma are common and often lead to missed opportunity in treating glaucoma patient in time. ONH appearance may vary greatly in normalcy and in disease, making it hard to pick up glaucoma. To acquire this skill takes time and practice as the learning curve is steep. But once acquired the accuracy of clinical glaucoma diagnosis in expert hands is quite high. There are a number of ways to systematically examine the optic disc and reach correct diagnosis. In this chapter we have primarily focused on assessing variations in the most important structure for visual function, the neural tissue of ONH. Delineating the neural tissue within the ONH by defining its outer and inner limits is the key skill to be learnt. Assessing the neural tissue for adequacy and abnormalities in all clock hours can help us differentiate disease from normal. Other aspects, such as peripapillary atrophy, asymmetry between fellow eyes, and vessel alterations may aid to differentiate normal from glaucomatous eyes. Progressive changes in the ONH or RNFL are best identified with serial optic disc photographs.

References

1. Greaney MJ, Hoffman DC, Garway-Heath DF, et al. Comparison of optic nerve imaging methods to distinguish normal eyes from those with glaucoma. Invest Ophthalmol Vis Sci. 2002;43:140–5.
2. Wollstein G, Garway-Heath DF, Fontana L, Hitchings RA. Identifying early glaucomatous changes: comparison between expert clinical assessment of optic disc photographs and confocal scanning ophthalmoscopy. Ophthalmology. 2000;107:2272–7.
3. Girkin CA, McGwin G Jr, Long C, et al. Subjective and objective optic nerve assessment in African Americans and whites. Invest Ophthalmol Vis Sci. 2004;45:2272–8.
4. Reus NJ, Lemij HG, Garway-Heath DF, et al. Clinical assessment of stereoscopic optic disc photographs for glaucoma: the European optic disc assessment trial. Ophthalmology. 2010;117(4):717–23.
5. O'Neill EC, Gurria LU, Pandav SS, et al. Glaucomatous optic neuropathy evaluation project: factors associated with underestimation of glaucoma likelihood. JAMA Ophthalmol. 2014;132(5):560–6.
6. Ramrattan RS, Wolfs RCW, Jonas JB, et al. Determinants of optic disc characteristics in a general population: the Rotterdam study. Ophthalmology. 1999;106:1588–96.
7. Jonas JB, Gusek GC, Naumann GOH. Optic disc, cup and neuroretinal rim size, configuration and correlations in normal eyes. Invest Ophthalmol Vis Sci. 1988;29:1151–8.
8. Jonas JB, Fernández MC, Naumann GO. Correlation of the optic disc size to glaucoma susceptibility. Ophthalmology. 1991;98(5):675–80.
9. Armaly MF, Sayegh RE. The cup-disc ratio. The findings of tonometry and tonography in the normal eye. Arch Ophthalmol. 1969;82(2):191–6.

10. Hoffmann EM, Zangwill LM, Crowston JG, Weinreb RN. Optic disk size and glaucoma. Surv Ophthalmol. 2007;52:32–49.
11. Fingeret M, Medeiros FA, Susanna R Jr, Weinreb RN. Five rules to evaluate the optic disc and retinal nerve fiber layer for glaucoma. Optometry. 2005;76(11):661–8.
12. Bayer A, Harasymowycz P, Henderer JD, Steinmann WG, Spaeth GL. Validity of a new disk grading scale for estimating glaucomatous damage: correlation with visual field damage. Am J Ophthalmol. 2002;133(6):758–63.
13. Zangalli C, Gupta SR, Spaeth GL. The disc as the basis of treatment for glaucoma. Saudi J Ophthalmol. 2011;25(4):381–7.
14. Wong EY, Keeffe JE, Rait JL, et al. Detection of undiagnosed glaucoma by eye health professionals. Ophthalmology. 2004;111:1508–14.
15. Malik R, Swanson WH, Garway-Heath DF. 'Structure-function relationship' in glaucoma: past thinking and current concepts. Clin Exp Ophthalmol. 2012;40(4):369–80.
16. Quigley HA, Dunkelberger GR, Green WR. Retinal ganglion cell atrophy correlated with automated perimetry in human eyes with glaucoma. Am J Ophthalmol. 1989;107:453–64.
17. Jonas JB, Budde WM, Lang P. Neuroretinal rim width ratios in morphological glaucoma diagnosis. Br J Ophthalmol. 1998;82:1366–71.
18. Spaeth GL, Lopes JF, Junk AK, et al. Systems for staging the amount of optic nerve damage in glaucoma: a critical review and new material. Surv Ophthalmol. 2006;51:293–315.
19. Morgan JE, Bourtsoukli I, Rajkumar KN, et al. The accuracy of the inferior>superior>nasal>temporal neuroretinal rim area rule for diagnosing glaucomatous optic disc damage. Ophthalmology. 2012;119(4):723–30.
20. Sihota R, Srinivasan G, Dada T, Gupta V, Ghate D, Sharma A. Is the ISNT rule violated in early primary open-angle glaucoma—a scanning laser tomography study. Eye. 2008;22(6):819–24.
21. You QS, Xu L, Jonas JB. Tilted optic discs: the Beijing eye study. Eye. 2008;22(5):728–9.
22. Sen SC, Bhattacharya P, Biswas PN. Situs inversus of the optic disc. Indian J Ophthalmol. 1988;36:44–5.
23. Ali BH, Logani S, Kozlov KL, Arnold AC, Bateman B. Progression of retinal nerve fiber myelination in childhood. Am J Ophthalmol. 1994;118:515–7.
24. Katz SE, Weber PA. Photographic documentation of the loss of medullated nerve fibers of the retina in uncontrolled primary open angle glaucoma. J Glaucoma. 1996;5(6):406–9.
25. Rinaldi E, De Rosa G, Severino R, Cennamo G. Morning glory syndrome with chronic simple glaucoma. Ophthalmic Paediatrics Genetics. 1986;7(1): 69–72.
26. Brodsky MC. Morning glory disc anomaly or optic disc coloboma? Arch Ophthalmol. 1994;112(2):153.
27. Kaur S, Jain S, Sodhi HBS, Rastogi A. Optic nerve hypoplasia. Oman J Ophthalmol. 2013;6:77–82.
28. Healey PR, Mitchell P. The prevalence of optic disc pits and their relationship to glaucoma. J Glaucoma. 2008;17(1):11–4.
29. Bochmann F, Ang GS, Azuara-Blanco A. Lower corneal hysteresis in glaucoma patients with acquired pit of the optic nerve (APON). Graefes Arch Clin Exp Ophthalmol. 2008;246(5):735–8.
30. Kaushik S, Ichhpujani P, Kaur S, Singh Pandav S. Optic disk pit and iridociliary cyst precipitating angle closure glaucoma. J Curr Glaucoma Pract. 2014;8(1):33–5.
31. Uzel MM, Karacorlu M. Optic disk pits and optic disk pit maculopathy: a review. Surv Ophthalmol. 2019;64(5):595–607.
32. Gramer G, Gramer E, Weisschuh N. Optic disc drusen and family history of glaucoma-results of a patient-directed survey. J Glaucoma. 2017;26(10):940–6.
33. Grippo TM, Shihadeh WA, Schargus M, et al. Optic nerve head drusen and visual field loss in normotensive and hypertensive eyes [published correction appears in J glaucoma. 2010;19(2):150]. J Glaucoma. 2008;17(2):100–4.
34. Drance S, Anderson DR, Schulzer M. Collaborative normal-tension glaucoma study group, risk factors for progression of visual field abnormalities in normal-tension glaucoma. Am J Ophthalmol. 2001;131:699–708.
35. Budenz DL, Anderson DR, Feuer WJ, et al. Ocular hypertension treatment study group, detection and prognostic significance of optic disc hemorrhages during the ocular hypertension treatment study. Ophthalmology. 2006;113:2137–43.
36. Airaksinen PJ, Mustonen E, Alanku HI. Optic disk haemorrhages precede retinal nerve fibre layer defects in ocular hypertension. Acta Ophthalmol. 1981;59:627–41.
37. Quigley HA, Katz J, Derick RJ, Gilbert D, Sommer A. An evaluation of optic disc and nerve fiber layer examinations in monitoring progression of early glaucoma damage. Ophthalmology. 1992;99:19–28.
38. Prum BE Jr, Lim MC, Mansberger SL, et al. Primary open-angle glaucoma suspect preferred practice pattern® guidelines. Ophthalmology. 2016;123(1):P112–51.
39. Hodapp E, Parrish RK II, Anderson DR. Clinical decisions in glaucoma. St Louis: The CV Mosby Co; 1993. pp. 52–61.
40. Allingham RR, Damji KF, Freeman S. Shields' textbook of glaucoma. 6th ed. Philadelphia, PA: Wolters Kluwer/Lippincott Williams and Wilkins; 2012.
41. Harizman N, Oliveira C, Chiang A, Tello C, Marmor M, Ritch R, et al. The ISNT rule and differentiation of normal from glaucomatous eyes. Arch Ophthalmol. 2006;124:1579–83.

8 How to Assess the Severity of Glaucoma Damage Accurately

George L. Spaeth and Parul Ichhpujani

8.1 Concept of Colored Zones

"Glaucoma" is a process in which an eye is damaged by an intraocular pressure (IOP) higher than the ocular tissues can tolerate. The manifestations of this process are multiple, including no pain to excruciating pain, corneal damage and loss of vision due to the death of retinal ganglion cells (RGCs). With the rare exception of newborns with primary congenital glaucoma, nobody starts with glaucomatous damage. The rate at which glaucoma worsens varies. For example, nearly 90% patients of primary open-angle glaucoma (POAG) are "slow progressors" and may never get any symptoms at all, even without treatment. Then there is another group, "rapid progressors" who deteriorate more rapidly, and are more likely to become blind. Patients with acute primary angle-closure glaucoma can progress so rapidly that a person can lose vision in hours. A condition is "severe: when (1) it has already become serious enough that it has already caused symptoms, or (2) when the rate at which it is worsening is rapid enough that it will cause symptoms.

In some people with glaucoma the severity is so serious that the people are almost blind when first seen and are rapidly worsening, in others much vision has been lost already, but continuing change is slow, in some the IOP is very high and yet the people feel fine and function well. In others the condition remains so mild as to be asymptomatic for years, yet all of these people have "glaucoma." That diagnostic term, then, does not mean anything specific in terms of how mildly or severely the "glaucoma" affects people's lives. We write this chapter in order to stress the importance of assessing this issue of severity, and, further, to share a method of how that can be done. This method applies to every type of glaucoma. In fact, it is useful when considering any condition.

Assessing the severity of a person's illness is necessary to understand what needs to be done for that person, both from the point of view of diagnosis and treatment. Let us first introduce two terms here: the "Green Zone" and the "Red Zone." [1] When people are in the "Green Zone" they are well and they feel well; when in the "Red Zone," they are diseased and feel sick (diseased). However, there is also a stage when a person has developed some pathology but is unaware of that because the pahology has not caused noticeable symptoms the "Yellow Zone." This applies to all conditions, so the concept is valuable to understand and utilize (Fig. 8.1).

When people are at the healthy end of the spectrum, in the "Green Zone," the harms associated with diagnostic procedures and interventions are usually far greater than the potential benefits of interventions employed to try to prevent development of symptoms. Phrased differently, "asymptomatic people cannot be made better, so interventions should be undertaken with that awareness in mind; however, asymp-

G. L. Spaeth (✉)
Glaucoma Service, Wills Eye Hospital, Philadelphia, PA, USA
e-mail: gspaeth@willseye.org

P. Ichhpujani
Department of Ophthalmology, Government Medical college and Hospital, Chandigarh, India

S. Pandav et al. (eds.), *The Optic Nerve Head in Health and Disease*,
https://doi.org/10.1007/978-981-33-6838-5_8

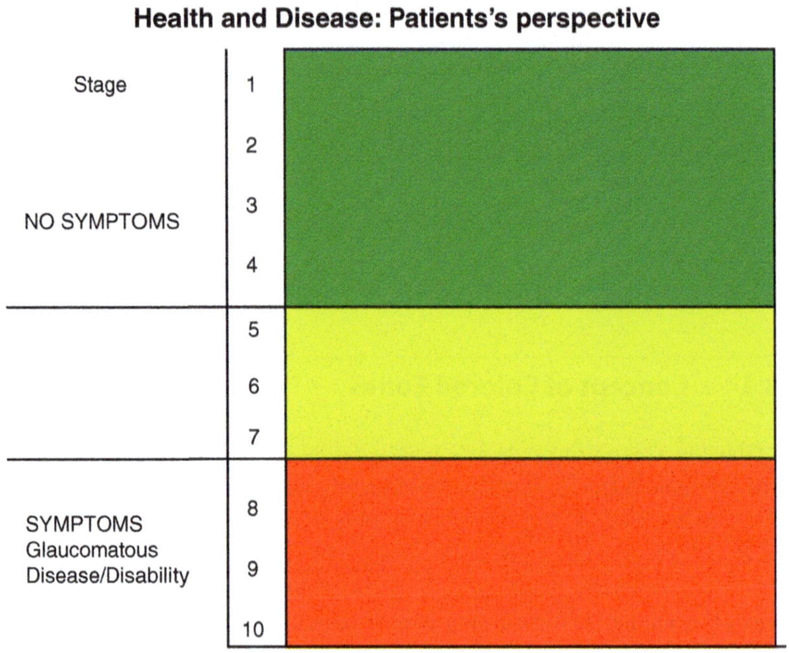

Fig. 8.1 Patients think in terms of how they feel and function, Well or Sick, Green or Red; with some awareness of a transition zone, Yellow. Numbers on the y axis refer to DDLS score (addressed later in the text)

tomatic people who have a reasonable likelihood of developing troublesome symptoms and losing the ability to function may, in some situations, need interventions, especially when the potential illness is severe and irreversible." In brief, when a person is doing well there must be clear justification for every intervention. The objective is to stop a person from deteriorating that he/she reaches the "Red Zone." The method is to assess the rate of changing stage and the risks associated with treatment for that particular person, so as to keep care as inexpensive, convenient, effective, and safe as possible by intervening only when necessary. It is when the patient's findings indicate that the development of a severe condition needs to be considered, so that deteriorating into the "Red Zone" is avoided, that interventions are needed.

Assessing stage must also consider the other end of the spectrum, specifically, when people are already in the "Red Zone," so they are already diseased, disabled in some way, and troubled by symptoms. Knowing that these people already feel bad, the proper objective is to help them feel better, or at the least to do what has the chance of preventing them from feeling worse. Some type of intervention then is always pertinent. In contrast, people in the "Green Zone" usually—but not always—are best followed without intervention.

So, just knowing the severity of a person's condition immediately provides needed information! There may be an advantage in using the term "stage" rather than severity, because "stage" carries with it the clearer implication of a changing process. And every process is changing. Every person is changing, even though we may not be able to detect the changes; also, to be remembered is the fact that not every change is of importance. Stability, worsening, and improving are not good or bad in themselves. Other factors always need to be considered, and the potential benefit of stability and the potential significance of worsening or improving need always to be evaluated in terms of relevance to what is being considered. No machine or algorithm can objectively provide the correct guidance.

Relevance, that is, the importance of an issue to an individual person is always subjective; it is never objective, and it is always relative. Thinking about the severity of the issue is essential.

Now let us add a third phrase, the "Yellow Zone." It is relatively easy to establish when people are in the Red Zone; all that is needed is thoughtful asking: "How are you? How do you feel?" It is also relatively easy to determine when people feel well and consider themselves healthy. However, a process may already be underway which is damaging them, a process of which they are unaware. The "Yellow Zone" is where this is occurring (Fig. 8.2).

A similar way physician's conceptualize disease is shown in Fig. 8.3. Here we now focus on a specific disease, glaucoma, though the concepts apply to all conditions. Risk factors are not the same as findings from the doctor's perspective. However, they tend to carry the same weight.

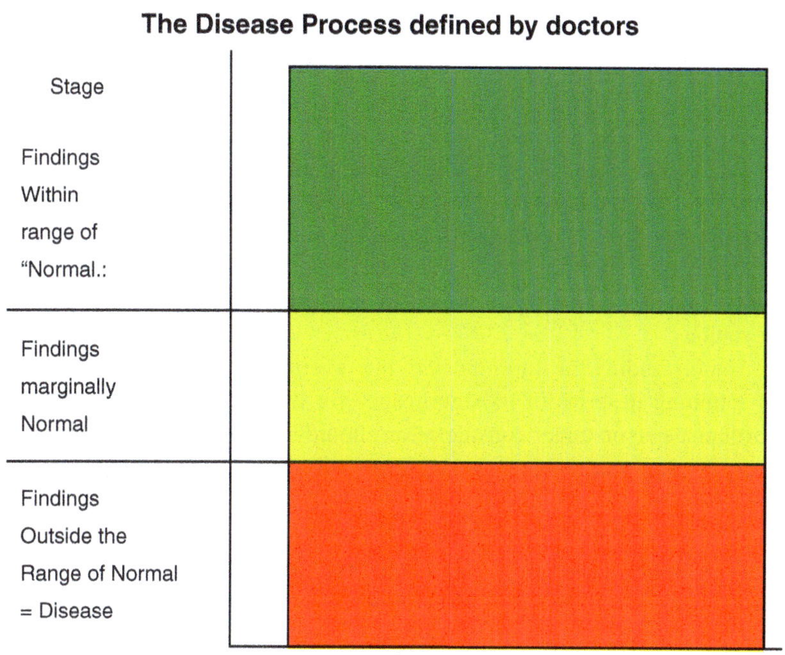

Fig. 8.2 The disease process as defined by Doctors. Health is present when findings are normal, that is within two standard deviations of the mean. Disease is present when findings are outside the range of normal. When findings are of uncertain statistical significance, or variable, the person is on the Yellow Zone

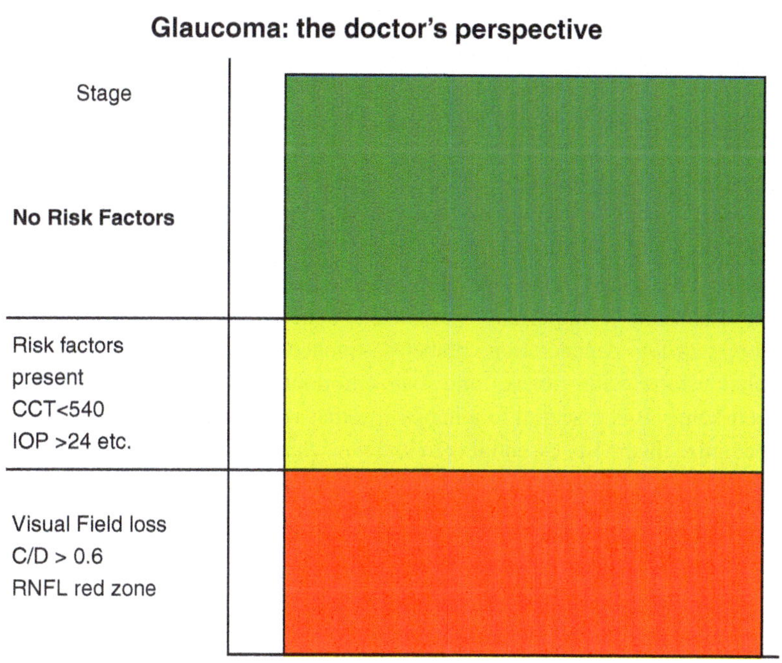

Fig. 8.3 The Doctors' vision of health and disease, is one in which the presence or absence of risk factors is a major consideration. However, risk is always relative, sometimes of importance and sometimes irrelevant. Furthermore, no person can be known to have no risk for developing glaucoma, so the Green Zone, using this system is meaningless

To be sure that a person is in the "Yellow Zone," it requires that we be relatively sure a damaging process is already underway. This is not always easy. A statistically abnormal finding, such as an IOP of 30 mmHg, does not ensure that a person is going to move into the "Red Zone," so this cannot be sufficient by itself to indicate a person is in the "Yellow Zone." On the other hand, a finding that is always indicative of an ongoing pathological process, such an IOP of 50 mm Hg, an afferent pupillary response or a definite field loss, is enough to say the person is in the "Yellow Zone." Findings are just that, findings, and their importance to the person in whom they are found must be evaluated in the context of that particular person, not as they relate to a group standard such as a mean, or standard deviation.

Understanding the importance of the severity of a finding in terms of its significance for the particular person under consideration should be clear, but is often not considered. That is, is the finding relevant? Moreover, is the finding important. A nearly full field is important to a basketball player but may matter little to a bed-ridden person who reads extensively. Wisely utilizing the concepts being explained here demands that data be evaluated in terms of considering (1) the validity (is the finding real), (2) the relevance (is the finding pertinent to the well-being of that patient), and the (3) importance (does it matter to the person).

The concept of understanding the importance of considering stage—severity—is clear. The practice of utilizing the concept wisely demands thinking that examines the validity, the relevance, and the importance of the data. Knowing one is in the "Red Zone" is important related to any condition, macular degeneration, diabetes, finances, relationships with others, and our emotional well-being. It is essential to a happy life that we recognize this. Also, essential is to know is when we have transitioned from being truly healthy in the "Green Zone," into an area which may or may not lead us to the "Red Zone."

The presence of sgtatisically abnormal findings, such as IOP or blood pressure or blood sugar does not prove the person with those "abnormal" findings is going to end up sick in the "Red Zone." Some markers are so ominous they almost always deserve attention and an intervention, even in the absence of symptoms. But many are merely irrelevant signs, like those on the side of the road telling us that at the next turn is a hotel or restaurant or service station; it is wise to be observant, but unwise always to act on what is observed. Here it is that a second purpose of staging is needed, specifically a method of determining *direction of change* and *rate of change*. We will discuss that in detail in a moment. At this point we want to introduce a framework that can be used for accurately assessing severity in those with glaucoma, or at considered to be at significant risk for developing glaucoma.

Appropriate care for a person with glaucoma, or at risk for glaucoma, must consider:

1. The current stage (severity) of the condition,
2. The rate and direction of change of the stage,
3. The duration the change will continue,
4. The reversibility of the change,
5. The importance to the affected individual of the change, and
6. The socioeconomic factors that influence the person's care.

Without knowing these factors care is not likely to be rational or appropriate. Knowing these six considerations is essential to the provision of good, cost-effective care.

8.2 Assessing the Severity: Physician Versus Patient Perspective

Severity must be understood from the affected person's perspective for diagnosis and treatment to be right for the patient under consideration. This often does not happen. Physicians are not often trained to appreciate the softness of data. This problem is made even worse by the incorrect belief that means, standard deviations from the mean, p values, and confidence limits can easily be validly generalized from group data to an individual. Further, great stress is frequently placed on the perceived importance of obtaining so-called objective findings, such as IOP, central corneal thickness, RNFL thickness or decibels of field loss, in contrast to "soft, subjective" data. But if we believe that what is of most importance to people is how they feel and how well they are functioning, then the only relevant measures are also subjective. Patients dare concerned about how they feel, what they can do, and the financial and pertinent socioeconomic considerations. Therefore, we need first to assess those things of importance to patients: feeling, function, and socioeconomic considerations. This can be done with standardized methods, such as the NEI-VFQ-25 quality of life survey and the Compressed Assessment of Ability Related to Vision (CAARV) [2]. However, using these tests of feeling and function increases the amount of time required to obtain data. Furthermore, they have the disadvantage of being standardized. A better understanding of how a particular person feels and functions, who he or she is, and what she or he can do and afford is gained by taking a proper history. It is these aspects that are the measure of severity from the patient's perspective, not the level of IOP or RNFL thickness, or any other finding or set of findings. The accuracy of the estimate of severity depends on the skill of learning how the person truly feels and about what he/she is most deeply concerned, and assessing functional ability by careful listening, observing and penetrating, compassionate, personalized asking.

What we are looking for is data regarding symptoms and function that are valid, relevant, and important: "valid," in agreement with reality, "relevant," meaningfully related to the issue being considered, and "important" of sufficient significance to the affected person that it deserves thinking about and acting on. The data also need to have a quantitative character, in order to designate stage in a way that relates to actual clinical condition, to determine whether symptoms and function are improving or deteriorating, to allow developing a valid rate of change, and to determine the duration change will continue. This can be presented as a "Colored Disease Process Graph." However, this is different from the Figs. 8.2 and 8.3, depicting health and disease from the medical professional's point of view. Here, in we illustrate what disease means from the patients' perspective, as we have already done. See Fig. 8.1. However, the "width" of the transition zone varies. It may be short or long. That is, the significance to the patient's well-being of the "Yellow Zone" varies, but tends to be underappreciated.

Therefore, we show Fig. 8.4, a more generic representation, though still grounded in the fundamental importance of symptoms.

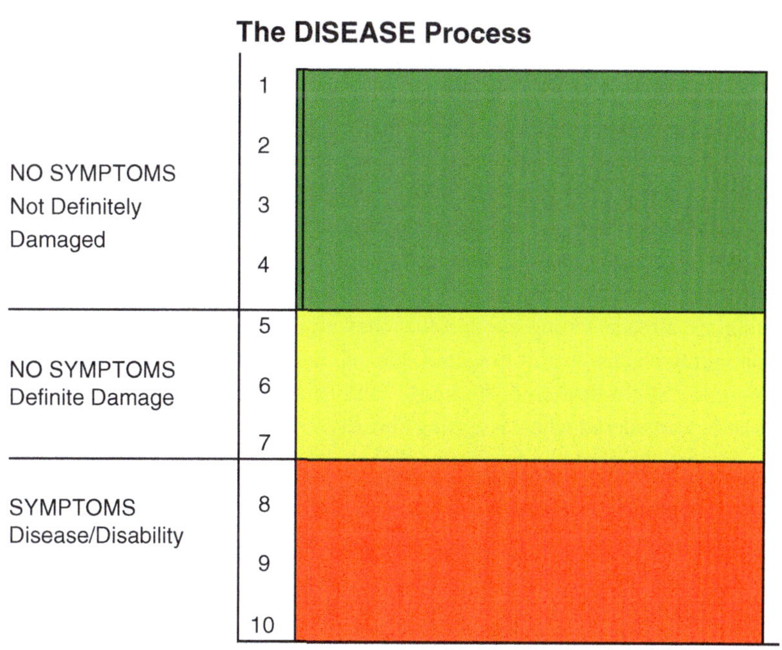

Fig. 8.4 A Generic depiction of how diseases change over time as considered by patients

At the top of the graph is the area where the person is healthy, feels well, and is able to do what he or she wishes to do. In order for this area to have an emotional impact on both the doctor and the patient, it is colored green. As mentioned already, this is called the "Green Zone." In contrast, at the bottom of the graph is the area in which a person knows that he or she is sick. That person already has troublesome symptoms. Again, so that a person viewing this will be affected viscerally, this area is colored red, and is called "The Red Zone." A person may feel and function well, that is, be asymptomatic and yet be at increased risk for becoming diseased. Any model of how any disease process relates to symptoms and changes must consider this zone of transition, in which establishing the certainty of worsening or improving is essential. That is the "Yellow Zone"; yellow is the universal color for caution. When a person still feels well, that is, has no symptoms, but has a finding proving that something is already biologically wrong, that person is in the "Yellow Zone." However, most of us have things that are biologically wrong, such as achy knees or slightly blurred vision or hearing poorly, but their presence does not mean we will need a wheel chair, or a white cane, or a hearing aid before we die. Phrased differently just because a person's health severity was worsened does not mean that person is going to become symptomatic.

While it is relatively straightforward to assign a person the "Red Zone," because such a person already has symptoms, deciding whether they are in "Yellow Zone" or the "Green Zone" takes thought, because patients are asymptomatic in both the Green and the Yellow zones and presence or absence of symptoms cannot be used to make the distinction. Findings indicating something are already wrong enough that they signal continuing change is now essential. We call these findings "supra-threshold findings" and these must be considered when assessing severity.

A supra-threshold finding is one that is always associated with the eventual presence of disease. For example, people with a blood pressure of 180/130 mmHg can still feel fine, but if the blood pressure remains at that level they will definitely become sick. A melanoma that has metastasized can occur in people who still feel healthy, but that finding is supra-threshold, indicating the person is transitioning to feeling sick. Supra-threshold findings in the field of ophthalmology include definite field loss, an afferent pupillary defect, IOP greater than 40 mmHg, asymmetry of IOP greater than 5 mmHg, an anterior chamber angle considered narrow enough to occlude with a characteristic peripheral anterior synechiae, other pathologic change in the anterior chamber angle, a rate of change of a finding such as rim width or RNFL thickness that always exceeds the rate of change in a healthy person, or a structural finding that never occurs in a healthy eye, such as an acquired pit of the optic nerve. The Cup: disc ratio (CDR) is **not** such a marker; it has NO supra-threshold significance. There is no point on the scale of 0.0–1.0 that, by itself, CDR that is always of concern, because there is no CDR that is always unhealthy. Noting a change from 0.2 to 0.3 may be a concern, but 0.3 by itself cannot be used to grade stage or severity.

CDRs are influenced by the size of the disc and the eccentricity of the cup. A CDR of 0.9 in a person with a disc with a diameter of 3 mm could be entirely healthy. Furthermore, CDRs do not consider the eccentricity of the cup. An average-sized disc with a CDR of 0.5 and a disc with a rim width that is the same in all areas, so that the outer edge of the cup is concentric to the other edge of the rim, will not have visual field loss due to glaucoma. That disc could have always been like that or perhaps only a year ago it was a disc with CDR of 0.1, one just does not know. But an average-sized disc with a CDR of 0.5 in which the cup is eccentric, so that in one area there is no NRR, will always have a visual field defect and is always abnormal. So single determinations of CDRs have no suprathreshold value and so cannot be used as a marker of damage to the ONH, because they do not consider disc size or rim irregularity (cup eccentricity).

Let us consider some other findings to see if they are of use in determining whether a person is in the Yellow Zone. A single measurement of RNFL thickness cannot be used to determine the severity of glaucoma damage because there is disagreement on the range of "normal," and, also, because many processes affect this tissue, so that the RNFL can be very thin as a result of a process other than glaucoma. Another example of a finding that can be of help in some ways, and is usually included in "risk calculators" is age. But there is no suprathreshold level for age. A person could have glaucoma at age 1 and not have glaucoma at age 101. So, age is not of diagnostic value because it lacks a suprathreshold level. However, the presence of asymptomatic field loss may mean a person is in the Yellow Zone. But, as with RNFL thickness, one must make sure the field loss is caused by glaucoma, not any of the many other reasons for field loss, especially in the elderly and those not intellectually sharp.

Is it possible to be sure field loss is real? We must discuss that as we consider how to assess severity accurately. The answer to the question is, No, it is not possible to be sure, that is certain, that what we consider field loss is field loss at all, much less field loss caused by glaucoma. However, it is possible to be adequately sure. Of what is it possible to be certain? very little. And of what is possible to be sufficiently certain that it is considered clinically valid? It is this latter question that must be answered. The answer to that is critical to providing good care to people. Being able to evaluate validity requires humility, honesty, and knowledge. The humility and honesty are just as important as the knowledge. There is no doubt that all of us see what we wish to see and do not see what we do not know how to see or do not wish to see. But the factors that affect validity are not mysterious. Careful consideration to the results of a machine-measured or even a confrontation field should be able to allow the observer to conclude with relative certainty that the field is adequately valid. That is, a subjective determination made by a skilled physician may be more likely to be accurate than the allegedly "objective" assessment made by the field machine, because the honest, humble, knowledgeable physician considers issues that affect validity, which machines cannot do as well. These issues include the known skill of the technician; is the patient told not to guess and only to press the button when absolutely sure, or told that the flashes are hard to see and if one seems to see one to press the button? Does the technician make sure the corrective lenses are clean and properly aligned? Is he/she the sort of person more likely to want to be productive or be accurate? The machine cannot evaluate the level or anxiety or fatigue of the patient, and how those aspects compare with the anxiety and fatigue at the time when the prior field was measured. If, in an area of variable energy supply, is the power to the machine standard? And on and on and on. Are all clinicians skilled at considering these aspects? The answer here is easy: No. Can they become skilled? The answer there is also easy—Yes. This particular chapter is about accurate assessment. Essential to understanding what results in accurate assessment is understanding that the validity of a determination is not based primarily on the type of assessment, but rather on the quality of the assessment. There is nothing intrinsically more likely to result in validity with a so-called objective test than one which is subjective. Properly designed, executed, and analyzed controlled clinical trials minimize bias better than anecdotal information. But that is unrelated to whether are "objective" or subjective." The most sophisticated controlled clinical trials possible are worse than a careful history in assessing whether a person truly has symptoms troubling him or her. Estimates of validity should be considered with all data, allegedly objective or subjective, and always put in the context of the entire situation; the data should never be assumed to be valid simply because they are on a "printout." The point of this discussion is that, when properly obtained and evaluated, a measurement of the visual field can sometimes be considered definite evidence of glaucomatous damage.

We have been discussing findings that indicate a person is in the Yellow Zone. Existing field loss is one of those findings. Establishing that a person previously without field loss has developed loss moves the patient from the Green into the yellow Zone. Such a patient has had a worsening of field, but the person may still be asymptomatic and still feel fine; in fact, that **person** has **not** gotten worse. We now discuss the second purpose of accurately assessing severity, specifically, determining the direction and the rate of change. It is obviously essential to establish whether glaucoma damage is lessening or worsening. It can do both, if worsening, the IOP is almost certainly too high, regardless of what it is measured to be. If lessening, the IOP is almost certainly low enough, regardless of what it is measured to be. No matter how carefully a target pressure is calculated, the target IOP is just a guess. It is a serious clinical mistake to assume that the guess is correct. It is whether the damage – structural damage or functional damage or both, – is improving or worsening that determines if treatment is correct.

Field loss is important to measure accurately when people are in the Yellow Zone, but cannot be used to monitor improvement or deterioration of glaucoma when the eye is in the Green Zone; the presence of real loss of visual field is always a sign of pathology and means that people are in the Yellow Zone, if asymptomatic, or the Red Zone if symptomatic. Symptoms cannot be used to monitor what is happening in the Green Zone, a because patients in the Green Zone have no symptoms. Let us consider a person who as an apparently healthy disc, with a Disc Damage Likelihood Score (DDLS) of 2. That person has no symptoms and is in the Green Zone. If the person develops ANY symptoms now he or she is in the RED zone. But the person's disc may show narrowing of the NRR so that the DDLS changes from 2 to 4, without the person developing any symptoms. The person has not gotten worse, but the person's disc has gotten worse. That person now has a "suprathreshold" finding showing worsening. That person, now, is in the Yellow Zone - no symptoms but something is definitely wrong. Some structural change always precedes a functional change; it is the structural change that causes the field loss to develop. To monitor change in all three zones a marker is needed that will indicate continuing change in all three zones. A good marker might be the number of retinal ganglion cells. However, establishing that at this time is not possible. Furthermore, loss of RGCs occurs as result of conditions other than glaucoma. A quantitative metric presently available, and shown to correlate with field loss better than Heidelberg Retinal Tomography (HRT) or Optical Coherence Tomography (OCT), is the DDLS [3]. At this time a suitable finding to use to monitor change for all three zones is the DDLS.

8.3 Disc Damage Likelihood Scale

The DDLS is based on three considerations:

1. The size of the disc, that is, the largest diameter of the optic disc (the distance in mm from the outer edge of the NRR to the outer edge of the NRR on the opposite side of the disc),
2. The narrowest width of the NRR,
3. The circumferential extent of rim absence (if there is an area where no rim is present).

8.3.1 Measuring the Disc Size (the Widest Disc Diameter)

The size of the disc can be measured using a high (+) lens and the biomicroscope, or using a direct ophthalmoscope. It is actually more accurate with a direct ophthalmoscope. To measure disc size with a direct ophthalmoscope one must first ascertain the size (diameter) in mm of the circular area of illumination of the beam on the fundus. This must be done because different ophthalmoscopes have different size beams. To do this one choses a person with an easily examined disc, with a small cup, and with a refractive error of less than three diopters. The size of that person's disc is then measured using a high (+) fundus lens at the slit lamp. A very narrow slit beam is directed onto the disc and the graticule above the oculars used to reduce the height of the beam until it corresponds in size to the disc. That is, the height of the slit beam is narrowed until its outer edges (top and bottom) coincide with the outer edges of the widest diameter of the disc (it may be necessary to rotate the arm). The mm indicated on the graticule is then read. If one is using a Volk +66D lens, the reading on the graticule will give a satisfactory indication of the disc size, as the Volk +66D lens only minimally underestimates the disc size (Fig. 8.5). This measurement can be done using a +60D, +78 D, or +90D lens but when using one of these lenses a corrective factor must be used to obtain the actual disc width.

Corrective factors for other lenses are: Volk 60D×0.88, 78D×1.2, 90D×1.33. Nikon 60D×1.03, 90D×1.63.

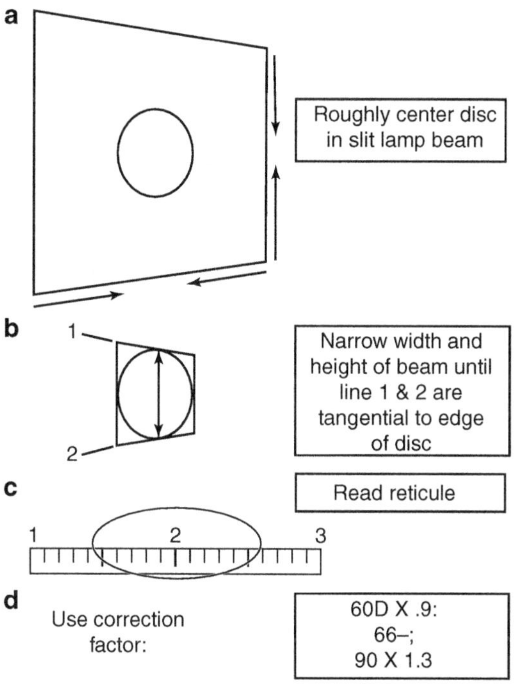

Fig. 8.5 Measurement of the disc size using a slit lamp graticule

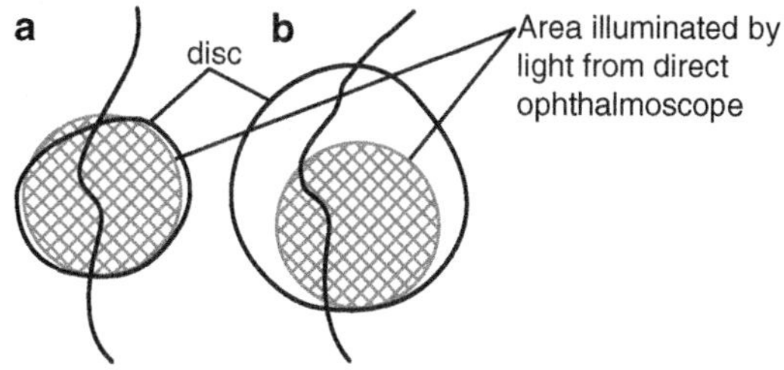

Fig. 8.6 Using a high + lens such as a 66D, the disc on the right has been determined to be 2 mm in diameter (widest diameter). The direct ophthalmoscope beam shines on an area about 2/3rds the diameter of this 2 mm disc. Therefore, the beam's diameter is 1.2 mm. Now one examines the disc on the left using the same direct ophthalmoscope. The examiner knows that this disc has a diameter of 1.2 mm

Having determined the size of that particular disc, by using the indirect ophthalmoscopic method with a high (+) lens, it is now necessary to do the next step. Let us say that the disc we have just measured has a 2.0 mm diameter (so it is a rather large disc). Now the examiner uses the direct ophthalmoscope. The beam size of that direct ophthalmoscope is selected so it is set on either medium or small. If the direct ophthalmoscope has settings that allow it to be used as a direct or an indirect ophthalmoscope, the "direct" setting is selected. The disc of that same person is then examined using that ophthalmoscope. The beam width must be small enough that the beam shines on the disc and only on the disc, and does not extend past the disc on to the retina. Phrased differently, the area on the disc that is illuminated by the light beam must be smaller than the entire size of the disc. If the beam is wider than the disc and also shines on the retina, a smaller beam must be chosen (Fig. 8.6). If the beam illuminates less than half the disc, a larger beam is chosen, but one still small enough that only the disc is illuminated.

Now, with the beam illuminating only part of the disc the examiner determines how much of that 2 mm-sized disc the beam illuminates (we know that disc has a 2 mm diameter because we have just determined that).

Let us say the beam shines on 2/3rds of the disc that is from the most inferior outer edge of the NRR to slightly above the center of the disc. If that were the case, then the examiner has determined that the beam width of the ophthalmoscope he or she is using is 1.2 mm in diameter. Knowing that, then one can use that ophthalmoscope with that same beam size selected to determine the disc size of all other discs. If, for example, the examiner notes that the beam illuminates the entire diameter of a disc of another disc, then that disc is 1.2 mm in diameter. This is the preferred method both for determining disc size and for examining the disc clinically. Few doctors now use the direct ophthalmoscope. The high (+) lens may be used to evaluate ONH size for eyes that have less the 3D of refractive error. The measurements become increasingly inaccurate as the refractive error increases beyond that. However, this is not a problem with the direct ophthalmoscope.

8.3.2 Measuring the Rim Width

The width of the NRR must be considered in terms of a Rim/Disc ratio (RDR) (Fig. 8.7). The nerve is inspected to find the area where the rim is narrowest. (Note, that we have used adjectives and nouns that refer to width or narrowness, not to thickness or thinness [4]). The narrowest pos-

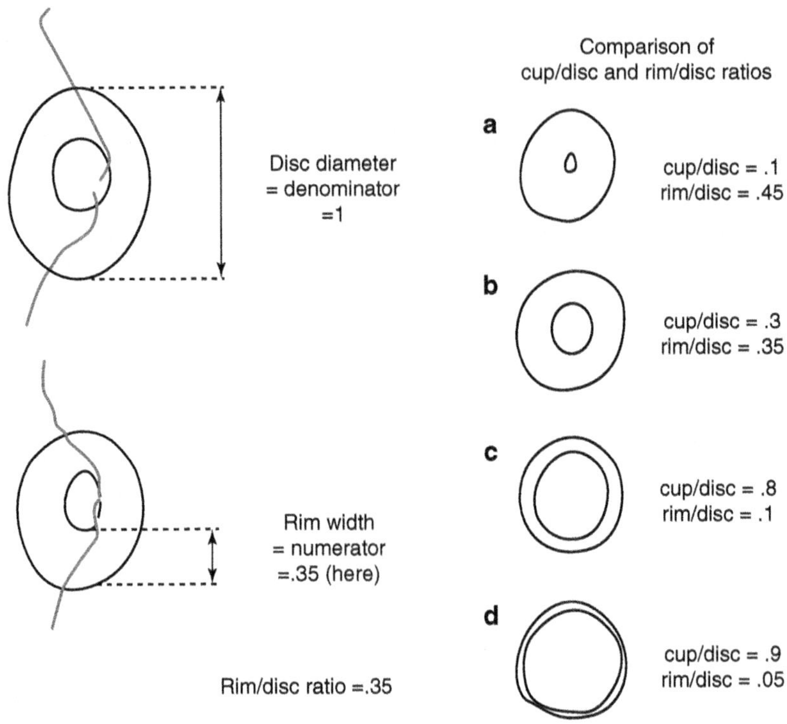

Fig. 8.7 Measurement of rim/disc ratio

sible RDR is 0.0 and the widest possible RDR is 0.5. A disc that has RDR of 0.5 for 360° would have no cup at all. If the cup was concentric so that the rim was the same width everywhere, then the RDR would be the same width everywhere.

Consider a disc with a concentric cup and a CDR of 0.6. The observer decides 0.6 is the CDR because the cup width is 6/10ths the width of the disc. That means the RDR is 0.2 everywhere. The RDR can be more easily and more accurately calculated than the CDR, because one only needs to consider one area of the rim, not two. Now, having measured the RDR, that RDR is used to start the determination of the DDLS. The various possibilities are shown in Fig. 8.3 for an average-sized disc one subtracts the narrowest rim disc ratio from 0.5. So, to calculate the DDLS of this eye, determine the narrowest RDR = 0.2, subtract 0.2 from 0.5 (0.5–0.2), which = 0.3. So, the DDLS of an eye with an average-sized disc with RDR of 0.2 is 3. The exception to that rule is when the NRR is extremely narrow, so that it is hard to be sure there is any rim at all. The RDR is less than 0.1. This ONH with rim still remaining in all areas, but rim that is extremely narrow is a DDLS of 5. An average-sized disc with such a narrow rim might have field loss or might not have field loss. It does not matter whether there is more than one "narrowest" area; whatever is the narrowest RDR is used to determine the DDLS.

8.3.3 When There Is An Area in Which There Is No NRR

In some cases of glaucoma, the damage has caused complete loss of the NRR in one or more areas. When that is the case one considers the circumferential extent of the rim absence, in degrees. If the rim is absent, for example, for three clock hours, perhaps from 3 o'clock to 6 o'clock, that is a rim absence of 90°; if absent from 5 o'clock to 6 o'clock that is a rim absence of 30°. When the rim absence in an average-sized disc is from 1 to 45°, that is a DDLS of 6. Such a disc will always have field loss. When there is no rim for >45° and <90° that is a DDLS of 7 for an average-sized disc (Fig. 8.8). If the rim loss totals more than 90° and less than 180° that is a DDLS of 8, if no rim for 181–270°, and if no rim for more than 270° the DDLS is 10 for an average-sized disc.

If the disc is of average size (1.5–2.0 mm), then one does not need to do anything further. The DDLS is what one has determined based on rim width or circumferential absence of rim. If the disc is smaller than 1.5 mm but larger than 1 mm, the scale must be modified, because the damage is more than appears to be the case based on cup/disc ratios. Thus, with a small disc one adds one DDLS unit; with a tiny disc—smaller than 1.0 mm—one adds two DDLS units. With a large disc the damage is less than appears to be the case based on cup/disc ratios; if the disc diameter is greater than 2.0 mm but smaller than 3.0 mm one subtracts 1 DDLS unit; with very large discs, greater in diameter than 3.0 mm subtracts two DDLS units. Figure 8.9 shows the DDLS nomogram.

Some examples:

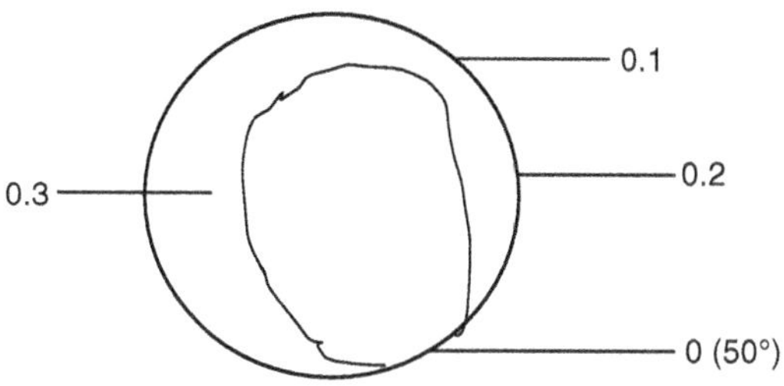

Fig. 8.8 This disc has a RDR of 0.1 at 1 o'clock, 0.2 at 3 0'clock, but 0 at 5 o'clock. As there is an area with no rim, the circumferential extent of rim absence is measured; here, that is 50°. This is less that 45 degrees. If this were a disc of average size, then the DDLS would be 6

1. A disc has a narrowest RDR of 0.01 and is 1.3 mm in size. This is a small disc. The DDLS for an average-sized disc is with a RDR of >0.1 is 5, but since this is a small disc

THE DISC DAMAGE LIKELIHOOD SCALE

	Narrowest width of rim (rim/disc ratio)					Examples	
New DDLS Stage	For Small Disc <1.50 mm	For Average size Disc 1.50-2.00 mm	For Large Disc >2.00 mm	Old DDLS Stage	1.25 mm optic nerve	1.75 mm optic nerve	2.25 mm optic nerve
1	.5 or more	.4 or more	.3 or more	0a			
2	.4 to .49	.3 to .39	.2 to .29	0b			
3	.3 to .39	.2 to .29	.1 to .19	1			
4	.2 to .29	.1 to .19	less than .1	2			
5	.1 to .19	less than .1	0 for less than 45°	3			
6	less than .1	0 for less than 45°	0 for 46° to 90°	4			
7	0 for less than 45°	0 for 46° to 90°	0 for 91° to 180°	5			
8	0 for 46° to 90°	0 for 91° to 180°	0 for 181° to 270°	6			
9	0 for 91° to 180°	0 for 181° to 270°	0 for more than 270°	7a			
10	0 for more than 180°	0 for more than 270°		7b			

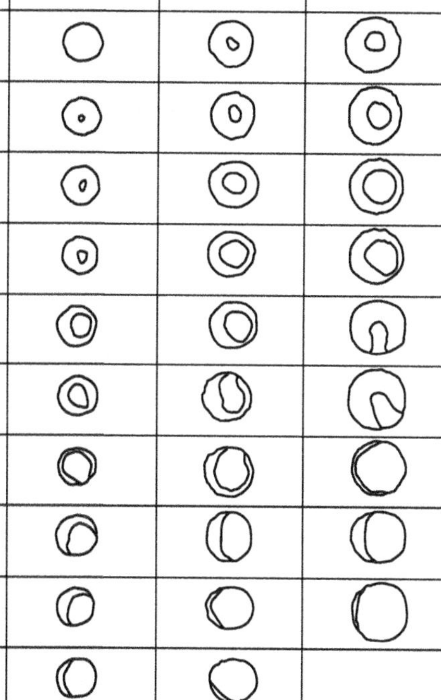

Fig. 8.9 This nomogram illustrates how to determine the DDLS. The central column titled "DDLS Stage" refers to the initial DDLS System and is included for those who learned that. That nomenclature has been replaced by the scores in the left-hand-most column. Not listed is a DDLS of 0, which would be applied when an average-sized disc had a rim/disc ratio of 0.5, or a large disc a rim/disc ratio of 0.1. (For the average-sized disc 5–5 = 0)

one adds one DDLS unit; the correct scores are DDLS = 6. Unlike an eye with a DDLS of 5, in which there may or may not be field loss, this person with a DDLS of 6 will have field loss. Even though that patient will have field loss, the amount of field loss will usually be so little that he/she is free of symptoms. But there is a definite finding of something of concern. No one starts with a DDLS of 6 so this patient's nerve at some point had to develop some disc damage. Thus, this asymptomatic person with a small disc and a DDLS of 6 is in Yellow Zone.

2. A disc has a narrowest RDR of 0.01 and is 2.3 mm in size. Again, that would be a DDLS of 5 for an average-sized disc but for this large disc the DDLS is 4. That patient will not have field loss and will be asymptomatic and will be in the Green Zone. Thus, a small disc and a large disc with the same RDR will be two DDLS units apart.
3. A disc has a RDR of 0.1 and a diameter of 1.75 mm. That is a DDLS of 4 (Remember, that to determine the DDLS when rim is present in all areas simply subtract the narrowest RDR from 0.5). That patient will be asymptomatic and in the Green Zone.
4. That same disc with a DDLS of 4 is now examined 2 years later. There is now no NRR for 95°, so it is a DDLS of 8. That patient now almost certainly has troublesome symptoms, and is in the Red Zone. Rims get narrower with age. The exact rate has not been established. Our guess, and it is just a hunch, is that rate of narrowing related to aging is about one DDLS unit every 40 years.
5. A healthy woman with an IOP of 45 mm Hg and around 50 years of life estimated to be remaining (YER) has a RDR 0.4 and a disc diameter of 1.6 mm. She has a DDLS of 1. She feels and functions well. She is in the Green Zone, but she almost certainly has glaucoma. She almost certainly needs treatment, so attempts are made to lower her pressure with medications and laser. They fail to lower her pressure more than a few mmHg. One year later she has a RDR of 0.2 despite maximal medicinal treatment. She still has no symptoms, and no field loss. She is still in the Green Zone. What does she need? She probably needs surgery, because her disc is worsening at a rate of two DDLS per year, and will continue to do so until her intraocular pressure is adequately lowered. Her rate of worsening is one DDLS per 1 year. It will probably take only 5 years before she has troublesome symptoms, and enough damage that the damage may be difficult to arrest. The ophthalmologist should consider surgical lowering of her IOP.

Figure 8.4 illustrates the relationship between symptoms and the DDLS. This is valid for the relationship between the Green Zone and a DDLS up through DDLS 4. Some patients with DDLS of 5 will have field loss, but it is usually minimal and not symptomatic. Such patients then are in the Yellow Zone. How much glaucoma damage a person must have in order to develop troublesome visual symptoms is not known. The relationship between field loss and Quality of Life of ability to perform the activities of daily living varies markedly from person to person, despite misleading comments to the contrary. Therefore, it is important to understand that the dividing line between the Yellow and the Red Zones will also vary from person to person. Some people may move into the Red Zone when one eye has a DDLS of 8 and the other DDLS 5, and some move into the Red Zone when both eyes are DDLS 6. So the line separating the Yellow from the Red Zone is not absolute. The patient who has troublesome symptoms due to visual loss caused by glaucoma is in the Red Zone, that is, already sick.

When discs are "atypical," as is often the case in eyes that are myopic, it can be impossible to determine a DDLS accurately. In such cases it is essential to acknowledge that difficulty. Misinformation is more problematic than no information.

The DDLS is of greatest use in those cases where decision making is most difficult, specifically the asymptomatic person. Here the DDLS provides highly valuable information about rate of change, which combined with duration of change is necessary to know in order to make rational, appropriate treatment decisions [5–7].

8.4 Summary

Knowing the severity and the stage of a person's condition, such as glaucoma, how rapidly that stage changing and the duration the stage will continue changing is necessary in order to give patients good care. The more accurately this is assessed the more valuable it is in influencing care. The most important aspect needing assessment is the patients' symptomatology. This establishes when a person is in the Red Zone of the Colored Disease Process Graph. When patients do not have symptoms, and so are either in the Green (Presumed Healthy) zone or the Yellow (Transition) zone of the Colored Disease Process Graph, physicians must rely on findings that are valid, relevant surrogates for severity, and that can indicate that change will occur. The DDLS can provide such information. As the DDLS correlates well with the severity of a person's glaucoma, is quantitative, and can be used to monitor direction and rate of change it works well as a marker to determine severity of glaucoma and to monitor change in severity.

References

1. Zangalli C, Gupta SR, Spaeth GL. The disc as the basis of treatment for glaucoma. Saudi J Ophthalmol. 2011;25(4):381–7.
2. Waisbourd M, Parker S, Ekici F, Spaeth GL, et al. A prospective, longitudinal, observational cohort study examining how glaucoma affects quality of life and visually-related function over 4 years: design and methodology. BMC Ophthalmol. 2015;15:91.
3. Spaeth GL, Reddy SC. Imaging of the optic disk in caring for patients with glaucoma: ophthalmoscopy and photography remain the gold standard. Surv Ophthalmol. 2014;59(4):454–8.
4. Spaeth GL, Jatla KK, Ichhpujani P. Do optic discs get "thinner" or "narrower?". J Glaucoma. 2010;19(5):288–92.
5. Spaeth GL, Henderer J, Liu C, Kesen M, Altangerel U, Bayer A, et al. The disc damage likelihood scale: reproducibility of a new method of estimating the amount of optic nerve damage caused by glaucoma. Trans Am Ophthalmol Soc. 2002;100:181–5.
6. Spaeth GL, Lopes JF, Junk AK, Grigorian AP, Henderer J. Systems for staging the amount of optic nerve damage in glaucoma: a critical review and new material. Surv Ophthalmol. 2006;51(4):293–315.
7. Kitaoka Y, Tanito M, Yokoyama Y, et al. Estimation of the disc damage likelihood scale in primary open-angle glaucoma: the glaucoma stereo analysis study. Graefes Arch Clin Exp Ophthalmol. 2016;254(3):523–8.

What Optic Nerve Head Conditions Mimic Glaucoma?

9

Gaurav Gupta, Surinder Pandav, and Sushmita Kaushik

9.1 Non-Glaucomatous Optic Disc Cupping

Optic disc cupping is always considered suspicious of glaucoma, but disc cupping is not necessarily caused due to glaucoma. There are conditions which may manifest as 'non-glaucomatous optic disc cupping'. We may not always be able to distinguish between glaucomatous and non-glaucomatous optic cupping based on the optic disc appearance alone [1], but a proper clinical examination always provides valuable clues to the diagnosis. One should always carefully look for cupping and pallor. If cupping is more than pallor, then it is likely to be glaucomatous, and if pallor is more than cupping, then one should always suspect non-glaucomatous causes of optic disc cupping. There are several conditions which can cause non-glaucomatous cupping and may mimic glaucoma. A few typical conditions are listed below:

1. Neurological diseases: compressive lesions,
2. Ischemic optic neuropathy,
3. Hereditary optic atrophy: Leber's Hereditary optic neuropathy (LHON); Autosomal dominant optic atrophy (ADOA),
4. Congenital conditions: Tilted disc, Coloboma, Hypoplasia,
5. Toxic optic neuropathy: Ethambutol, Methanol,
6. Nutritional optic neuropathy: Vit B12, Folic Acid,
7. Traumatic optic neuropathy,
8. Inflammatory diseases: Optic neuritis,
9. Others: syphilis, radiation, shock.

9.1.1 Differentiating Non-Glaucomatous Cupping from Glaucomatous

9.1.1.1 Fundoscopy

Cupping is more profound in eyes with glaucoma, whereas non-glaucomatous eyes with cupping have greater degrees of neuroretinal rim (NRR) pallor (Fig. 9.1) [2]. The depth of the cup is considered one of the most critical objective findings of the optic nerve head (ONH) and may help to differentiate glaucoma from non-glaucomatous optic neuropathy. Shallow form of cupping is usually seen in non-glaucomatous optic neuropathies [3]. Table 9.1 enlists the funduscopic features favouring Non-glaucomatous cupping and the associated conditions.

9.1.1.2 Visual Field Defects

Glaucomatous field defects typically respect the horizontal meridian owing to the arrangement of the retinal nerve fibres of the superior and inferior hemisphere meeting at the horizontal raphe

G. Gupta · S. Pandav · S. Kaushik (✉)
Glaucoma Service, Advanced Eye Center, PGIMER, Chandigarh, India

S. Pandav et al. (eds.), *The Optic Nerve Head in Health and Disease*,
https://doi.org/10.1007/978-981-33-6838-5_9

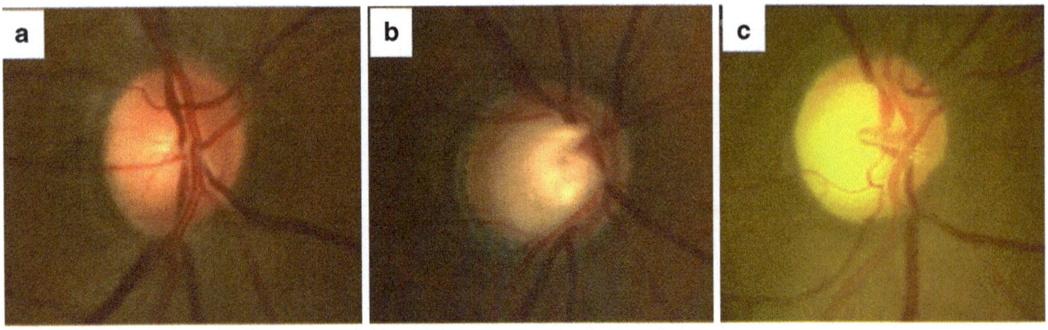

Fig. 9.1 (**a**) Normal disc; (**b**) Glaucomatous cupping with inferior notch; (**c**) Non-glaucomatous cupping with temporal pallor

Table 9.1 Funduscopic features favouring non-glaucomatous cupping [4]

Finding	Conditions
• Generalized disc pallor	Ischemic Optic neuropathy; Optic neuritis,
• Sectorial pallor	Ischemic Optic neuropathy
• Retinal arteriolar narrowing	Ischemic Optic neuropathy; CRAO; trauma; radiation optic neuropathy
• Bilateral, symmetrical, temporal, segmental disc pallor	Hereditary optic neuropathy, toxic or nutritional optic neuropathy
• Unilateral, segmental temporal pallor:	Optic neuritis
• Severe optic pallor with arteriolar attenuation:	CRAO

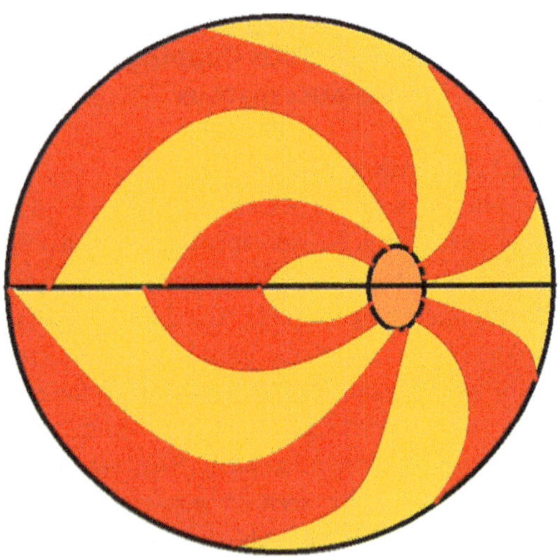

Fig. 9.2 Diagram showing normal arrangement of retinal nerve fibre layers

(Fig. 9.2). The resultant visual field defects in glaucoma are classically manifest as Bjerrum's scotoma or an arcuate scotoma (Fig. 9.3a). Visual field defects due to neurological compressive optic neuropathy do not respect the horizontal meridian and may be oriented vertically such as seen in hemianopia or quadrantanopia (Fig. 9.3b).

9.1.1.3 Optical Coherence Tomography (OCT)

Figure 9.4a shows a normal OCT scan. On OCT, the Retinal Nerve Fibre Layer (RNFL) loss in non-glaucomatous optic disc cupping is not typically in the superior and inferior quadrants, as reported in glaucoma (Fig. 9.4b), rather more varied depending upon the aetiology (Fig. 9.4c). Also, for a similar average RNFL thickness, the macular volume is reduced significantly in patients with non-glaucomatous cupping compared to patients with glaucomatous cupping [5]. Anterior laminar depth is deeper in glaucoma than in non-glaucomatous eyes and measurements of the Anterior laminar depth has a good ability to differentiate non-glaucomatous from glaucoma [2].

9.1.1.4 Neuroimaging

Magnetic Resonance Imaging (MRI) and Computed Tomography (CT) scans are the neuroimaging modalities available, which can help in diagnosing neurological causes of optic nerve head cupping. Indications for neuroimaging are enlisted in Table 9.2.

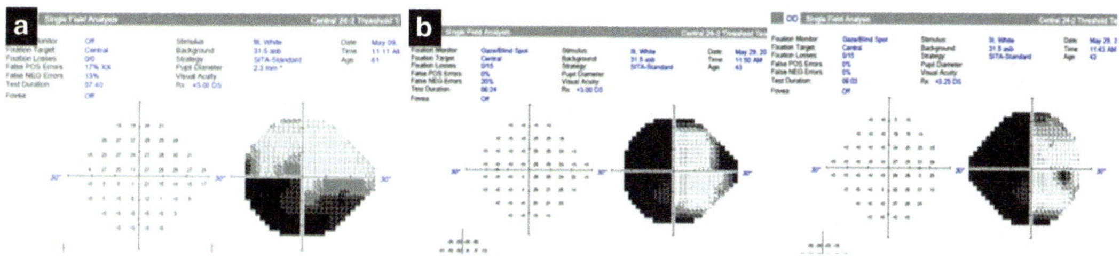

Fig. 9.3 (**a**) Defect respecting the horizontal meridian resulting in an Arcuate scotoma and (**b**) defect respecting the vertical meridian resulting in hemianopia

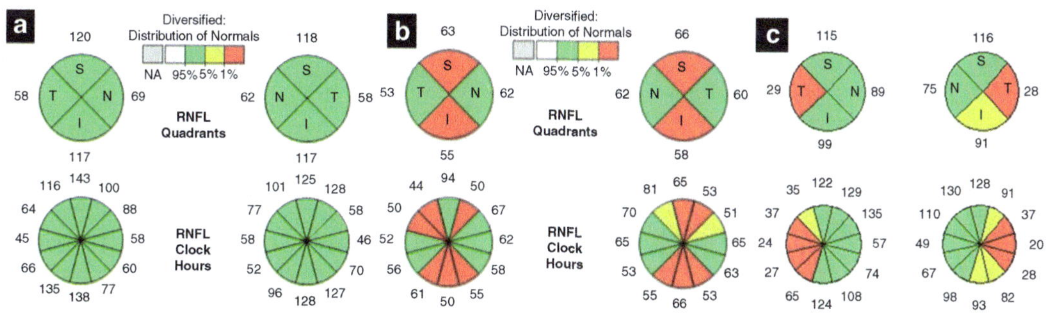

Fig. 9.4 (**a**) Normal RNFL scan on OCT, (**b**) superior and inferior quadrant loss on OCT in glaucoma, (**c**) varied RNFL loss on OCT, depending upon the aetiology

Table 9.2 Indications of neuroimaging

Age < 50 years
New-onset or increase in severity of headaches
Colour vision abnormality
Pallor of neuroretinal rim
Neurological field defects, respecting vertical meridian
Lack of correlation in visual field and disc changes

9.2 Neurological Cupping

There are various neurological conditions in which the ONH may mimic like that of glaucoma. These are usually compressive lesions, compressing the anterior visual pathway [6], such as:

- Tumours: pituitary adenomas, gliomas, meningiomas
- Aneurysm: fusiform aneurysms of the intracranial carotid arteries
- Cyst
- Chiasmatic arachnoiditis

Among these, pituitary adenoma and meningioma are the most common causes of compressive optic neuropathy. Compressive optic neuropathy in such cases may sometimes be clinically indistinguishable from glaucomatous optic neuropathy.

In cases of Pituitary adenoma, on fundoscopy, there is bilateral temporal pallor of the optic disc with cupping. On perimetry, there is bitemporal hemianopia in chiasmatic lesions (Fig. 9.2). Figure 9.5 shows a case of 72 years old man with pituitary macroadenoma with bilateral non-glaucomatous optic disc cupping with temporal pallor and visual field shows early bitemporal hemianopia. Figure 9.6 shows the reversal of field defects of same patient after tumour mass resection.

9.3 Ischemic Optic Neuropathies

Ischemia at the optic nerve head is known as anterior ischemic optic neuropathy (AION). Optic nerve head infarction occurring due to short posterior ciliary artery vasculitis is called arteritic AION (AAION). If this infarction occurs due to insufficiency of optic nerve circulation exacerbated by structural crowding at ONH, it is called non-arteritic AION (NA-AION).

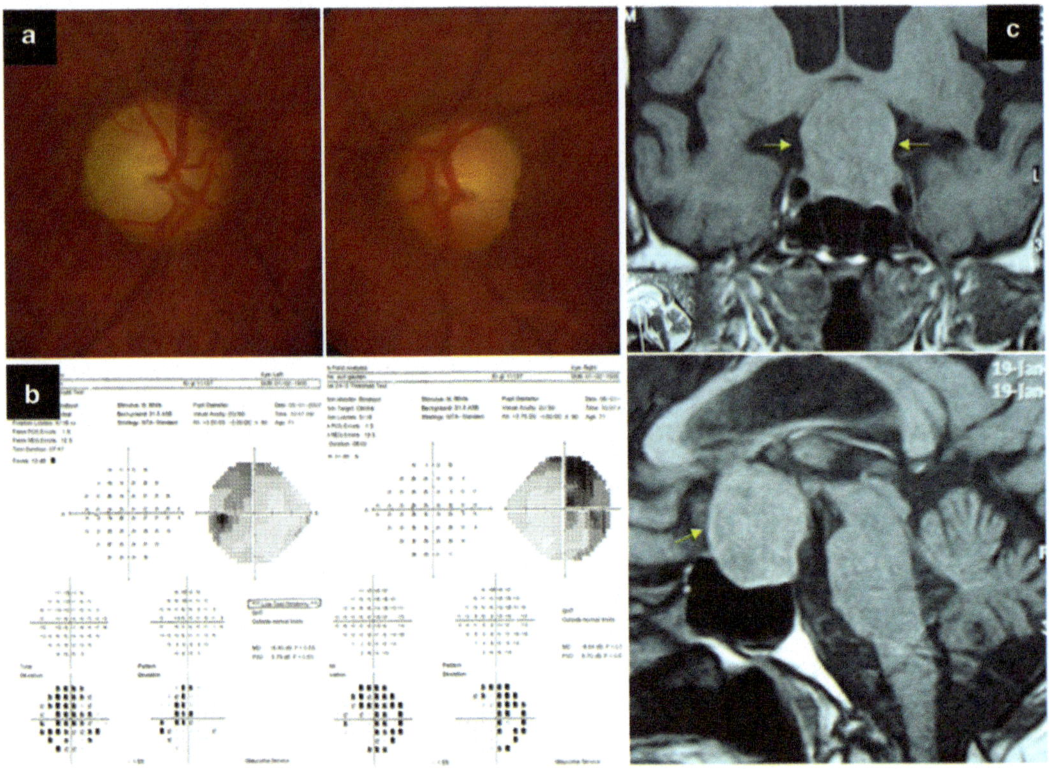

Fig. 9.5 A case of 72 years old man with pituitary macroadenoma. (**a**) Disc pictures showing bilateral non-glaucomatous optic disc cupping with temporal pallor; (**b**) Visual field shows early bitemporal hemianopia, (**c**) MRI images showing a mass in pituitary region suggestive of pituitary macroadenoma (yellow arrows)

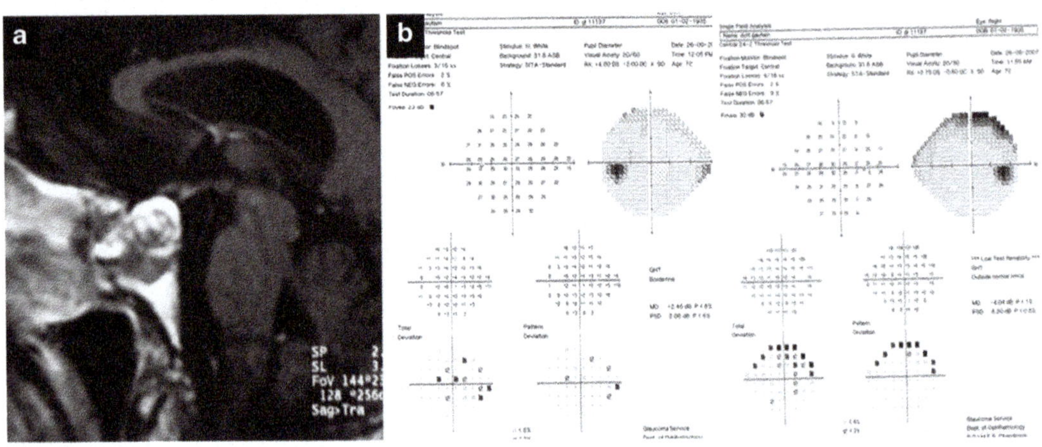

Fig. 9.6 Postoperative images of the same patient as in Fig. 9.5 after tumour mass resection. (**a**) MRI images shows no residual mass and (**b**) visual field shows reversal of field defects

Hayreh [7] has stated that AAION provides a telescoped natural course of cupping that closely resembles that of glaucoma and normal-tension glaucoma, owing to similarities in underlying pathogenesis. He believes that acute AAION produces acute hypoperfusion of the optic nerve, whereas glaucoma produces a chronic hypoperfusion state. Infarction of the anterior optic nerve in AAION destroys neural tissue and connective tissue. Further, in AAION, the retrolaminar optic nerve infarcts and may become fibrotic, which can lead to backward traction on the lamina cribrosa inciting maximal cupping at approximately four months. Thus, the destruction of neural tissue and backward bowing of the lamina are the key factors contributing to disc cupping in AION.

In AION, optic nerve head cupping is usually unilateral and has sectoral or generalized chalky-white pallor of the disc. On visual field testing, mostly altitudinal field defects are seen, but generalized depression, broad arcuate scotomas, and ceco-central defects can also be seen. In cases of NA-AION, the examination of the other eye can help in distinguishing it from glaucomatous cupping. The disc in the contralateral eye is typically smaller in diameter and may have small or absent physiological cup (crowded disc).

Cupping may also occur as a sequala of central retinal artery occlusion, which may occur likely due to death of just ganglion cells in the retina (with delayed death of their axons) without necrosis of the optic disc's glial and connective tissue (as opposed to glaucoma and AION).

Figure 9.7 shows a 64-year-old woman, who presented with left eye diminution of vision and normal intraocular pressure and a Relative Afferent Pupillary Defect (RAPD).

9.4 Leber's Hereditary Optic Neuropathy (LHON)

It is an inherited disorder occurring due to point mutation in the mitochondrial DNA. It manifests in young age as a distinct heredodegenerative optic neuropathy and patient present with subacute onset of dyschromatopsia with bilateral visual loss.

This alteration in complex I causes a decrease in ATP production, but more significantly, contributes to a build-up of reactive oxygen species (ROS). The increased ROS can lead to a cascade resulting in cell death. The primary cell type that is lost in LHON is the retinal ganglion cell, which is highly susceptible to disrupted ATP production and oxidative stress [8].

At the clinical examination in early stage, the fundus may look entirely normal, while the optic disc is more commonly hyperemic with peripapillary telangiectasias and vascular tortuosity of the central retinal vessels and OCT shows swelling of the retinal nerve fibre layer (RNFL), which gradually subsides once optic atrophy develops. There is characteristic loss of papillomacular nerve fibre layer leading to temporal thinning of RNFL and then there is progressive generalized RNFL thinning on OCT [9]. Visual field defect consist if centrocecal scotoma that begins nasal to blind spot and extends to involve fixation on both sides of vertical meridian.

Figure 9.8 shows a case of 43 years old woman, who presented with decreased vision and normal IOP and positive family history. She had symmetrical temporal disc pallor with non-glaucomatous optic disc cupping and thinning in temporal quadrant on OCT. Ganglion cell thickness map also shows decreased ganglion cells in complete macular region and all features are suggestive of LHON.

9.5 Nutritional and Toxic Optic Neuropathies

Nutritional deficiencies of certain vitamins (B12 or folic acid) and toxins such as methanol or ethambutol may lead to optic neuropathies.

These vitamins are involved in pathways of mitochondrial metabolism so their deficiency lead to defective metabolism and ATP deficiency. Similarly, these toxins also interfere in the mitochondrial metabolism pathways leading to deficiency of ATP. Decreased ATP leads to damage of retinal ganglion cell and papillomacular bundles are the most commonly affected part [10].

These patients present with slowly progressive bilateral loss of central vision. There is defect of colour vision as well. Disc findings are similar to LHON as both have similar pathogenesis. OCT has temporal RNFL thinning due to

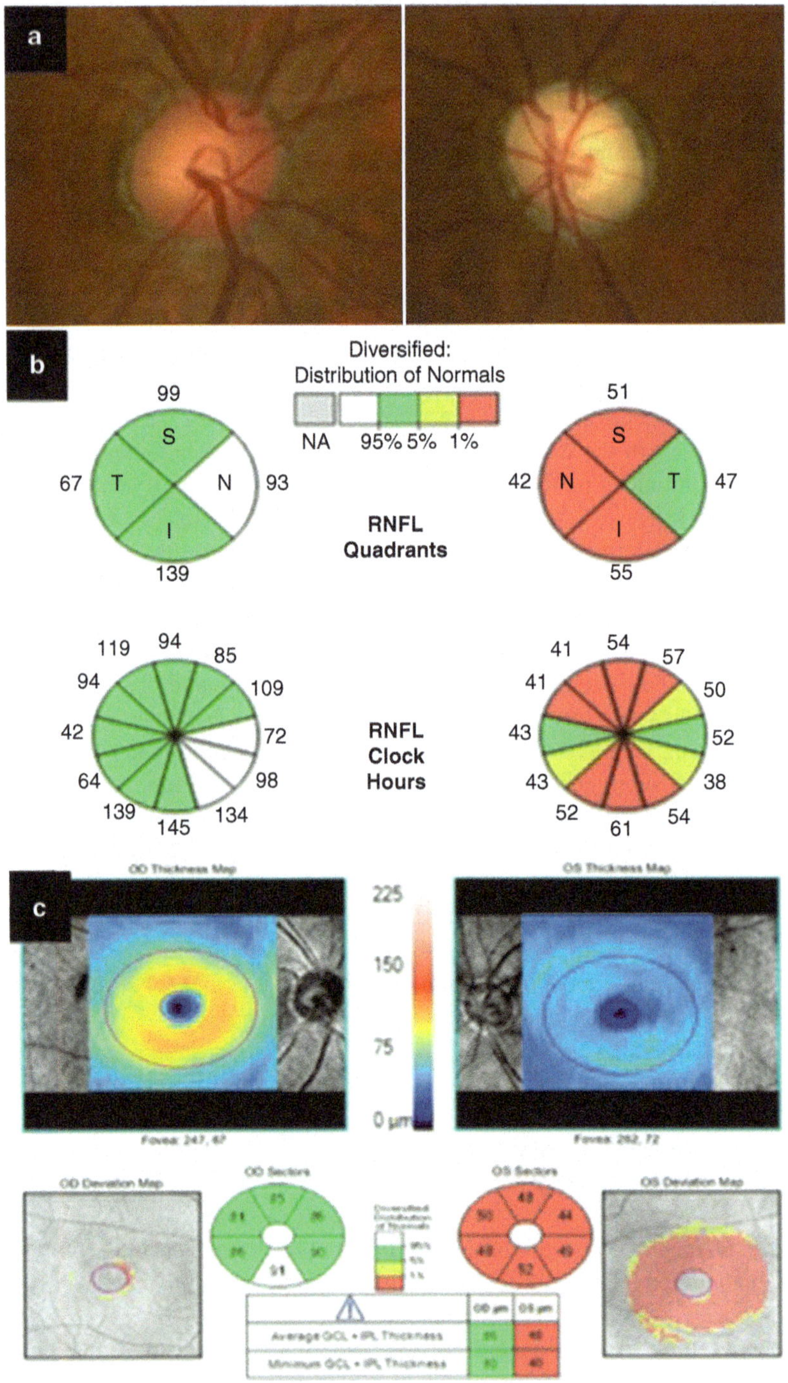

Fig. 9.7 (**a**) Disc photographs show optic disc cupping in left eye with pallor of NRR and there is crowded disc in right eye, features suggestive of old AION; (**b**) OCT RNFL in left eye shows thinning in three quadrants; whereas in right eye we can see RNFL is thickened than normal suggesting crowding of nerve fibre layers. (**c**) Ganglion cell thickness map shows decreased ganglion cells in macular region in left eye

loss of papillomacular bundle and visual field testing shows centrocecal scotoma that extends to involve fixation on both sides of vertical meridian.

Figure 9.9 shows images of a 40-year-old male, known smoker and alcoholic, having vitamin-B 12 deficiency who presented with complaint of diminution of vision with normal

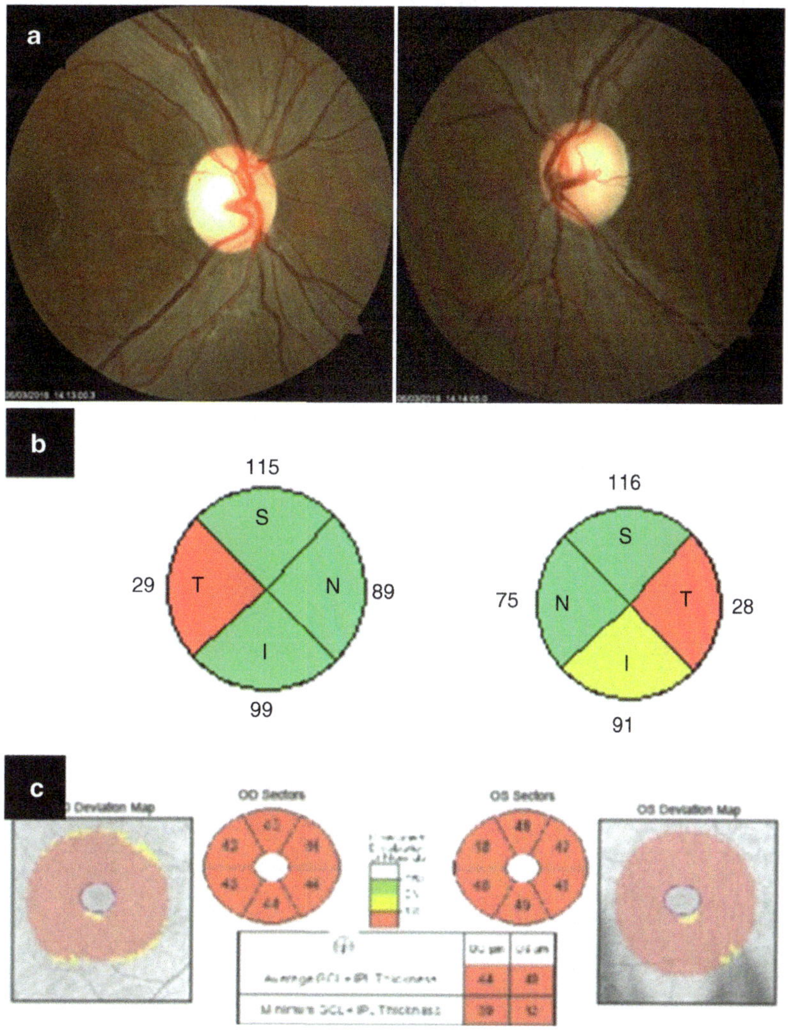

Fig. 9.8 (**a**) Disc photographs of both the eyes show symmetrical temporal disc pallor with non-glaucomatous optic disc cupping; (**b**) OCT RNFL shows thinning in temporal quadrant; (**c**) Ganglion cell thickness map shows decreased ganglion cells in the entire macular region

IOP. He had temporal pallor of NRR, OCT RNFL showing borderline thinning in temporal region in right eye and left eye also has an area of borderline thinning. Ganglion cell analysis shows loss of ganglion cells in the macular region suggesting loss of papillomacular bundle. All features are suggestive of combined toxic and nutritional optic neuropathy.

9.6 Congenital Disc Anomalies

Optic disc anomalies that may produce focal depressions of the normal surface topography include tilted disc and disc colobomas.

9.6.1 Tilted Disc

It is common and may mimic as glaucomatous disc and there may be localized associated RNFL defect, but there is usually no visual field defect in these cases. It is just an anatomical various due to oblique insertion of disc. It has been addressed in detail in a previous chapter (Chap. 7).

9.6.2 Optic Disc Coloboma

Coloboma confined to the disc is rare. In these cases, the cupping is deepest inferiorly, with a corresponding nonprogressive visual field defect [11].

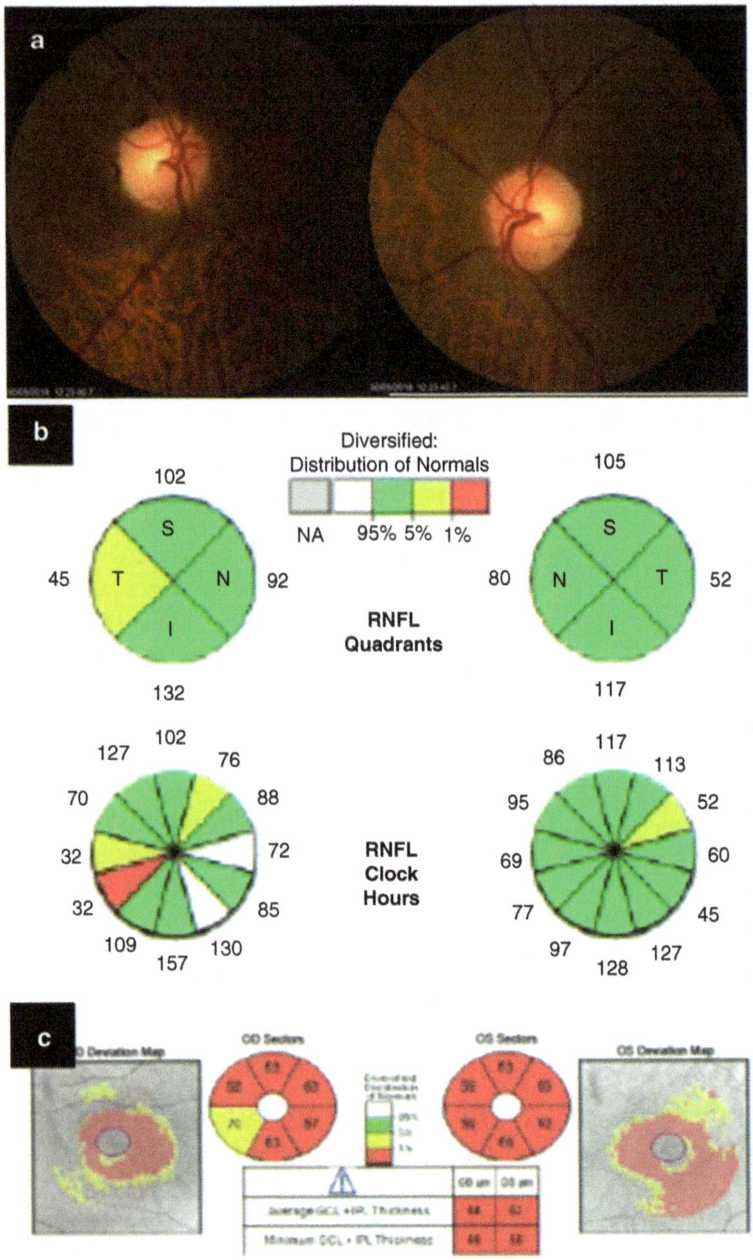

Fig. 9.9 (**a**) Disc photographs show temporal pallor of NRR; (**b**) OCT RNFL showing borderline thinning in temporal region in right eye and left eye has an area of borderline thinning; (**c**) Ganglion cell analysis shows loss of ganglion cells in the macular region suggesting loss of papillomacular bundle

Another anomaly that can produce cupping is a variant of optic nerve hypoplasia in children with periventricular leukomalacia [12]. In preterm babies with anoxic brain damage, axonal disruption in the optic radiations may occur (with corresponding visual field defects), leading to transsynaptic retrograde degeneration across the geniculate body. The resulting loss of optic nerve axons may give rise to cupping. Cupping in this situation occurs only if the anoxic insult occurs at between 29 and 34 weeks of gestation, prior to full development of the optic nerve and after the time when scleral plasticity leads to a small disc in cases of optic nerve hypoplasia.

Figure 9.10 shows a cases of 40 years old male who was referred to us for suspected discs. Disc photograph shows the presence of disc pit in temporal part of disc, which is better appreciated on red free image. Visual fields show scattered defects. Figure 9.11 shows a case of 43 years old

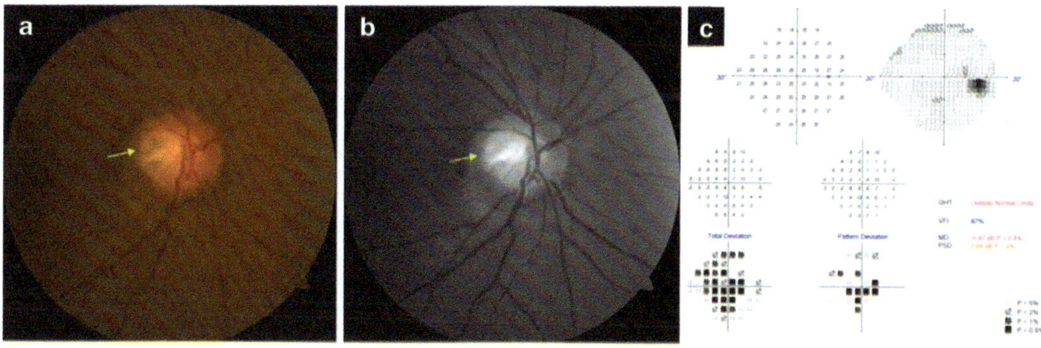

Fig. 9.10 A 40-year-old male with suspicious discs. (**a**) Disc photographs show presence of disc pit in temporal part of disc (yellow arrow). (**b**) Pit is better highlighted in the Red free image better (yellow arrow). (**c**) Visual filed shows scatter filed defects

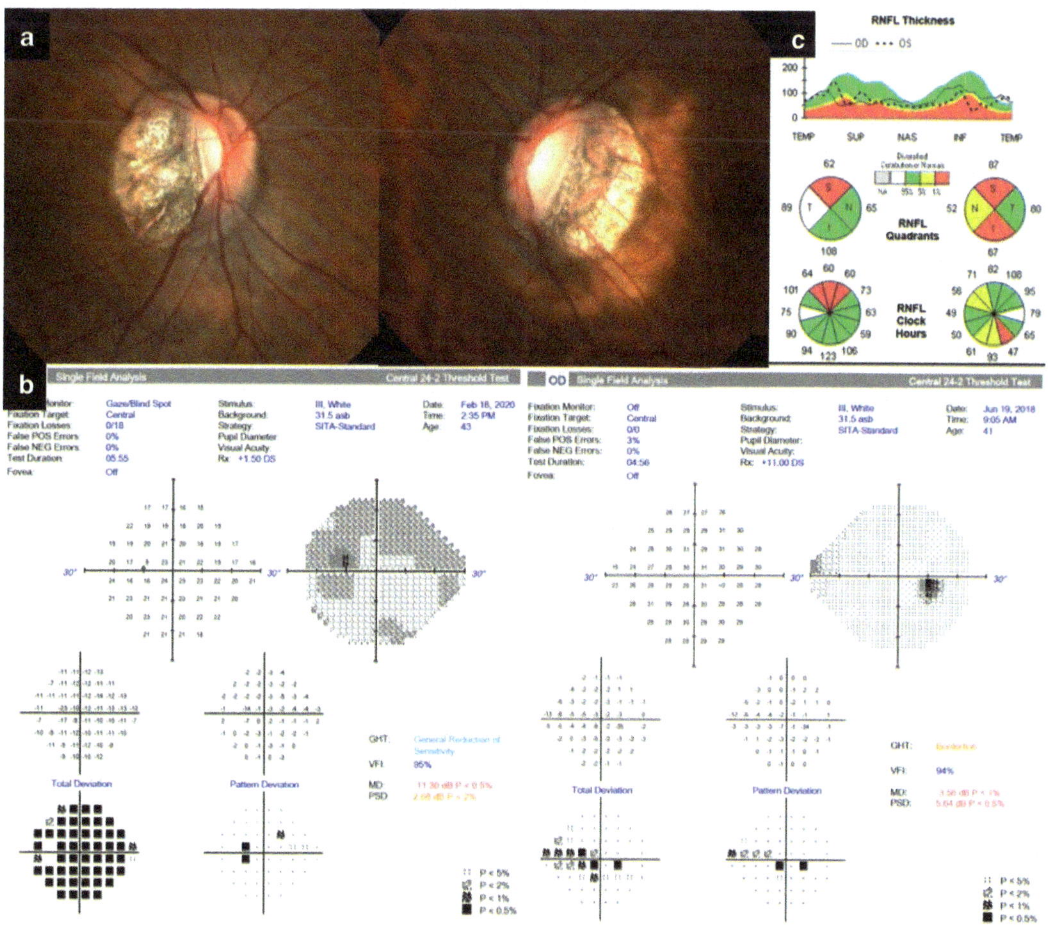

Fig. 9.11 A case of 43 years old female who presented with suspected discs and normal IOP. (**a**) Disc photos show a bilateral tilted disc due to oblique insertion of optic nerve head. (**b**) Visual fields are within normal limits. (**c**) OCT RNFL shows localized RNFL thinning

female who presented with suspected discs and normal IOP. Disc photos show a bilateral tilted disc due to oblique insertion of optic nerve head. Visual fields are normal but the OCT RNFL shows localized RNFL thinning.

9.7 Conclusion

Optic disc cupping is a consequence of many disorders causing neural loss at the optic nerve head. The clinical features and careful examination of the anatomy and vasculature of the optic disc can provide valuable insights into why and how optic nerve head cupping occurs in various conditions. The clues to distinguish glaucomatous from nonglaucomatous optic disc cupping depend largely upon a careful patient history, clinical finding of the optic nerve head, and visual fields assessment. It is important to remember that cupping can be seen with neurological processes, including many benign tumours that are treatable. The vigilant clinician can detect uncommon but potentially threatening forms of non-glaucomatous optic disc cupping, and ensure appropriate investigations and management.

References

1. Trobe JD, Glaser JS, Cassady J, et al. Nonglaucomatous excavation of the optic disc. Arch Ophthalmol. 1980;98:1046–50.
2. Fard MA, Moghimi S, Sahraian A, et al. Optic nerve head cupping in glaucomatous and nonglaucomatous optic neuropathy. Brit J Ophthalmol. 2019;103:374–8.
3. Ing E, Ivers KM, Yang H, Gardiner SK, Reynaud J, Cull G, Wang L, Burgoyne CF. Cupping in the monkey optic nerve transection model consists of prelaminar tissue thinning in the absence of posterior laminar deformation. Invest Ophthalmol Vis Sci. 2016;57:2914–27.
4. Ambati BK, Rizzo JF 3rd. Nonglaucomatous cupping of the optic disc. Int Ophthalmol Clin. 2001;41:139–49.
5. Gupta PK, Asrani S, Freedman SF, El-Dairi M, Bhatti MT. Differentiating glaucomatous from nonglaucomatous optic nerve cupping by optical coherence tomography. Open Neurol J. 2011;5:1–7.
6. Kupersmith MJ, Krohn D. Cupping of the optic disc with compressive lesions of the anterior visual pathway. Ann Ophthalmol. 1984;16:948–53.
7. Hayreh SS. Pathogenesis of cupping of the optic disc. Br J Ophthalmol. 1974;58:863–76.
8. Kwittken J, Barest HD. The neuropathology of hereditary optic atrophy (Leber's disease). Am J Pathol. 1958;34:185–9.
9. Meyerson C, Van Stavern G, McClelland C. Leber hereditary optic neuropathy: current perspectives. Clin Ophthalmol. 2015;9:1165–76.
10. Grzybowski A, Zülsdorff M, Wilhelm H, Tonagel F. Toxic optic neuropathies: an updated review. Acta Ophthalmol. 2015;93:402–10.
11. Rintoul AJ. Colobomatous cupping of the optic disc. Br J Ophthalmol. 1971;55:396–9.
12. Jacobson L, Hellström A, Flodmark O. Large cups in normal-sized optic discs. Arch Ophthalmol. 1997;114:1263–9.

Getting Better: Learning, New Tools and Risk Management

10

Zhichao Wu, Michael A. Coote, and Keith R. Martin

10.1 Improving Learning and Education

It is well-recognised that early intervention in glaucoma is a cost-effective strategy due to the increasing costs of managing this condition as the disease worsens [1]. Despite this, half of those with glaucoma still remain undiagnosed despite having accessed eye health service within the last 12 months [2]. There is thus an urgent need to ensure a high level of performance for detecting a glaucomatous optic nerve head (OHN) for the entire eye health workforce. This is especially crucial given the large degree of variation in the performance of qualified eyecare practitioners.

Two previous studies that included more than 450 practitioners reported that their accuracy for discriminating between healthy and glaucomatous optic discs spanned from approximately 67% to >88% in 95% of the participants [3, 4]. For ophthalmologists, those who completed their residency more recently performed better than more senior colleagues [3], whilst factors for better performance in optometrists related to working in a hospital setting and having additional qualifications related to glaucoma [4]. Improved learning and education for those currently in, or entering, the eye health workforce thus remains central to minimising the impact of glaucoma.

Numerous studies have reported, however, that traditional didactic approaches to teaching show limited or minimal improvement for improving the evaluation of the optic nerve for glaucoma. One study reported that a one-hour lecture resulted in a minimal improvement in performance of nearly 100 doctors [5]. Two different studies of approximately 50 optometrists in Australia [6] and the United Kingdom [7] both also showed that lecture-based or predominantly lecture-based programs had little influence on the overall accuracy of glaucoma diagnosis.

To provide eye health practitioners with a tool for self-assessment of their performance in optic disc examination for glaucoma, the Glaucomatous Optic Nerve Evaluation (GONE) project was developed [8]. In this project, a set of 42 monoscopic optic disc photographs were selected to capture a range of optic disc morphologies, levels of glaucomatous damage, and perceived level of difficulty with its assessment (As discussed in detail in Chap. 5). These images were uploaded onto an online platform, which asked each participant to assess nine topographic features and an overall subjective likelihood of glaucoma

Z. Wu
Centre for Eye Research Australia, University of Melbourne, Melbourne, Australia

M. A. Coote (✉)
Centre for Eye Research Australia, Royal Victorian Eye and Ear Hospital, Melbourne, Australia

K. R. Martin
Managing Director, Centre for Eye Research Australia, Royal Victorian Eye and Ear Hospital, Melbourne, Australia

S. Pandav et al. (eds.), *The Optic Nerve Head in Health and Disease*,
https://doi.org/10.1007/978-981-33-6838-5_10

presence for each image. In the latest version of the website (https://gone-project.com/newgone/), deficiencies in aspects of optic disc examination based on a baseline self-evaluation test of 15 images will be identified and targeted teaching will be provided. Through this process of training and with repeated self-assessment, clinicians can ensure that their performance for identifying glaucomatous optic discs are optimised.

10.2 Artificial Intelligence and Implications for Clinical Practice

Recent advances in the field of artificial intelligence (AI), especially in the area of machine learning (ML), have led to the development of artificial neural networks that can powerfully learn to recognise complex patterns and features in tasks similar to those required in the assessment of the optic nerve head for glaucoma. ML models learn such patterns and features based on the training data it is provided, and it can either seek to replicate the labels associated with the data (e.g. healthy or glaucoma; described as supervised learning) or to discover patterns in the data by itself (described as unsupervised learning). One such approach is deep learning (DL), an approach that automatically learns representations of images based on features present on multiple layers of abstraction [9], which can either be supervised or unsupervised.

Deep learning has shown promise for being a powerful approach in ophthalmic conditions, with one recent landmark study demonstrating its high level of performance for distinguishing between optic discs with and without papilloedema, and also from those with other optic disc abnormalities [10].

Numerous studies have now also shown that a DL approach can perform comparably or superiorly to eye care practitioners in the discrimination of optic nerve photographs from those with and without glaucoma [11–13] or in the assessment of optic nerve photographs that would be deemed referable for glaucoma [14]. The power of this approach stems from a computer's ability to learn automatically from large amounts of data and through its consistent application of the learned information, without variations in mental acuity expected from humans.

The full implications of AI on the clinical management of glaucoma, but also more broadly in healthcare, remain to be fully established. Of note, regulatory approval of the first autonomous AI diagnostic system by the Food & Drug Administration (FDA) was in eye care—a software called IDx-DR that performs screening for diabetic retinopathy using digital colour fundus photographs. Following image analysis, the software provides a recommendation for further evaluation without the input from a clinician.

However, these technological advances are accompanied by a wealth of new complexities that surround the legal, ethical, and regulatory issues regarding the use of AI in healthcare. This include discussions around whether a health practitioner could be held liable when relying on algorithmic recommendations [15]. Nonetheless, these advances show tremendous promise for assisting eye care practitioners with the assessment of the optic nerve for glaucoma, which forms a crucial—but nonetheless only one part of—eye health care.

10.3 Advances in Imaging and Visualisation

Technological advances have also led to the development of novel tools to visualise the loss of retinal ganglion cells (RGCs) that characterise glaucomatous optic neuropathy. Optical coherence tomography (OCT) imaging is an example of a tool that has become increasingly ubiquitous in clinical practice for visualising the retina with near-cellular resolution and three-dimensionally. Whilst there has been a predominant reliance on summary quantitative measures derived from imaging modalities like OCT, there is an increasing recognition that substantial improvements in performance can be achieved by scrutinising the raw imaging data [16]. This is a similar approach taken when evaluating the optic nerve appearance clinically or on a colour fundus photograph, which considers known patterns of glaucomatous damage and normal anatomical variation [17].

Other innovations being explored include the incorporation of adaptive optics to OCT imaging to improve image resolution and quality, which can enable visualisation of subtle changes in the individual RGC axonal bundles and changes in the lamina cribrosa architecture [18]. The direct visualisation of RGC apoptosis through fluorescent labelling and imaging with confocal scanning laser ophthalmoscopy is also currently being explored [19]. Rapid advances in biomedical optics also show promise of enabling a greater ease of visualising RGC loss and optic nerve head changes. More applicable methods for clinical electrophysiology, such as through the use of a handheld stimulation device along with self-adhering skin electrodes placed below the lower lid margin [20], may enable objective functional measurements of RGC function.

10.4 Uncertainty and Risk Management

Despite the promises of AI and novel imaging for improving the detection of glaucomatous optic neuropathy in the future, a definitive diagnosis of glaucoma remains difficult to establish in the early stages. This is because as much as 50% of RGCs would need to be lost before visual field loss can be reliably detected [21], yet the clinical assessment of the optic nerve appearance can be highly subjective and challenging due to the large degree of interindividual variability. Indeed, a previous study has demonstrated that a glaucomatous appearing optic nerve is a weak predictor of future visual field loss [22].

The challenges of accurately identifying eyes experiencing glaucomatous optic neuropathy based on the optic nerve appearance are apparent by the fact that approximately one in 13 people over 50 years of age would be deemed as having possible or probable glaucoma based on the optic nerve appearance. This is five times as many people who would be considered as having definite glaucoma [2], and such individuals are often considered "glaucoma suspects".

Since one in eight of these glaucoma suspects will develop glaucoma within a two-year period [23], there is a need to identify those at high-risk of progression to target for careful surveillance and potentially preventative treatments. However, current tools will only correctly identify up to 30% of people who actually develop glaucoma, whilst having an unacceptably high false-positive rate of about 25% [24]. A previous health economic modelling study reported that the cost-effectiveness of screening for glaucoma is highly dependent on its expected prevalence in the population being screened [25]. Therefore, optimal methods for accurately identifying high-risk individuals (where the prevalence of glaucoma development will be higher) are needed to enable a cost-effective early identification of glaucoma.

The careful assessment of the optic nerve appearance and its progressive change over time remains one of the most important factors for predicting the development of glaucoma amongst suspects [22]. This assessment is considered alongside all the other available clinical evidence to form an overall assessment of the risk of a glaucoma suspect for developing glaucoma. The determined level of risk is then used to guide the management of glaucoma suspects, such as whether to initiate preventative treatment [26]. This framework based on risk assessment seeks to minimise the risk of direct functional disability from developing glaucoma [27, 28], and to avoid indirect disability from the adverse effects of treatments [29]. The former remains a key area of research based on using self-reported outcomes and real-world functional assessments [30].

Our ability to refine the process of risk assessment will continue to improve as novel diagnostics and analytics become established. Nonetheless, the assessment of the optic nerve appearance will still remain a vital part in this process as we await the development of these novel approaches.

References

1. Lee PP, Walt JG, Doyle JJ, et al. A multicenter, retrospective pilot study of resource use and costs associated with severity of disease in glaucoma. Arch Ophthalmol. 2006;124:12–9.

2. Keel S, Xie J, Foreman J, et al. Prevalence of glaucoma in the Australian national eye health survey. Br J Ophthalmol. 2019;103:191–5.
3. Reus NJ, Lemij HG, Garway-Heath DF, et al. Clinical assessment of stereoscopic optic disc photographs for glaucoma: the European optic disc assessment trial. Ophthalmology. 2010;117:717–23.
4. Hadwin SE, Redmond T, Garway-Heath DF, et al. Assessment of optic disc photographs for glaucoma by UK optometrists: the Moorfields optic disc assessment study (MODAS). Ophthalmic Physiol Opt. 2013;33:618–24.
5. Andersson S, Heijl A, Boehm AG, Bengtsson B. The effect of education on the assessment of optic nerve head photographs for the glaucoma diagnosis. BMC Ophthalmol. 2011;11:12.
6. Yoshioka N, Wong E, Kalloniatis M, et al. Influence of education and diagnostic modes on glaucoma assessment by optometrists. Ophthalmic Physiol Opt. 2015;35:682–98.
7. Myint J, Edgar DF, Murdoch IE, Lawrenson JG. The impact of postgraduate training on UK optometrists' clinical decision-making in glaucoma. Ophthalmic Physiol Opt. 2014;34:376–84.
8. Kong YXG, Coote MA, O'Neill EC, et al. Glaucomatous optic neuropathy evaluation project: a standardized internet system for assessing skills in optic disc examination. Clin Exp Ophthalmol. 2011;39:308–17.
9. LeCun Y, Bengio Y, Hinton G. Deep learning. Nature. 2015;521:436–44.
10. Milea D, Najjar RP, Jiang Z, et al. Artificial intelligence to detect papilledema from ocular fundus photographs. N Engl J Med. 2020;382:1687–95.
11. Shibata N, Tanito M, Mitsuhashi K, et al. Development of a deep residual learning algorithm to screen for glaucoma from fundus photography. Sci Rep. 2018;8:14665.
12. Liu S, Graham SL, Schulz A, et al. A deep learning-based algorithm identifies glaucomatous discs using monoscopic fundus photographs. Ophthalmol Glaucoma. 2018;1:15–22.
13. Jammal AA, Thompson AC, Mariottoni EB, et al. Human versus machine: comparing a deep learning algorithm to human gradings for detecting glaucoma on fundus photographs. Am J Ophthalmol. 2020;211:123–31.
14. Phene S, Dunn RC, Hammel N, et al. Deep learning and glaucoma specialists: the relative importance of optic disc features to predict glaucoma referral in fundus photographs. Ophthalmology. 2019;126:1627–39.
15. Price WN, Gerke S, Cohen IG. Potential liability for physicians using artificial intelligence. JAMA. 2019;322:1765–6.
16. Wu Z, DSD W, Rajshekhar R, Ritch R, Hood DC. Effectiveness of a qualitative approach toward evaluating OCT imaging for detecting glaucomatous damage. Trans Vis Sci Tech. 2018;7:7.
17. Hood DC. Improving our understanding, and detection, of glaucomatous damage: an approach based upon optical coherence tomography (OCT). Prog Retin Eye Res. 2017;57:46–75.
18. Dong ZM, Wollstein G, Wang B, Schuman JS. Adaptive optics optical coherence tomography in glaucoma. Prog Retin Eye Res. 2017;57:76–88.
19. Yang E, Al-Mugheiry TS, Normando EM, Cordeiro MF. Real-time imaging of retinal cell apoptosis by confocal scanning laser ophthalmoscopy and its role in glaucoma. Front Neurol. 2018;9:338.
20. Wu Z, Hadoux X, Hui F, Sarossy MG, Crowston JG. Photopic negative response obtained using a handheld electroretinogram device: determining the optimal measure and repeatability. Trans Vis Sci Tech. 2016;5:8.
21. Harwerth R, Wheat J, Fredette M, Anderson D. Linking structure and function in glaucoma. Prog Retin Eye Res. 2010;29:249–71.
22. Medeiros FA, Alencar LM, Zangwill LM, et al. Prediction of functional loss in glaucoma from progressive optic disc damage. Arch Ophthalmol. 2009;127:1250.
23. Miki A, Medeiros FA, Weinreb RN, et al. Rates of retinal nerve fiber layer thinning in glaucoma suspect eyes. Ophthalmology. 2014;121:1350–8.
24. Weinreb RN, Zangwill LM, Jain S, et al. Predicting the onset of glaucoma: the confocal scanning laser ophthalmoscopy ancillary study to the ocular hypertension treatment study. Ophthalmology. 2010;117:1674–83.
25. Burr JM, Mowatt G, Hernández R, et al. The clinical effectiveness and cost-effectiveness of screening for open angle glaucoma: a systematic review and economic evaluation. Health Technol Assess (Winchester England). 2007;11:1–190.
26. Appropriateness of Treating Glaucoma Suspects RAND Study Group. For which glaucoma suspects is it appropriate to initiate treatment? Ophthalmology. 2009;116:710–6.
27. Ramulu P. Glaucoma and disability: which tasks are affected, and at what stage of disease? Curr Opin Ophthalmol. 2009;20:92.
28. Jammal AA, Ogata NG, Daga FB, et al. What is the amount of visual field loss associated with disability in glaucoma? Am J Ophthalmol. 2019;197:45–52.
29. Janz NK, Wren PA, Lichter PR, et al. The collaborative initial glaucoma treatment study: interim quality of life findings after initial medical or surgical treatment of glaucoma. Ophthalmology. 2001;108:1954–65.
30. Skalicky SE, Lamoureux E, Crabb D, Ramulu P. Patient reported outcomes, functional assessment and utility values in glaucoma. J Glaucoma. 2019;28:89–96.

The manufacturer's authorised representative in the EU is Springer
Nature Customer Service Centre GmbH, Europaplatz 3, 69115 Heidelberg,
Germany. If you have any concerns regarding our products, please
contact ProductSafety@springernature.com

Printed and bound by CPI Group (UK) Ltd, Croydon, CR0 4YY
30/09/2026
02225266-0005